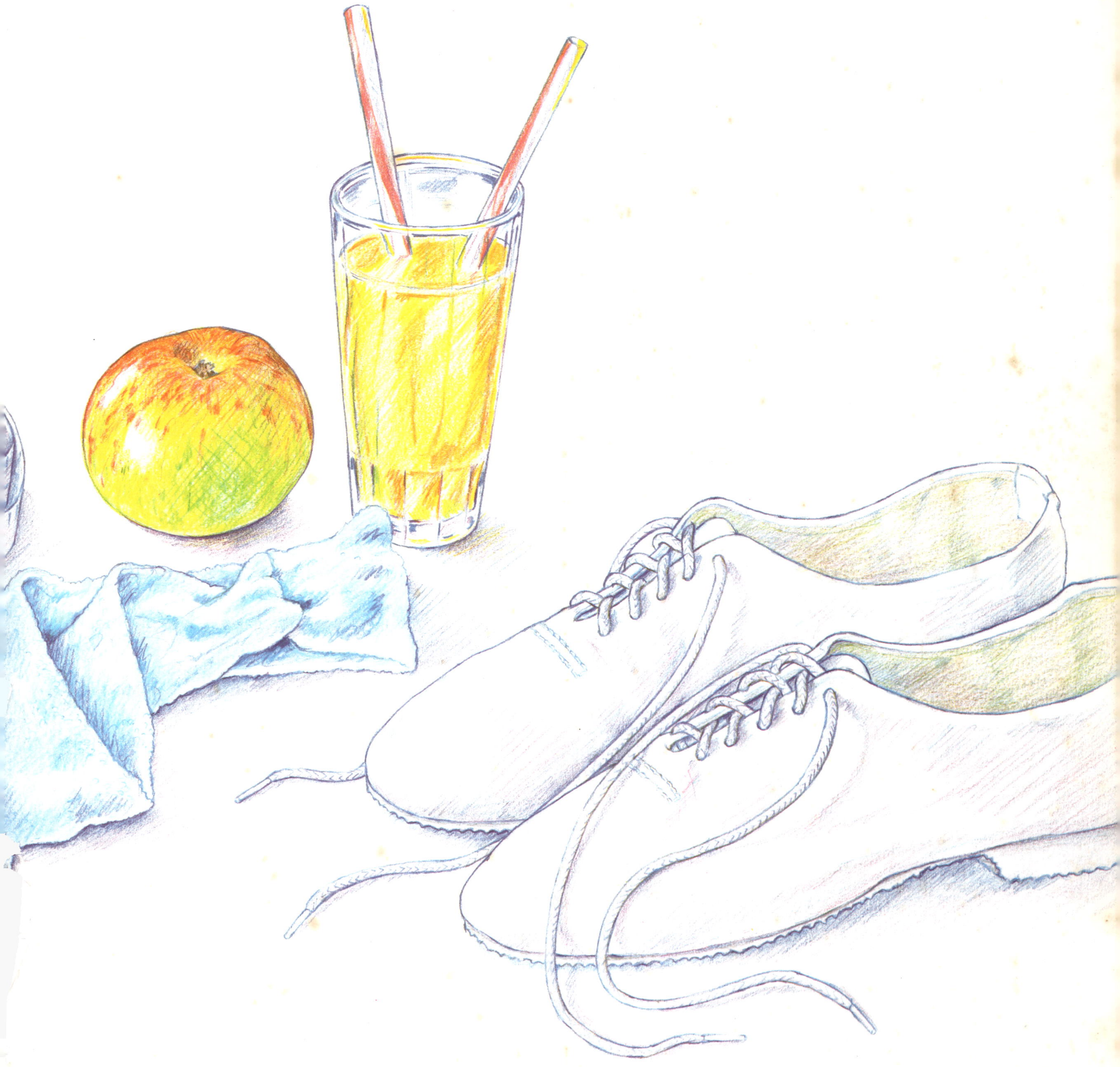

Slimming Magazine
HOME HEALTH FARM

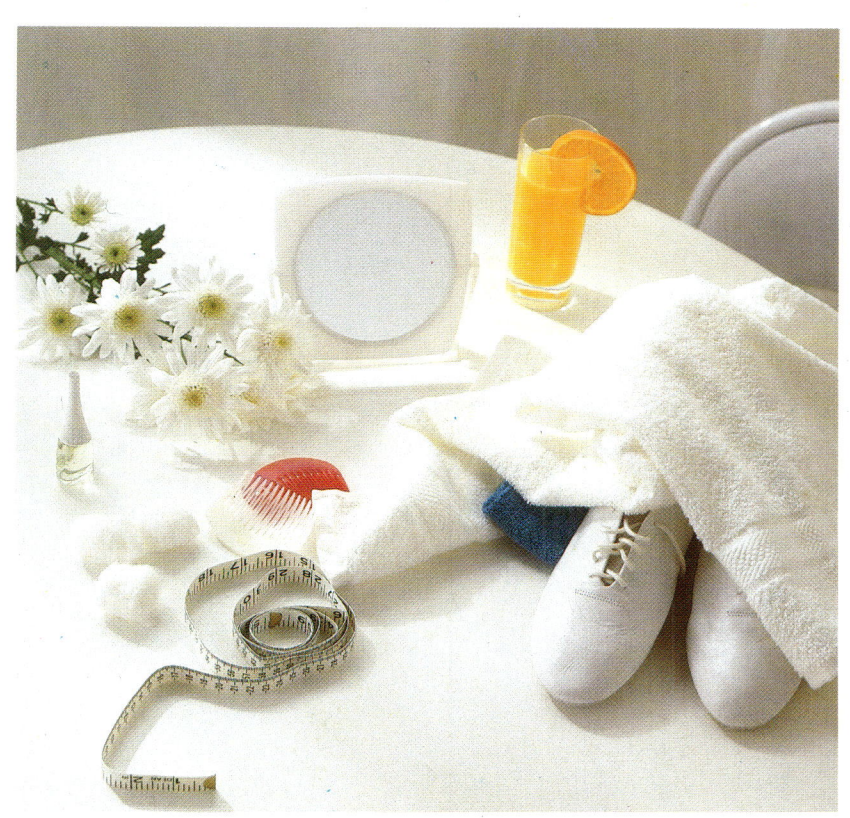

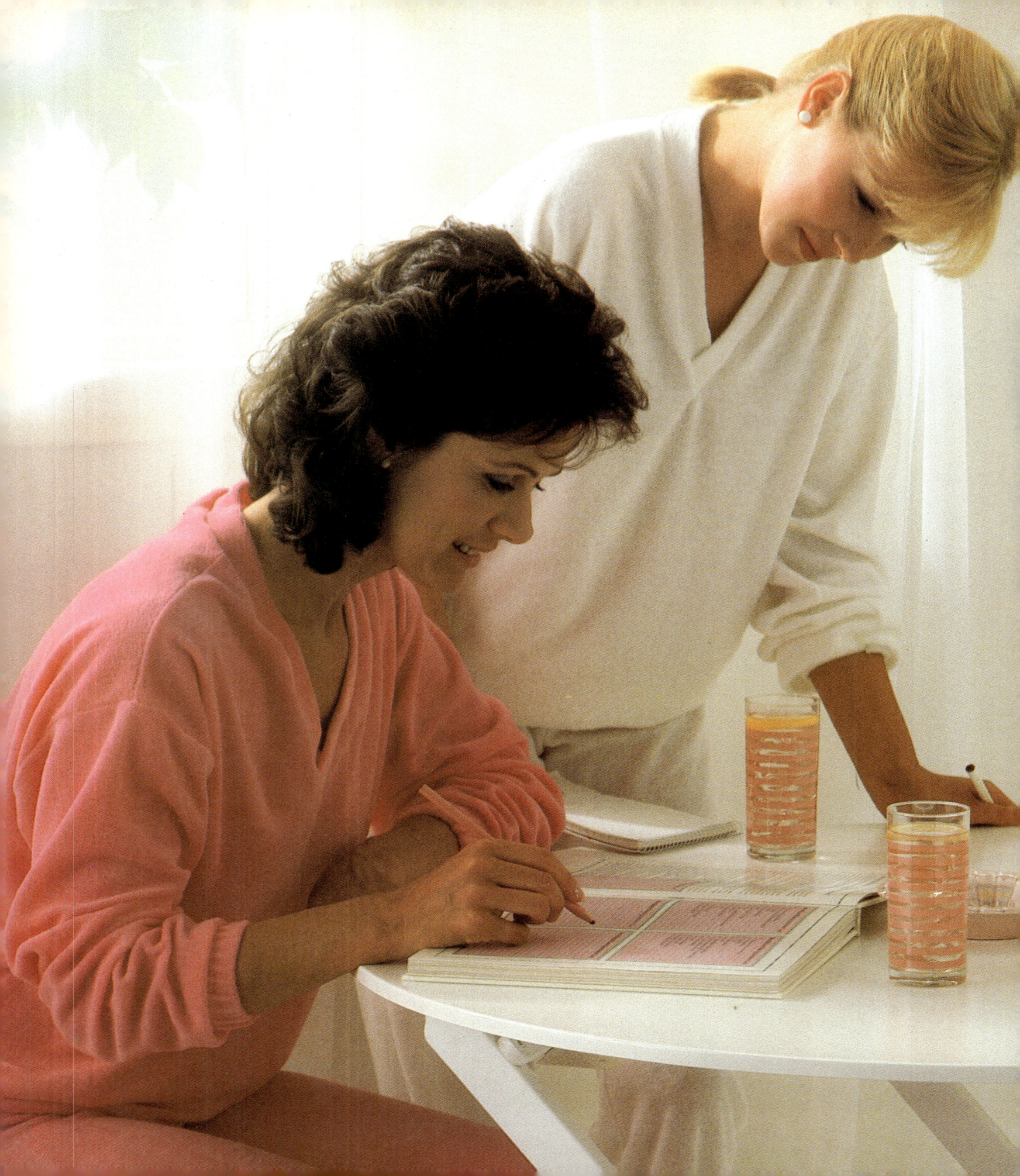

CONTENTS

YOUR PROGRAMME

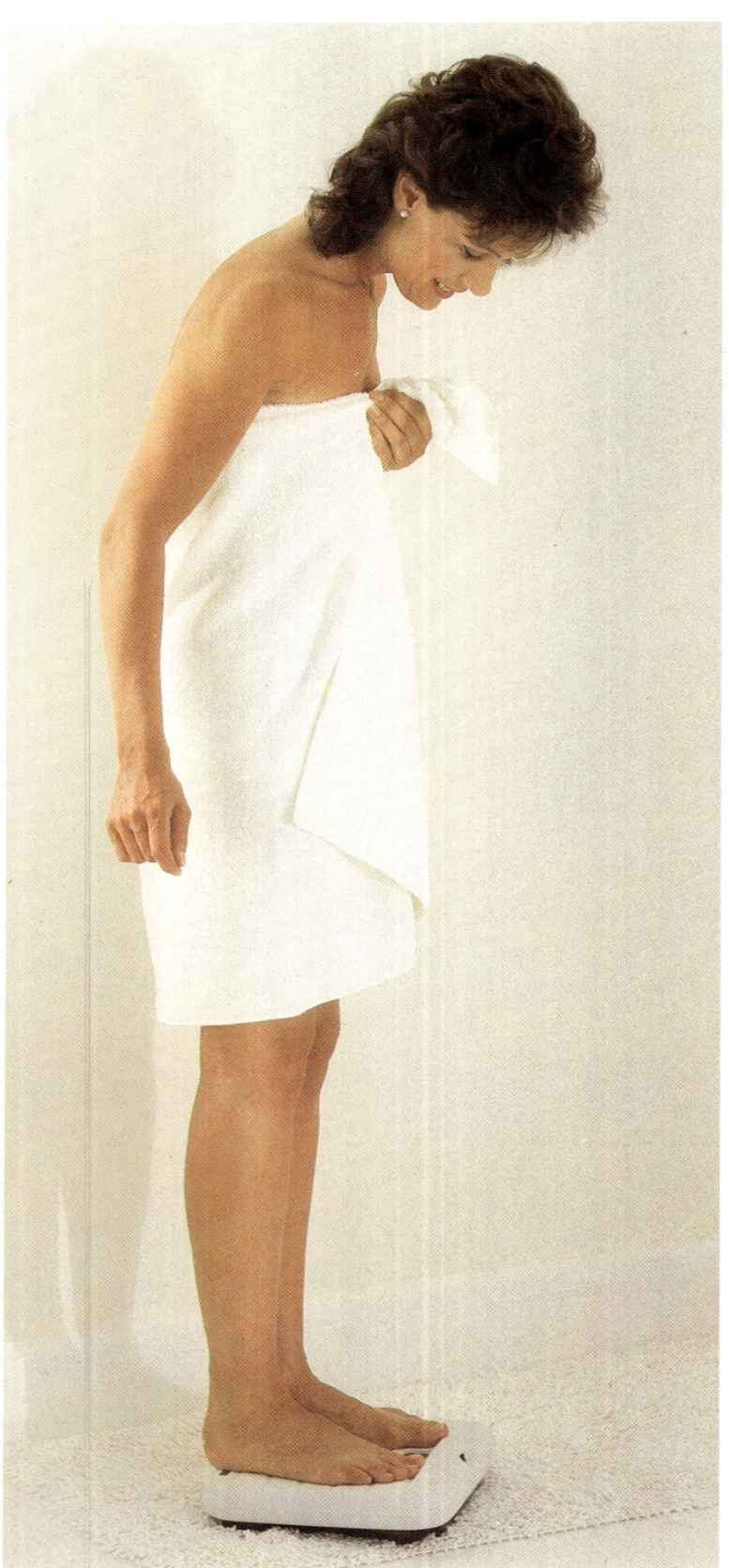

Introduction

Most women, at some stage of their lives, dream of spending time at a health farm – to achieve a substantial weight loss and trim away extra inches, to obtain a new look, or to simply indulge in total relaxation. This book makes that dream come true. We give you a selection of diets, exercise work-outs and beauty therapy, the treatments you would expect to enjoy at any exclusive health farm. But they have all been carefully designed so that you can treat yourself to them in your own home. All you have to do is find the time to enjoy them.

Whether you have a few hours a day, can spoil yourself for an entire weekend or plan an even longer-term trim, tone and beauty care programme, you will find this book has everything you need for a period of luxurious home pampering.

The programmes in the book are colour coded for easy reference. If you have tended to neglect your body you will probably start with the blue programmes. The yellow programmes are for women who are quite active and a stone or two overweight, and the pink programmes will appeal to those who are fit with only a slight weight problem. The Home Health Farm Questionnaire (page 14) and the Beauty Planner (page 11) will lead you to the programmes most suited to your needs.

Before you begin, though, spend some time assessing your needs and carefully plan the days or hours you wish to spend at your Home Health Farm. Do you mainly want to relax, to recuperate from the stresses of work or family responsibilities? Or, do you want a programme of self-improvement – to make a sprinting start to a weight programme, take a new look at your hair and makeup, or firm up flabby muscles? This book gives you the opportunity to tackle all these areas if you wish, or you can just concentrate on the ones you feel will be of most benefit.

Once you have decided on your purpose, write it down. No matter what change you are considering or what success you want to achieve, seeing it in writing will help clear your mind, bring objectives into sharp focus and make it more manageable. If you need to lose weight write down exactly how much weight you need to shed by filling in the Slim Speed Chart on page 8. This is the stage at which you can clarify your position and be realistic. You can then work out the actions you must take to get to your goal.

The following pages will tell you how to choose your treatments, then all you have to do is fill in your 'Appointments Card' (page 12) and start your Home Health Farm pampering programme.

Diet

Every health farm pays great heed to diet and yours should be no exception. We have six long-term diets from which you can choose. Each is designed to suit a particular lifestyle or need. We also have a four-day Super-speedy Health Farm Diet for

First published 1984 by
Octopus Books Limited
59 Grosvenor Street, London WI

© Text: Slimming Magazine
© Illustrations: Octopus Books Ltd 1984
ISBN 0 7064 2172 8

Reprinted 1987

Produced by Mandarin Publishers Limited,
22a Westlands Road,
Quarry Bay,
Hong Kong
Printed in Spain by Cayfosa, Barcelona
Dep. Legal. B-28964-1984

Editor: Sybil Greatbatch
Beauty: Rosalyn Chissick
Diets: Glynis McGuinness, Victoria Anthony,
Alison Graham
Nutritionist: Dr Nigel Dickie

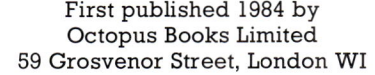

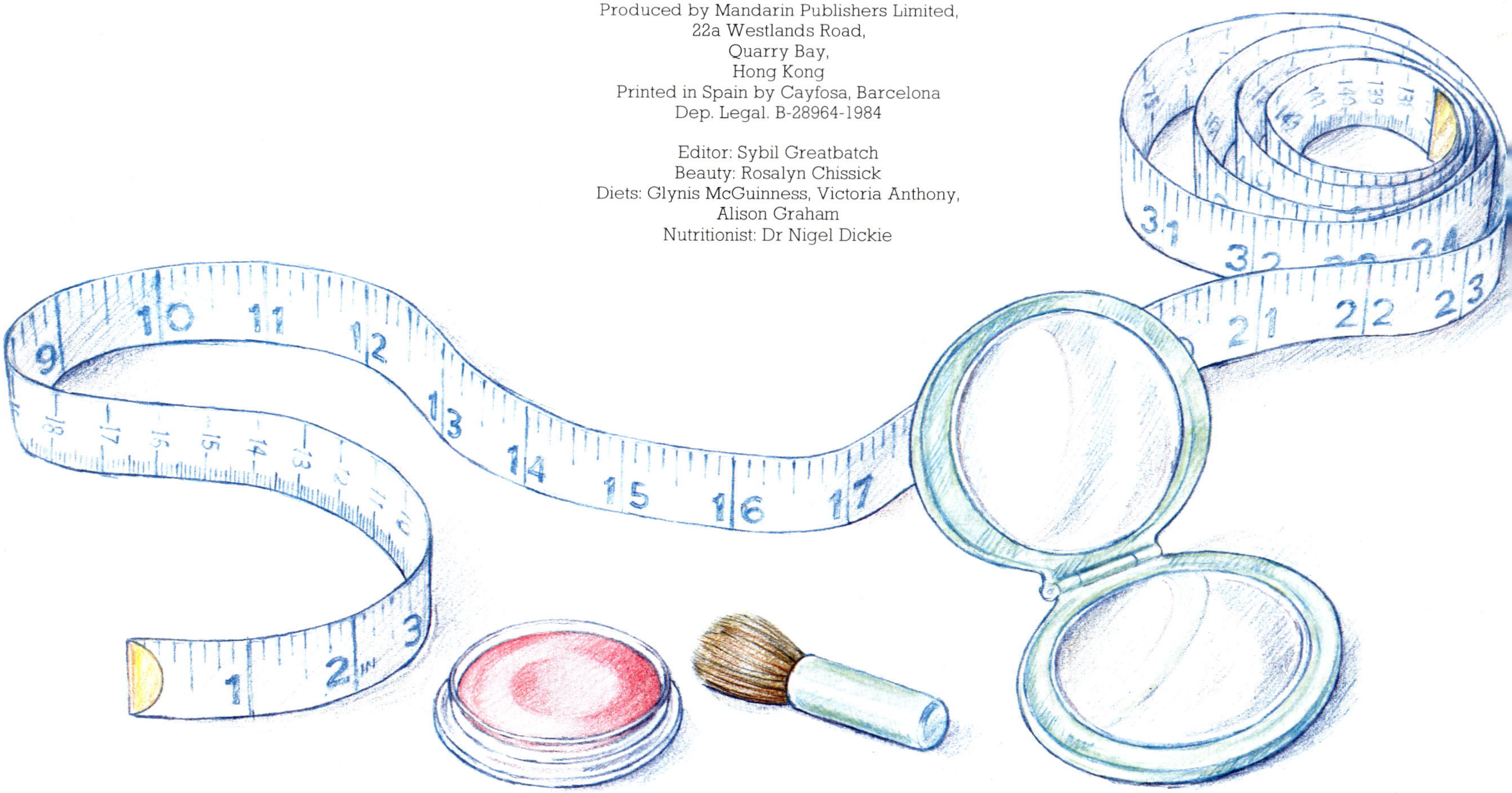

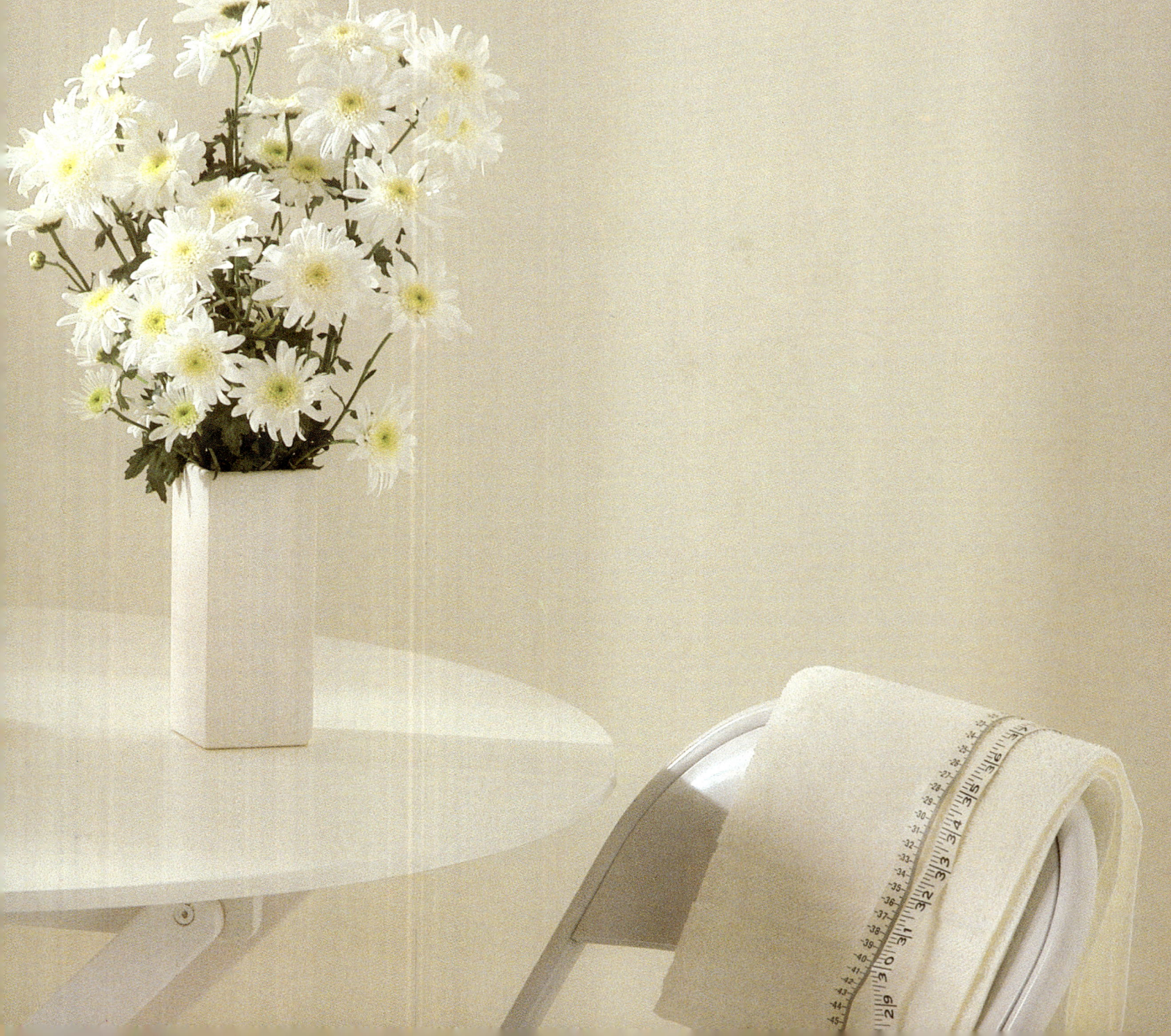

Slimming Magazine
HOME HEALTH FARM

those who have only a pound or so to lose. Choose the most suitable one for you from the questionnaire on page 14.

All diets work because they feed you less calories than your body needs so that it is forced to fall back on its fat reserves. The number of calories you require each day will depend on how much you weigh. The heavier you are, the more calories your body uses up just moving around.

If you have over 3 stone (19 kg/42 lb) to lose, you can start your diet at 1,500 Calories a day, but you may find you need to cut down to a strict 1,000 Calories as you near target weight.

If you don't have any weight to lose but just want to get yourself into a healthier way of eating, select a 1,500 Calorie a day diet and add an extra 250 or 500 Calories daily.

There is no special merit in keeping your calories below your requirement unless you have weight to lose. And don't be fooled by other dietary fallacies. The idea, for example, that sipping lemon juice all day will somehow flush out your system is nonsense. Your body doesn't need flushing out like a drain any more than any of your vital organs needs to be given a rest.

Fibre is important in this respect and The Extra Fibre Formula (see page 90) will ensure you are having a healthy amount of dietary fibre while keeping your intake of fats and sugar low. Another health recommendation is that most people need to cut down their consumption of salt (sodium). So wherever we mention seasoning you can use a potassium salt substitute.

Exercise

The other side of the 'get slim and healthy' story is activity and all health farms concentrate on exercise as well as diet.

Physical activity burns up calories and the more energetic that activity, the more calories you will use. In the course of an average working day Ms Today may well be using up fewer calories than her predecessors. Scientists now suspect that there are many women who burn up rather less than 2,000 Calories, which used to be considered an almost universal level. Labour-saving devices in the home and at work mean that today's woman just doesn't spend as much time or energy on chores and jobs as did her mother or grandmother. So if you find your weight loss is not as high as you had expected – 1 kg/2 lb loss a week is a good average – then you need to increase your activity level.

Physical activity is a term which embraces all bodily movement and includes walking across the room to switch on the television as well as taking part in sports or games. Every time we move, we are burning up calories. The more of our bodies we move the more calories we are burning. Hence, moving the whole body from place to place by walking will burn up considerably more calories than simply moving one arm to do the ironing or two hands to do the typing. The faster we move, the greater the calories used.

The exercise workouts in this book are primarily designed to tone up muscles, and are suitable for exercise experts as well as beginners; but if you are keen to burn up as many extra calories as possible, build some walking, skipping or indoor mountaineering into your day as well. (More about these in Planning Your Programme, page 8).

Whatever you plan to achieve with your Home Health Farm programme, remember there is plenty of work to be done before you start feeling the full benefit. If you slip up on your diet from time to time, it isn't the end of the world or the end of your diet. Just make up for a binge by being super-strict the next day. You may feel disappointed that you can't master all the exercises you try at once, but don't give in. Gradually you will improve and the exercises will seem easier.

Beauty – Inside and Out

Diet and exercise are perhaps the 'hard work' aspects of a health farm. But equally important is the indulgent pampering every woman needs. So do not neglect this. Looking as good as you can, even if you do have some excess weight, is going to make you feel so much better and so much more in command of yourself that you will find it easier to start a diet and stick to the changed habits it entails.

Before you start your Home Health Farm programme sit in front of the mirror and experiment with your make up and your hairstyle. Then go through your wardrobe and be ruthless about chucking out every item that doesn't make you look good. Don't keep a 'best' outfit under wraps. Wear it.

Doing things that make you feel good is a wise kind of self love because it is nourishing the part of you that wants to achieve things and enjoy life. It is an essential part of making you a happy person, able to cope with everything that life throws in your direction. It's a sad fact that many women are so eager to keep everybody happy that they don't have any time to think about themselves and their needs.

You can gain maximum benefit from your Home Health Farm by making it a top priority to do at least one positive thing that you enjoy every single day and have the courage to demand time for yourself now and again. If you always cook a big meal on Sundays, for instance, decree that you are taking the day off and suggest the family or partners make do with baked beans on toast or something just as simple.

Stop expecting others to think you are wonderful just because you keep doing things for them. They are more likely to take your efforts for granted, if they think about it at all. Do expect others to respect you for finding satisfaction in doing things that make you feel good and insist that they shoulder their full responsibilities to make such outlets possible.

At the end of each day ask yourself: "What have I done that was nice for me? What little treat have I enjoyed?" Even if the answer to begin with is 'nothing' this habit will encourage you to plan one of the best things you can do for your morale and your well being: finding time for your own needs. And this includes setting aside time for a visit to your Home Health Farm.

Planning Your Programme

Spend time assessing your needs and planning your programme for the days or hours you wish to spend at your Home Health Farm. The questionnaire on page 14 will help you choose the diet which will get you down to your target weight in the fastest possible time. It will also guide you to your most effective exercise work-out. Just answer 'Yes' or 'No' to the questions and follow the arrows until you reach your personal exercise and diet plan. All the diets, exercises and beauty treatments are colour coded: blue are the more relaxed programmes, yellow will get you working a little harder, and pink is for the determined self-improver.

Before starting your programme you will need to make sure that you have all the food required for the diet you intend to follow and any lotions or equipment for your beauty treatments. You won't need anything very special for the exercise work-outs, but wear clothing that will allow you to move freely, such as a leotard or tracksuit.

Your Diet Plan

In order to choose your diet, your first step has to be on to the bathroom scales. Make sure the scales are standing on a flat surface (preferably not on a carpet). Stand straight with your feet evenly placed on the scales and resist rocking backwards or forwards to make the needle drop lower! Now write down your weight.

The chart below gives a guide to your ideal weight, but you could easily be around 4.5 kg/10 lb more or less than that. Every individual differs a little in bone structure and muscle format which both affect weight. So use our chart as a guide and not as gospel.

If you are overweight now the weight you were when you were slim should be your ideal weight. It doesn't matter if that was 20 years ago. Ideal weight levels do not vary as you get older, although if you want to concede just a few pounds to your age, there is no real harm done.

If you have always been overweight, set yourself a target that is not too low. When you have reached this weight assess how you look. Are there still plump places? If so, you probably need to lose a little more. Remember, too, that bulges – particularly those around the tummy – can be caused by slack muscles as well as surplus fat. So if you are at your ideal weight but still less than firm, exercise is probably what you need.

Heights are minus footwear; but these medium-frame weights include an allowance of about 1 kg (2 to 3 lb) for light indoor clothing.							
4ft 10	1.47m	7st 7	47.5kg	5ft 5	1.65m	9st 0	57kg
4ft 11	1.50m	7st 9	48.5kg	5ft 6	1.68m	9st 5	59.5kg
5ft 0	1.52m	7st 12	50kg	5ft 7	1.70m	9st 9	61kg
5ft 1	1.55m	8st 1	51.5kg	5ft 8	1.73m	9st 13	63kg
5ft 2	1.57m	8st 4	52.5kg	5ft 9	1.75m	10st 3	65kg
5ft 3	1.60m	8st 7	54kg	5ft 10	1.78m	10st 7	66.5kg
5ft 4	1.63m	8st 11	56kg	5ft 11	1.80m	10st 11	68.5kg

Your Slim Speed Chart

Now that you've checked your ideal weight, mark your personal finishing post on the chart below. Counting one square for every kilogram (or pound) you have to lose, count back from the finish and mark your starting square. Then follow your diet formula faithfully and you'll soon be speeding along to your target weight. If you have more kilos or pounds to lose than our chart allows, you can start again once you have reached the finishing post. It is best to set yourself goals which allow you to see the results quite quickly.

Weigh yourself once a week only. Daily alterations in body weight are largely meaningless as far as measuring fat is concerned. Most people find they are lightest if they step on the scales first thing in the morning. To get an accurate measure of your weight loss always weigh yourself at the same time of the day each week and wear similar clothing.

40	39	38	37	36	35
					34
28	29	30	31	32	33
27					
26	25	24	23	22	21
					20
14	15	16	17	18	19
13					
12	11	10	9	8	7
					6
FINISH	1	2	3	4	5

Which Diet?

The diet which will be most successful is the one that closely follows your regular eating habits and your food likes and dislikes.

If you know you can't get through the day without raiding the refrigerator or resorting to a nibble of some sort, you won't be happy with a diet that asks you to stick strictly to three meals a day and nothing else. The questionnaire on page 14 will lead you to a diet that fits your tastes and one that takes into account the size of your weight problem.

If you have just a few pounds to shift, or want to balance out a few days of over-indulgence, the Super-speedy Health Farm Diet is ideal (see page 150). It is designed to be followed for no more than four days at a time but is very effective as an emergency plan. You can choose to have a liquid day, or one that allows you a bowlful of salady stuff that you can dip into whenever you wish. Either can be prepared first thing in the morning so that it won't be necessary to cook anything for the rest of the day.

If you opt to follow any of the longer-term diets you should select simple meals on your health farm days. Choose recipes which need the minimum of preparation and cooking so that you have lots of time to spend on your beauty treatments and exercise sessions.

Step by Step to Slimness

Here are some totally painless adjustments you can make to your eating habits that will make dieting easier and keeping in trim simple.

SHOPPING
Prepare your shopping list when you are not hungry and shop when you are not hungry. That way you should find yourself less vulnerable to the impulse-buying of 'high temptation' foods which you are trying not to eat.

COOKING
If you are in the habit of nibbling while preparing meals, try to cook in batches and freeze dishes in advance to cut down on the time you spend in the kitchen.

WHERE YOU EAT
Make it a rule to eat only if you are sitting at your dining table. Even if you are just having a snack, make sure you sit down at the table. This should curb the impulse to nibble while doing other things such as watching television or reading a book.

It has been proved medically that the more we concentrate on pain the more we feel it. The same goes for hunger or what we may think is hunger. Don't sit around thinking about the food you are trying not to eat. Do something instead that will take your mind off it, such as one of the Home Health Farm exercise workouts or going for a walk.

LEFTOVERS
Plan ahead how you will dispose of any leftovers, otherwise you may find yourself nibbling them. Are there enough to provide another meal? If so, set them aside for that purpose. If leftovers are identified in your mind as being reserved for a special purpose you are less likely to pick at them. Don't feel guilty about throwing away any food.

EATING ALONE
Try to avoid eating alone. Most overweight people eat most of their excess calories when they are alone: the same applies to between-meal snacks. For many people a single resolve not to eat anything unless in the company of at least one other person could in itself result in a gradual weight loss.

EATING PROCEDURE
Many people are in the habit of saving the best on the plate for last. Don't! Eat the best first. If you save the food you like best for last, you're going to make room for it. If you eat it first, you may leave some of the other food, thus lowering your calorie intake.

Action Planner for a Down Day

Remember that dieting successfully isn't just a matter of cutting down or cutting out foods. Your mental attitude to your weight loss programme is of vital importance. If you are feeling down, it is much harder to stick to a strict diet than when you are feeling really good about the world. If you suddenly find the blues descending, try this Action Plan:

GET MOVING
Get out of doors and get moving. A really brisk walk in the fresh air can make you feel better at any time. Ten minutes is better than nothing, half an hour better still. It's impossible to mope when you're on the move and hard to go on moping when you come back full of fresh air – as you'll discover.

LOOK GOOD
Maybe this is just another ordinary day and you feel every surplus pound is showing. But you're meeting misery more than halfway if you give in and don't bother about your appearance. Clothes you enjoy wearing, good grooming, flattering make up and hairstyle give your spirits a lift.

BE FRIENDLY
Be more open and friendly towards others – and they will be more responsive to you.

CATCH UP
Do something you have been putting off for ages. Procrastination is the thief of time and the biggest guilt and anxiety-maker ever. Do not be haunted by lurking thoughts of tasks undone – write the letter, pay the bill, make the phone call. You will feel terrific when you've done it.

Your Exercise Plan

The questionnaire on page 14 will guide you to the most suitable exercise work-out for you to follow. The work-outs are devised to help tone muscles and can do a great deal to improve your appearance if slack muscles are spoiling a new slim shape.

Virtually every exercise benefits certain muscles more than others; and some will trim certain areas by toning muscles there. But you cannot spot-reduce in the sense of removing fat from a particular area at a greater rate than elsewhere. When you are following a successful slimming plan, fat is lost evenly from all over your body despite the pounding you may be giving one particular area in an attempt to slim it down.

When you are filling-in your Home Health Farm appointment card (see page 12), allow yourself one or two work-outs each day. If you are not as young as you were or if you are very overweight, 'easy-does-it' must be your exercise motto. Be sure to consult your doctor before embarking on any exercise plan if you have health worries of any sort.

Don't think only strenuous exercise such as an hour on a squash court or 20 strenuous lengths of the nearest swimming pool will burn up the calories. Research has shown that, for practical purposes, by far the most beneficial exercise is walking. Although walking doesn't burn up as many calories as some of the more energetic pursuits, it's something that can conveniently become an everyday habit. Cycling is another good way to burn up calories; or you can borrow a skipping rope or try – see below – indoor mountaineering.

Build one of these calorie-burning activities into your Home Health Farm day. Not only will the exercise burn up calories, it will also make you feel good. Exercise helps ease stress and raise morale, so it's a first-class way to beat a weight problem.

WALKING

Walking is so familiar and gentle an exercise that you may never have regarded it as a method of losing weight. Certainly when compared with a vigorous activity like running or playing squash it may appear to be of little importance. But don't underrate its value.

When it is done the correct way, walking can be a very effective calorie-burner and when you walk uphill you burn up even more calories because you're not only moving your whole body weight, but moving it against the force of gravity.

Of course, how you walk will make a difference to the number of calories you burn up. The faster you walk the more calories you burn up. If you walk on a rough surface like a country track you will use more calories than if you walk on a smooth flat footpath.

If you are unused to exercise, half an hour's brisk walking to achieve the maximum calorie expenditure might very well make you feel thoroughly puffed out – and even unable to maintain the pace or the length of time aimed at.

Well, there's a solution to that: you can walk at a number of different paces. Spend two minutes getting into your stride in a slow walk. For the next thirty minutes do alternate five-minute periods of brisk and standard walks. Then spend a couple of minutes tapering off in a slow walk again. Or you can work out any other permutations of varying-pace walking that could add up to the same effect.

Walking Chart		Cycling Chart	
Ms Average will burn up the following number of calories in 5 minutes.		Here's how many calories on average you'll burn up in 5 minutes.	
	Calories		*Calories*
Strolling	10–15	Easy pace	25
Comfortable pace	20	Fast cycling	40
Purposeful pace	25	Uphill	50
Walking uphill slowly	25	Downhill	5–10
Brisk walking	30	Pushing bike	20

CYCLING

Consider borrowing a bike if you don't have one. Hard uphill pedal work eats calories, but you won't burn up many by just sitting on the bike and letting it roll downhill. For maximum calorie expenditure pedal up hills, then get off your bike and push it down the other side. If you haven't cycled for a long time, don't go too far on your first trip. You are aiming to return from your cycle trip feeling invigorated, not too tired to carry on with your Home Health Farm programme.

SKIPPING

A skipping-rope is an excellent calorie-burning slimming aid. When you jump up and down, as in skipping, you are moving the whole body weight against the pull of gravity. That takes extra energy and burns up extra calories.

A person just sitting around doing nothing energetic will usually burn up about 1 Calorie per minute, 10 Calories in 10 minutes. If you skip energetically for 10 minutes you can burn up about 90 Calories on top of this. Skipping is not an exercise for anyone heavily overweight or for anyone less than fit. So don't overdo it – concentrate on short sessions and work up gradually to longer sessions.

INDOOR MOUNTAINEERING

Walking up and down stairs repeatedly and briskly is one of the best calorie-burning exercises there is – you burn from 6 to 12 calories a minutes. (But again we would not recommend it for anyone heavily overweight or with health worries.) The walking up part accounts for most of the calorie expenditure. Your own weight determines whether you burn up nearer 6 or 12 calories a minute – the heavier you are the higher you score. If you have a stone (7 kg/14 lb) or less in excess weight you can increase your calorie expenditure by carrying a pack on your back like a mountaineer. Follow another mountaineering tactic and divide your session into a series of pitches – perhaps each about three or four minutes long.

Your Beauty Plan

Study the Beauty Planner below and select those treatments you would like to tackle on your Home Health Farm days. We tell you how long each treatment will take, consider this when filling in your Appointment Cards (see page 12). You can choose to concentrate on bare essentials such as caring for your hands and feet with a careful manicure or pedicure, or opt to take time for things like shaping your eyebrows and getting your hair and skin into tip-top condition.

When tackling the Complete Makeover you are asked to make an honest appraisal of any face faults so that you can learn how to camouflage problem areas. But never dwell on beauty faults. Remember that it's not how naturally good-looking you are that matters, it's how good-looking you feel.

RELAXATION

Not only will our basic beauty treatments make you feel good when they are finished, but they make you sit down and relax while you are doing them.

Relaxation is something we don't always make enough time for in our busy lives, which is why tension can build up. So whatever other treatments you plan during your Home Health Farm stay, make sure that you do spend some time with your feet up, or soaking in a luxurious bath.

Nothing is more relaxing than a warm bath, scented with your favourite bath essence. Make your bathroom a totally delightful place to spend half an hour or so. Ensure that it is comfortably warm and have a soft, thick bath towel ready to wrap around yourself as you step out of the water. If you find music relaxing, put on a favourite record or tape before you start. If you wish, you can apply a face mask while you soak; and if your skin is dry, massage yourself with body cream after you have dried off.

Even on the busiest of days allow yourself half an hour or so in which to relax in a way that makes you feel peaceful and contented. Relaxation does not have to mean lying flat on your back deliberately unwinding all the physical knots of tension (though if you are tense, this isn't a bad idea). It can mean doing anything that makes you feel calm and gives you mental and spiritual refreshment . . . savouring a cup of coffee while you read your favourite magazine . . . sitting by the fire and stroking the cat . . . listening to music with your eyes peacefully closed . . . knitting or sewing while you tune in to a radio programme. There are lots of different ways to enjoy a quiet, relaxing time.

INNER BEAUTY

Generally speaking, a woman is as attractive as she believes herself to be.

Someone with regular features and a good shape may lack confidence to such a degree that her insecurity comes over as stand-offishness, or even arrogance. On the other hand, a woman who is obviously attractive to other people may be less than perfect in shape and appearance, but what she does have is an excellent body image. She is reasonably satisfied with her body's good points and happily philosophical about any faults; she projects a positive 'I'm nice to know' aura. Almost invariably people will take her at her own unspoken evaluation and respond in a positive way.

Wearing a new dress also illustrates the point. Worn on the first occasion it is quite likely to bring you compliments on how pretty the dress is, or how nice you are looking. Worn a year later it is unlikely to attract compliments. The dress looks exactly the same, you look the same, but your feelings about the dress and consequently your appearance in it have changed.

It is rather more difficult to alter how you feel about yourself than alter how you look. And unless you can banish a feeling of inferiority, you won't enjoy the full rewards of being an attractive woman.

Beauty Planner

BARE ESSENTIALS	Manicure page 62 *Allow 30 minutes*	Applying False Nail Tips page 63 *Allow 1 hour*	Pedicure page 64 *Allow 40 minutes*	Bleaching Body or Facial Hair page 65 *Allow 30 minutes*	Facial page 65 *Allow 1 hour*	Eyebrow Shaping page 67 *Allow 20 minutes*	
COMPLETE MAKEOVER	Professional Makeup page 68 *Allow 45–60 minutes*	Applying False Eyelashes page 72 *Allow 30 minutes*	Colouring your Hair page 72 *Allow 5–60 minutes*	Conditioning your Hair page 76 *Allow 10–30 minutes*	Eyelash Tinting page 78 *Allow 30 minutes*	Eyebrow Tinting page 78 *Allow 20 minutes*	Eyebrow Bleaching page 79 *Allow 20 minutes*
PROFESSIONAL TREATMENTS	Paraffin Wax Treatment for Hands and Feet page 81 *Allow 30 minutes*		Wax Treatment for Unwanted Hair page 81 *Allow 1–2½ hours*		Body Massage page 84 *Allow 1 hour*		

ASSESSING YOUR WARDROBE

You can achieve a new look by simply being more selective about what you wear.

If you have asked a friend to help you with the body massage you can take the opportunity while she is with you to go through your wardrobe and discuss which clothes suit you best.

Everyone makes fashion mistakes sometimes, even the world's most well-dressed women. Get a second opinion on the outfits you are a little doubtful about. If there is no way to turn the mistakes into something you feel comfortable in, get rid of them. You may be able to swop clothes with your friend or give rejects away to a charity shop or jumble sale.

Here are some tips to help you select the styles that are right for you:

1 No matter how 'in' a fashion is, keep it out of your wardrobe unless it flatters.

2 If you and your face are very round, a round neck just adds unkind echoes. A collared style dipping into a lengthening V will flatter more.

3 To add height, make sure the clothes above your waist tone with those below. A dark skirt with a light-coloured blouse chops a figure in half and makes a small person look squat.

4 With surplus pounds to hide, never pick anything peasanty – the gathers and frills will only make you look plumper.

5 Very few unwaisted styles look better for a belt: the fullness invariably gathers up ungracefully.

6 Big belts are for small waists – with not a lot above and below.

7 A high choker collar or polo-neck sweaters may seem an ideal disguise for a not-so-young throat, but it only works for someone with a swan-like neck and nicely shaped bosom.

8 A soft stretchy fabric is only for trim torsos. Anything that is strained, tight and crumpled is sheer cruelty.

9 Bright white alone is cruel unless you've a terrific tan, pearly teeth and gallons of glow.

10 Shine adds emphasis and the illusion of extra inches. Darker, matt surfaces will do the opposite. You can use this rule to improve proportions, boosting a small bust, for instance with a pale silky-sheened shirt above a dark-toned skirt or trousers with a discreet dull surface.

11 Plain court shoes with a comfortably high heel flatter the legs. Don't buy shoes with straps if you have thick ankles and never buy shoes that have too high a heel for you to walk comfortably.

12 Anyone over 30 must expect under-arm slackness. The top of your arms can be a woman's least attractive part and elbows can run a close second. Sleeveless and strapless tops are for the young – more mature arms are better covered up.

One of life's lousiest laws decrees that you always meet an old flame, a worst enemy or your future boss when looking your worst. The lesson is never get behind with grooming and never think: 'No one will see me'. Always make an effort with your appearance. Knowing you are looking good will give you the confidence to deal with all sorts of encounters.

Home Health Farm Appointment Cards

Plan the hours or days you intend to spend at your Home Health Farm well in advance and fill in an appointment card for each day. (We suggest you use a pencil so that you can alter the programme next time you want to pamper yourself with a visit to the Home Health Farm.)

We tell you how long each beauty treatment or exercise session is likely to take and this enables you to plan your programme to the minute. Remember to allow extra minutes to change into your exercise gear or gather together any cosmetics you will require. Leave yourself plenty of free time in which to relax (see page 11) and also allow yourself time to prepare your diet dishes for the following day. Complete your appointment card a few days in advance so that you have time to buy food and beauty items you will need.

The sample appointment cards opposite illustrate programmes which would be ideal to follow if you can steal two days for a self-pampering programme. Use them as a guide, making small changes for your personal requirements. Stock up on food and potions, shift any family responsibilities on to other shoulders and set about indulging yourself . . . at your Home Health Farm. . . .

HOME HEALTH FARM *Appointment Card*

HOME HEALTH FARM *Appointment Card*

Day 1

8.00 Wake up and do a few stretches
8.30 Wash, dress and get into something comfortable
9.30 Breakfast
10.30 Manicure
11.30 First exercise work-out
12.30 Lunch
1.30 Go for a walk for 30 minutes
2.30 Pedicure
3.30 Drink or snack from allowance and relaxation
4.30 Condition hair
5.30 Second exercise work-out
6.30 Dinner
8.00 Facial
9.00 Drink or snack
10.00 Prepare next day's diet meals
11.00 Bath and relaxation

HOME HEALTH FARM *Appointment Card*

Day 2

8.00 Wake up and do exercise work-out
9.00 Wash and dress
10.00 Breakfast
11.00 Facial
12.00 Shape eyebrows
1.00 Lunch
2.00 Dye eyelashes or lighten facial hair
3.00 Get out skipping rope and do 30 minutes exercise
4.00 Drink or snack from allowance
4.30 Complete makeover
6.30 Dinner
8.00 Plan hair changes
9.00 Drink or snack
10.00 Second exercise work-out
11.00 Bath and relaxation

HOME HEALTH FARM *Appointment Card*

HOME HEALTH FARM *Appointment Card*

Home Health Farm Questionnaire

By simply answering Yes or No to the following questions we will lead you to the exercise work-out and diet-plan that is best suited to your needs and lifestyle. Complete the questionnaire each time you visit your Home Health Farm.

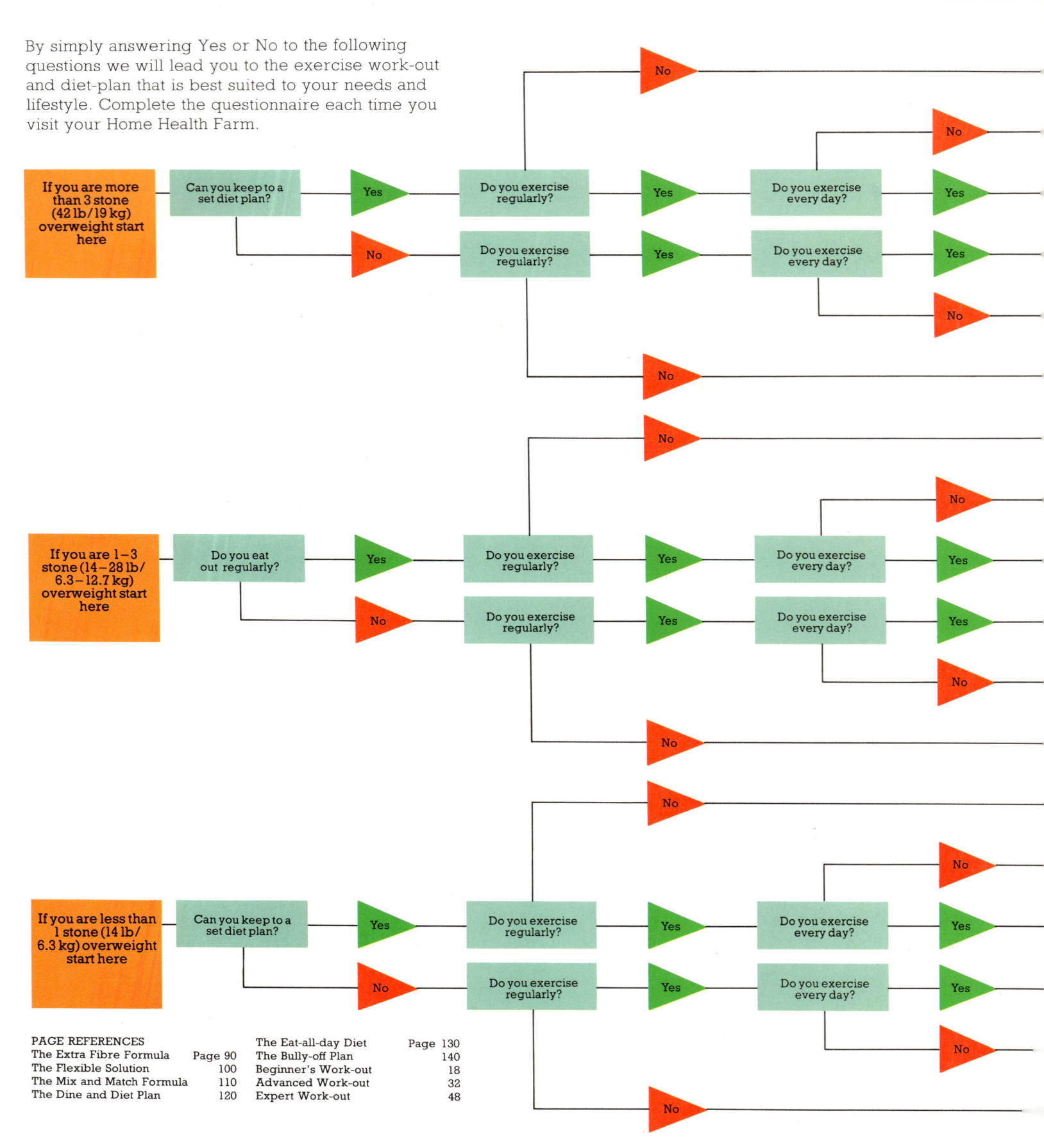

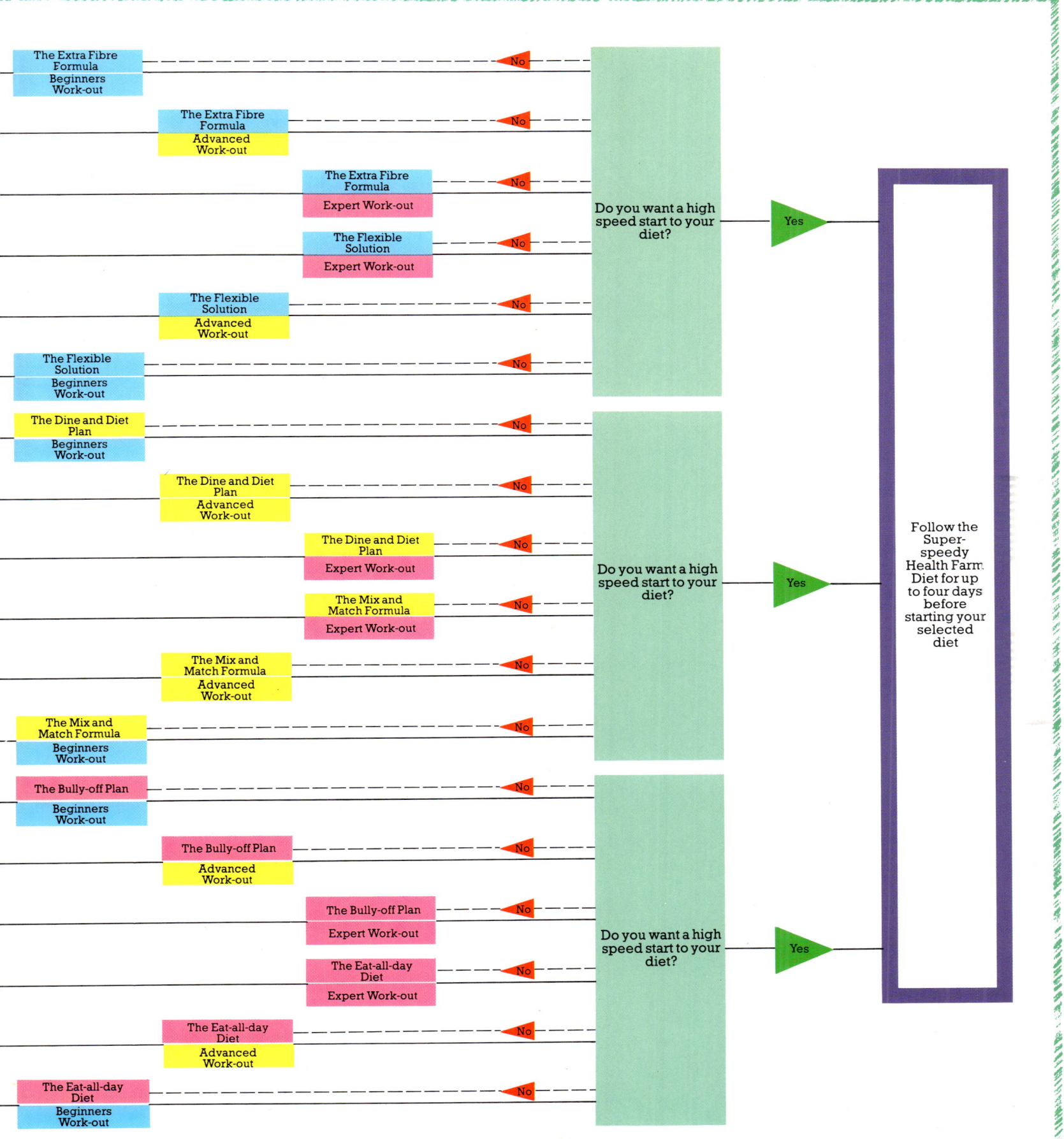

The Extra Fibre
Formula
Beginners
Work-out — — — No

The Extra Fibre
Formula
Advanced
Work-out — — — No

The Extra Fibre
Formula
Expert Work-out — — — No

The Flexible
Solution
Expert Work-out — — — No

The Flexible
Solution
Advanced
Work-out — — — No

Do you want a high speed start to your diet? Yes

The Flexible
Solution
Beginners
Work-out — — — No

The Dine and Diet
Plan
Beginners
Work-out — — — No

The Dine and Diet
Plan
Advanced
Work-out — — — No

The Dine and Diet
Plan
Expert Work-out — — — No

The Mix and
Match Formula
Expert Work-out — — — No

Do you want a high speed start to your diet? Yes

The Mix and
Match Formula
Advanced
Work-out — — — No

The Mix and
Match Formula
Beginners
Work-out — — — No

The Bully-off Plan
Beginners
Work-out — — — No

The Bully-off Plan
Advanced
Work-out — — — No

The Bully-off Plan
Expert Work-out — — — No

The Eat-all-day
Diet
Expert Work-out — — — No

Do you want a high speed start to your diet? Yes

The Eat-all-day
Diet
Advanced
Work-out — — — No

The Eat-all-day
Diet
Beginners
Work-out — — — No

Follow the Super-speedy Health Farm Diet for up to four days before starting your selected diet

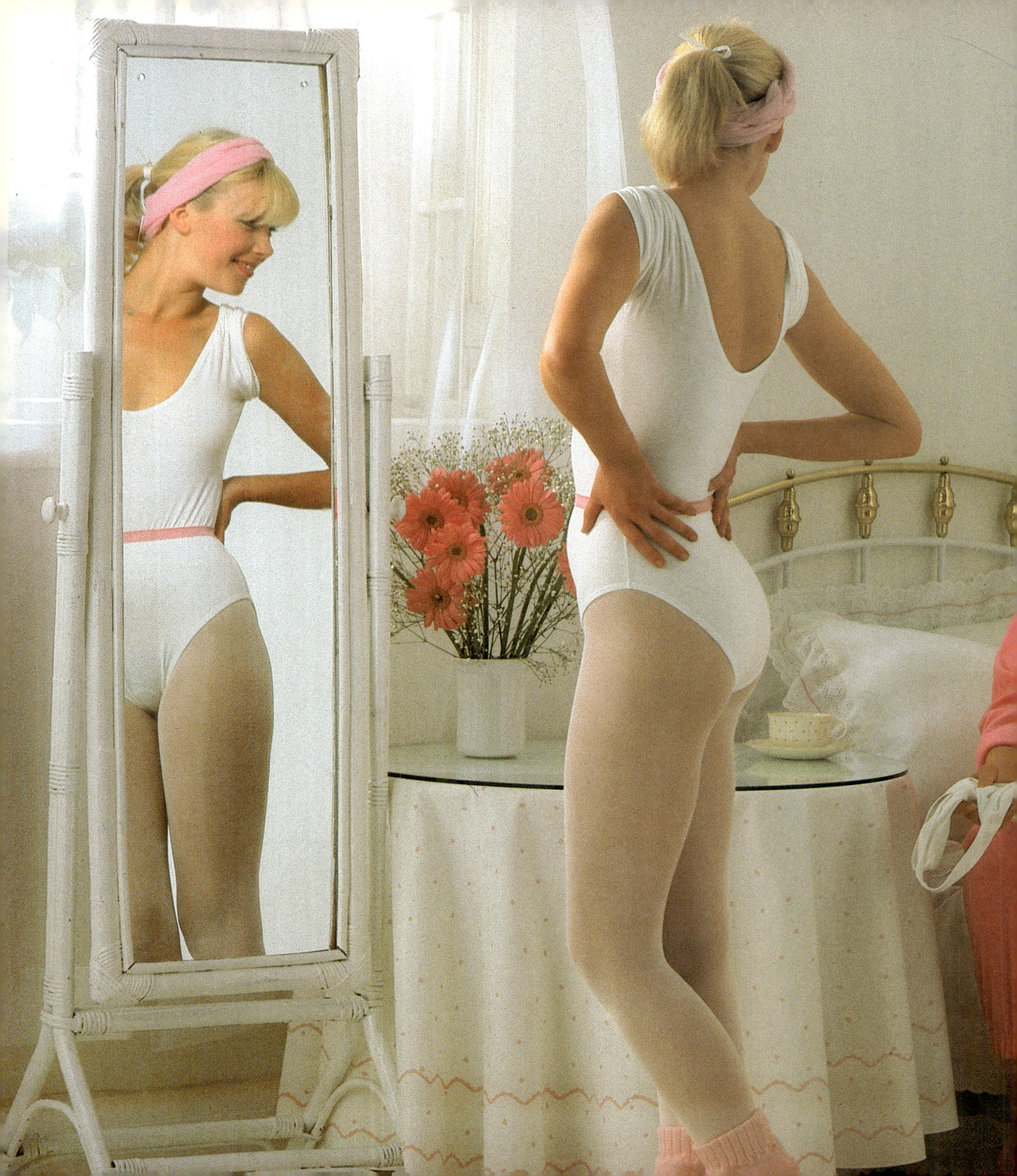

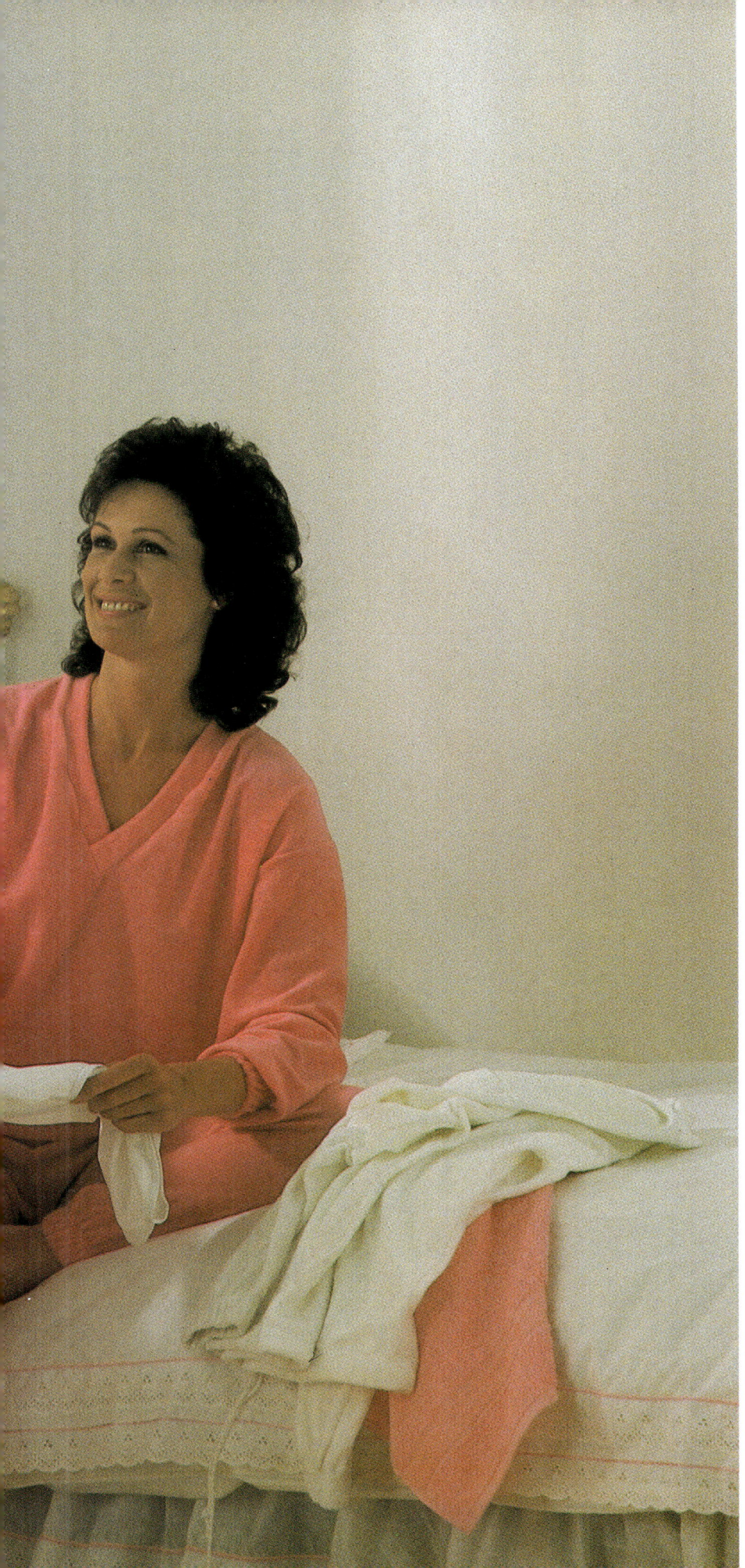

EXERCISE

Exercise is always a total tonic but if you have excess pounds to lose, diet combined with exercise is definitely the most effective way for you to get into shape.

Complete the Home Health Farm Questionnaire on page 14 and get started on your personal exercise programme. Each exercise work-out is devised to help tone up muscles all over the body.

Build regular exercise sessions into your week, for best results you need to do a work-out at least two or three times a week. To really see results though you must be patient, if your muscles have become flabby and slack it may be several months before they tone up enough to noticeably trim you down.

If you are very much out of condition, and/or more than 6 kg/14 lbs or so overweight, launching suddenly into a punishing physical programme does not make sense. Even professionl dancers, gymnasts and athletes respect the importance of limbering up before attempting anything demanding. So always start your work-out with the warmup exercise given.

Beginner's Work-out 1

Allow 30 minutes for this session

Exercise can be fun and enjoyable so don't be put off if you've never bothered to exercise much. You are certainly not alone! Many women rarely exercise. They would . . . if they had the time . . . if they had the energy . . . or if they thought they could keep it up. Don't use these 'ifs' as an excuse to give up before you begin. It's amazing how much better you will feel after even a short exercise session. And it's at those times when you least feel like making the effort that the best results can be obtained. Just try it and see for yourself.

If you have never exercised since school or haven't done a session for a long time, take it very easy at first. Copy the family cat. You never see her rush off after lying still or asleep without first doing some long, long stretches. Each of the following exercise sessions starts with a stretch. Take your time and really work at this and you will feel an immediate benefit. It will improve your posture, too.

Before you start your exercises make sure you have plenty of space to stretch upwards, downwards, to the side. If necessary move furniture to the outside of the room to make your own mini work-out studio. Music helps to keep the rhythm going, so switch on the radio or choose an up-tempo record or tape.

Exercise should be done slowly and rhythmically and at no point should you strain to reach a position. But that doesn't mean you don't have to work hard: the harder you work, the more your figure will benefit.

If you have ever had any kind of back trouble, blood pressure problems or a serious illness, please check with your doctor before undertaking an exercise campaign.

This first work-out will take about half an hour. If you want to do more than one session (two is the most you should attempt on your first day) you can either repeat this session or go on to Beginner's Work-out 2.

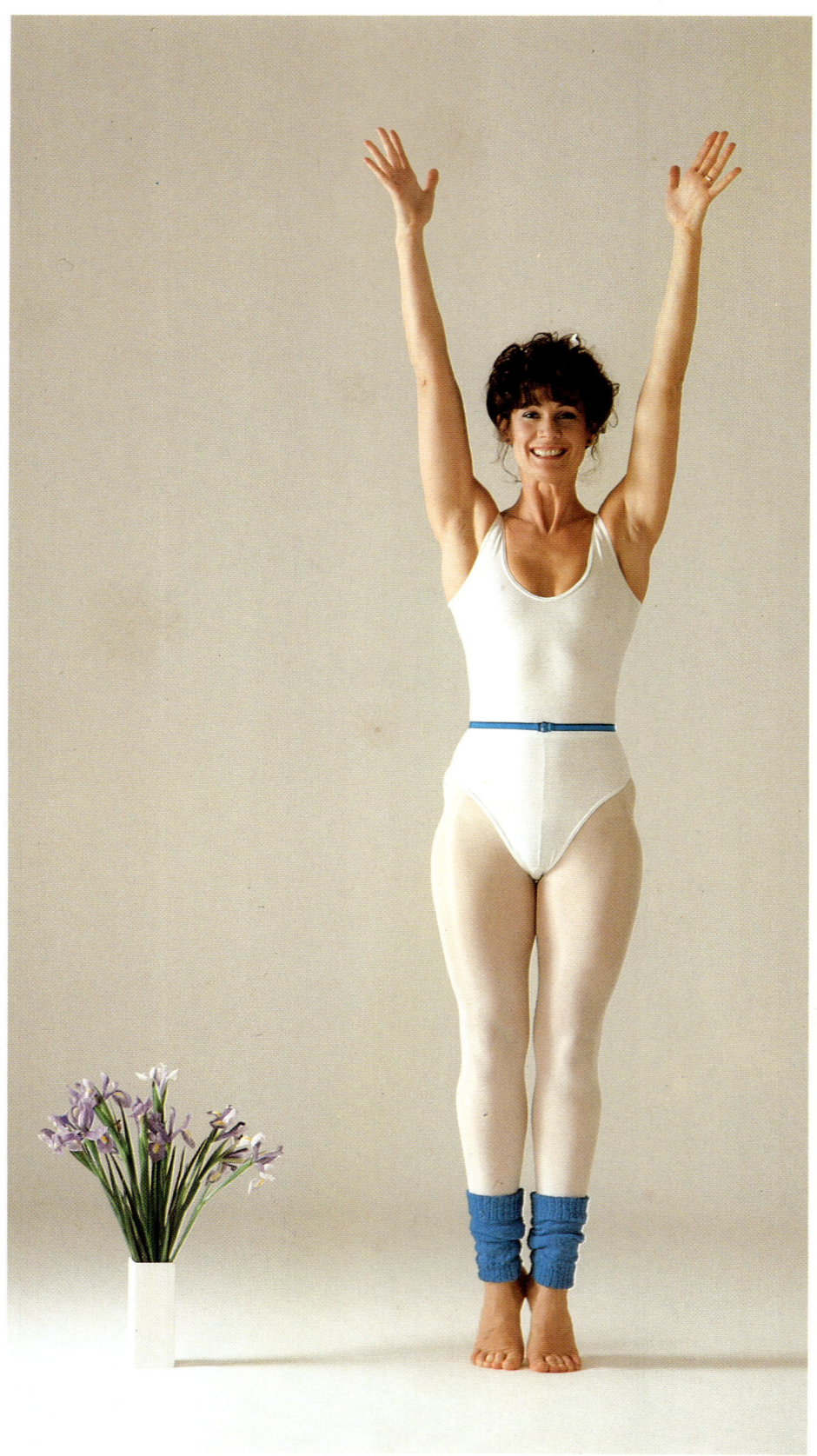

Exercise 1

What it does
Stretches and tones the whole body

How you do it
1 Do this exercise very slowly and deliberately. Stand up straight, feet together (1).
2 Go up on tiptoe, raising arms from sides.
3 Push up, trying to make fingertips touch the ceiling.
4 Lower arms and heels.
5 Repeat the whole exercise five times.

Exercise 2

What it does
Stretches the body and works on the stomach and hips.

How you do it
1 Stand up straight, feet apart, hands by sides, fingers pointing towards ground (2a).
2 Raise arms above head (2b), breathe out as you bend to the right and grasp right ankle with right hand (2c).
3 Breathe in and stretch up.
4 Repeat to the left.
5 Repeat the whole exercise eight times.

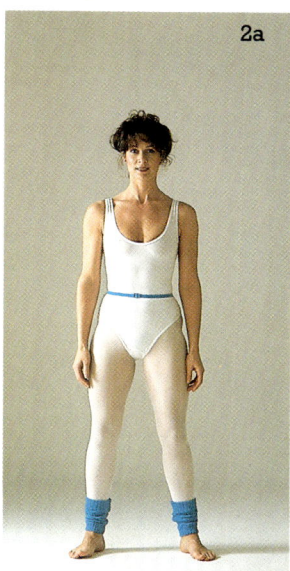

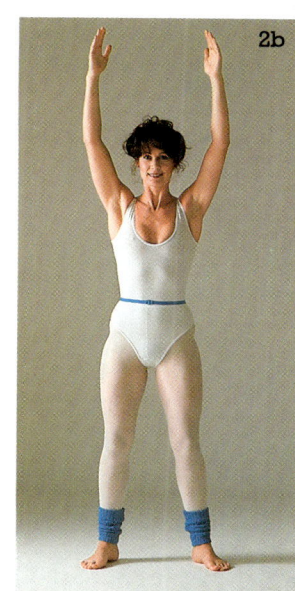

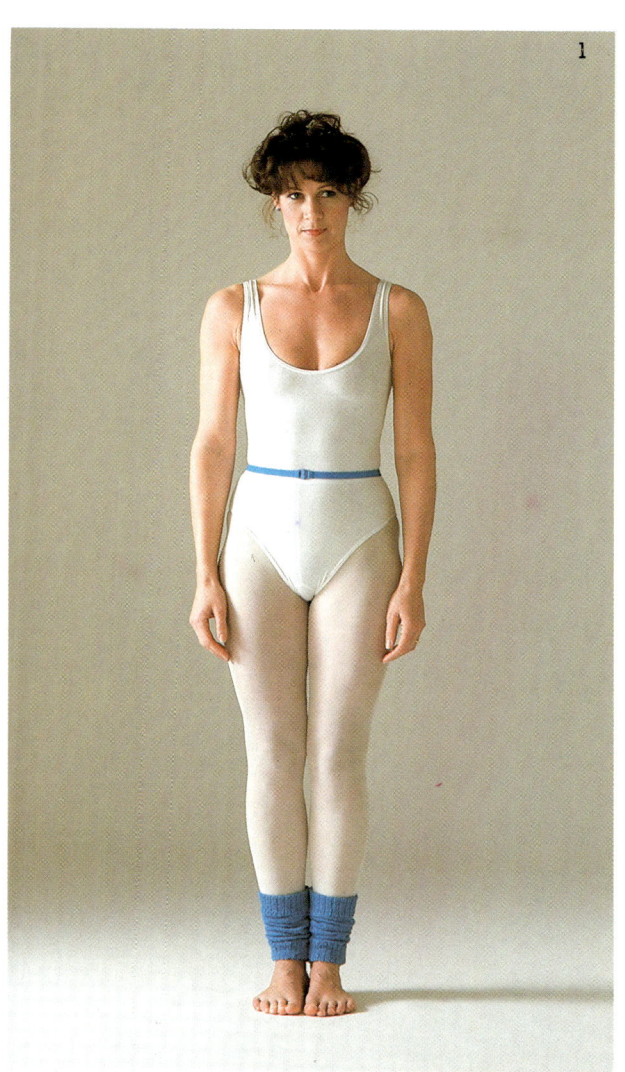

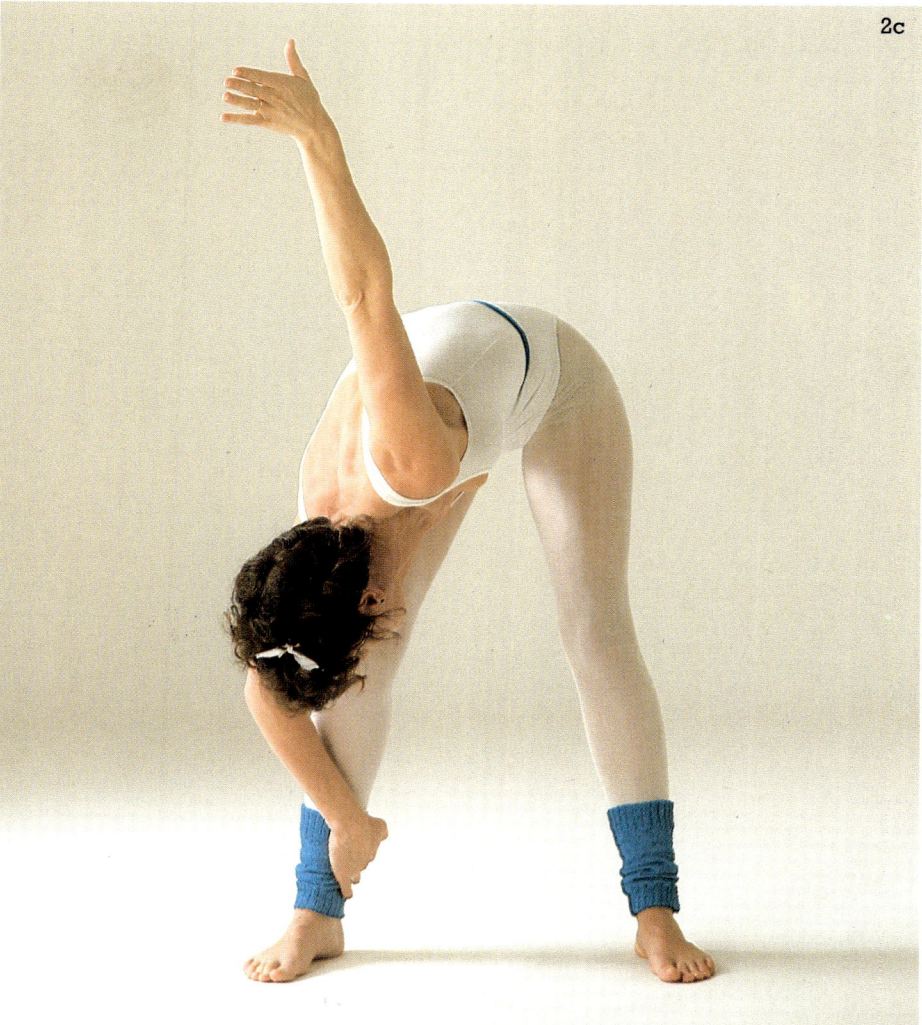

Exercise 3

What it does
Relaxes the neck and shoulders, easing away tension

How you do it
1 Sit or stand, shoulders relaxed and chin at right angles to neck.
2 Drop head forwards so that chin rests on chest (3a).
3 Now circle head to the right (3b) and open mouth as you gently circle head backwards (3c).
4 Circle round to the left, closing mouth as you return to starting position.
5 Repeat these circles four times to the right, then reverse and circle five times to the left.

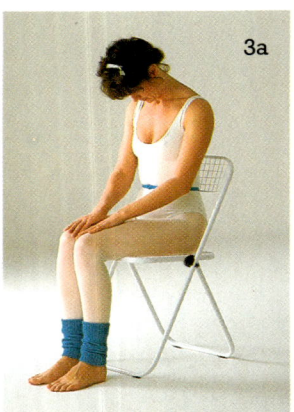

3a

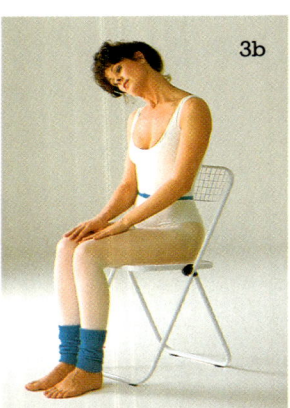

3b

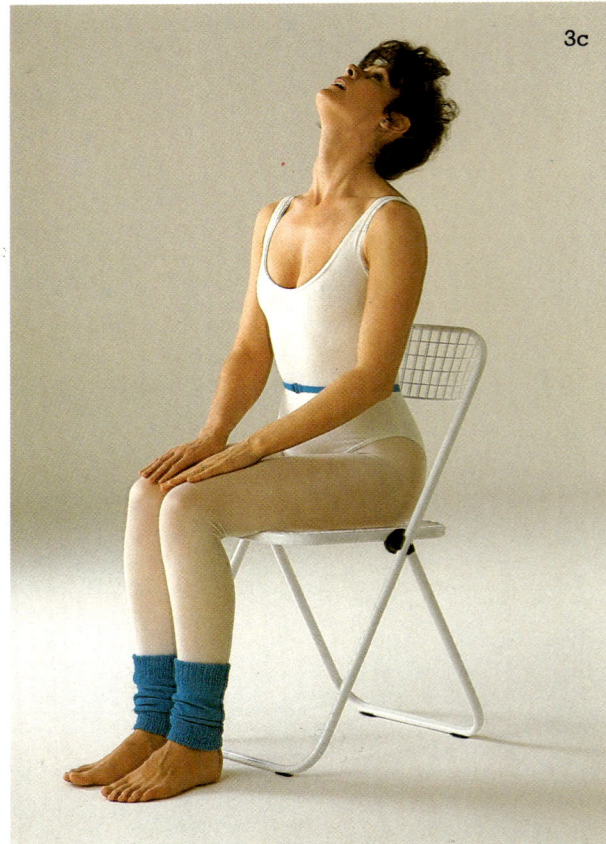

3c

Exercise 5

What it does
Exercises the hip joints and firms up thighs

How you do it
1 Stand up straight and hold on to a chair with right hand (5a).
2 Keeping right leg straight and foot flat on floor, swing left leg forwards (5b) and back 10 times (5c). Keep standing upright and do not bend forwards as you swing.
3 Turn round and hold chair with left hand, swing right leg forwards and back 10 times.

Exercise 4

What it does
Tones the upper arms, firming under-arm sag

How you do it
1 Stretch arms out straight horizontally from shoulders, palms down (4a).
2 Twisting palms upwards, bend arms at elbows and keeping forearm at right angles to upper arm, shake arms up and down 10 times (4b).
3 Stretch arms out straight again and turn palms downwards. Tighten muscles as you shake arms up and down 10 times in shallow jerks – the faster the better.
4 Repeat the whole exercise once.

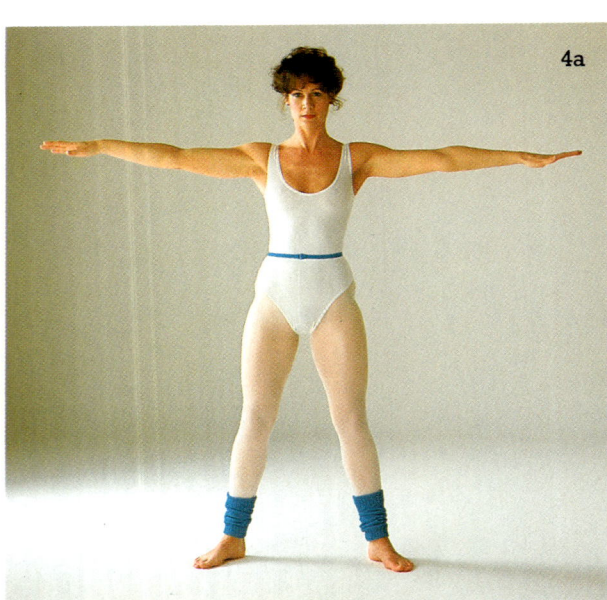

4a

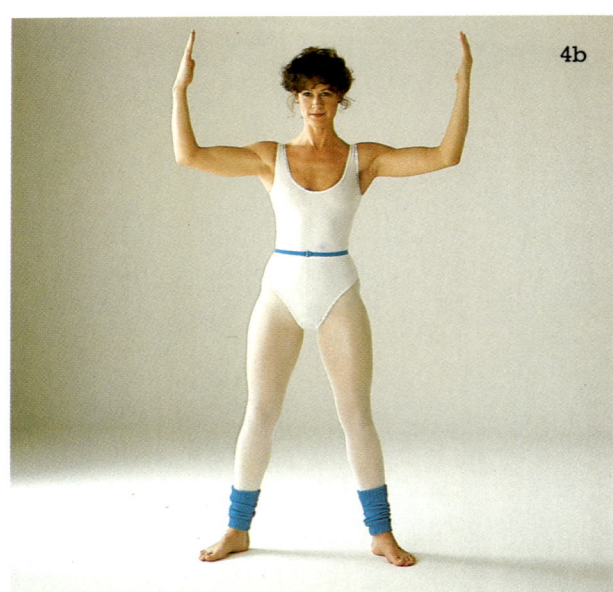

4b

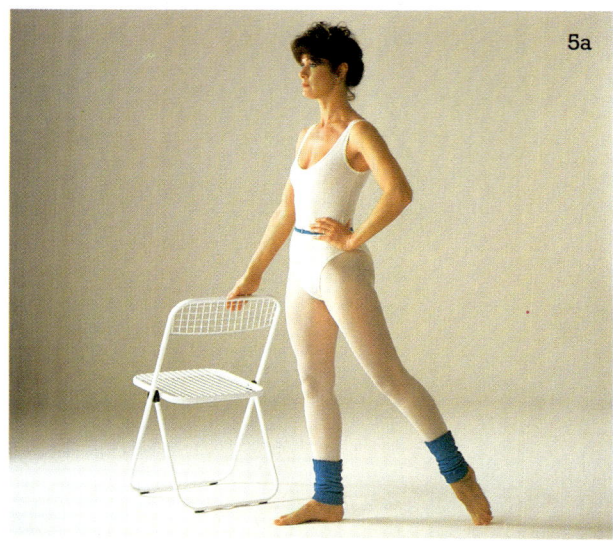

5a

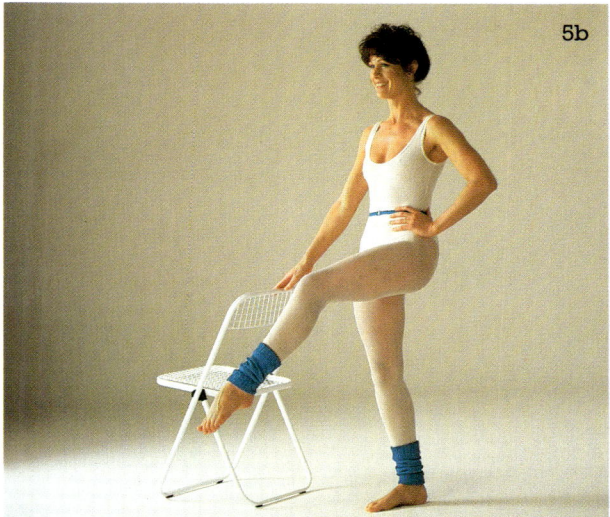

5b

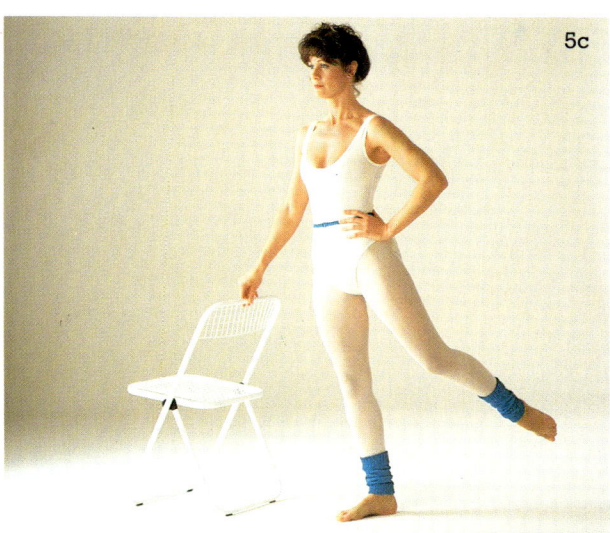

5c

Exercise 6

What it does
Lifts the bustline and tones upper arms

How you do it
1 Lie flat on your back on the floor.
2 Bend knees up halfway, keeping feet flat on floor.
3 Press palms of hands together in prayer position in front of chest.
4 Breathe in. Breathe out. As you breathe out, press hands together as hard as you can, keeping chin down and nape of neck pressed firmly against floor (6).
5 Repeat the exercise slowly five times.

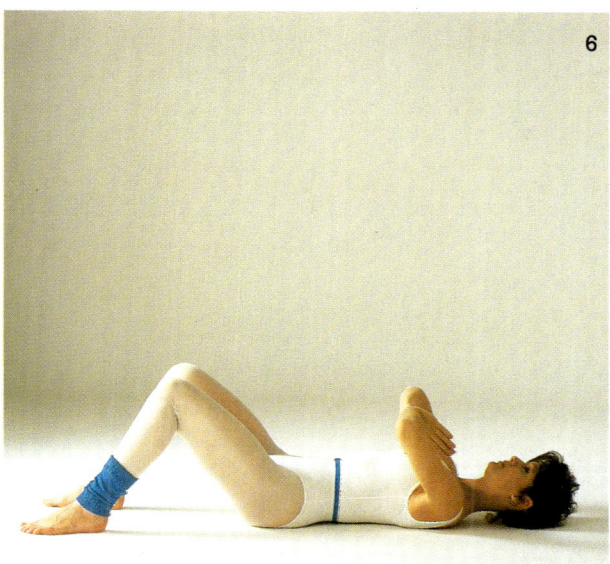

6

Exercise 7

What it does
Goes to work on thigh flab

How you do it
1 Lie flat on your back on the floor, knees bent, feet flat on floor, arms outstretched at shoulder level.
2 Raise left leg in the air, then lower (7). Repeat with right leg.
3 Repeat these alternate lifts 10 times.

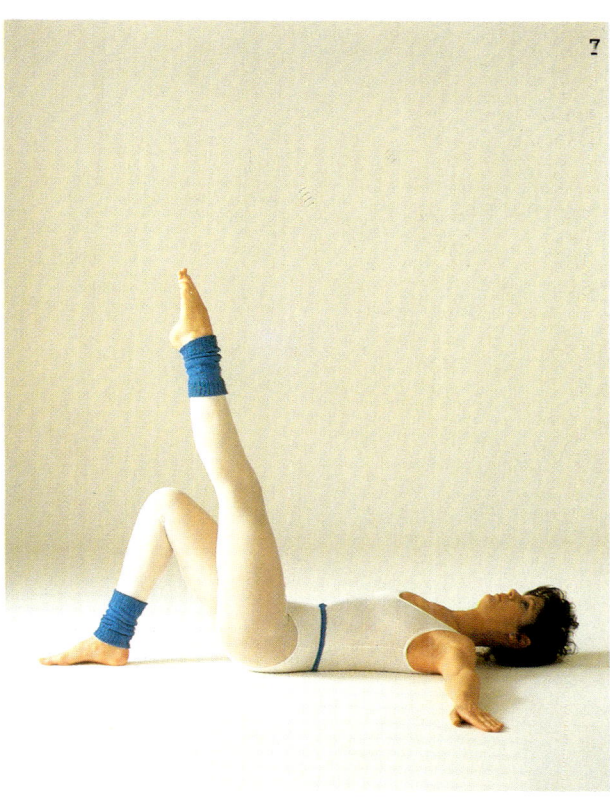

7

Exercise 8

What it does
Works the stomach muscles

How you do it
1 Stand up straight, feet apart, arms stretched above head (8a).
2 Slowly bend over to touch toes, allowing knees to bend, letting head and hands relax but pulling in stomach quickly, then releasing it (8b).
3 Straighten up. Stand with hands on hips and pull stomach in, then release it (8c).
4 Repeat the whole exercise five times.

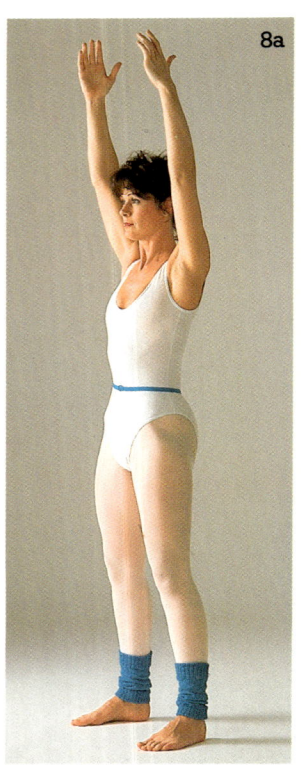

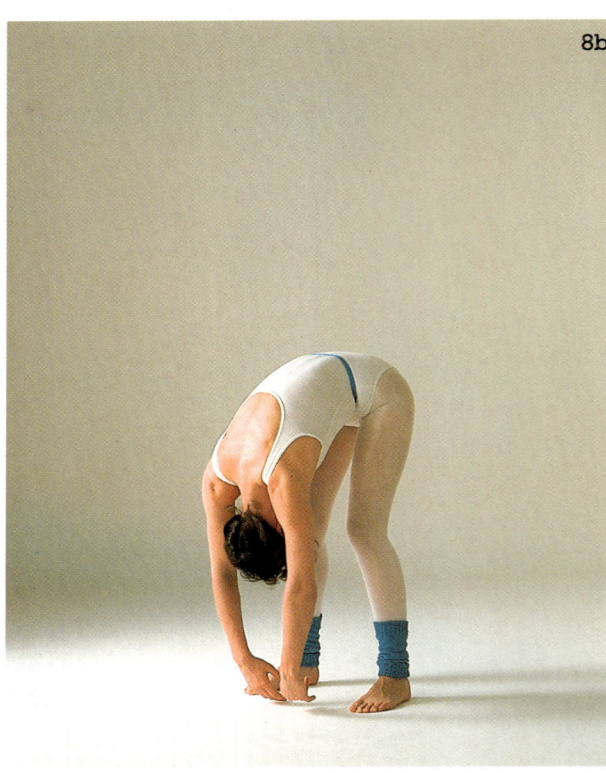

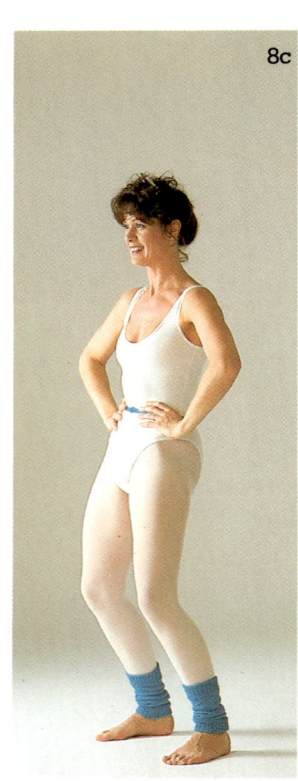

Exercise 9

What it does
Trims the waistline and helps make you supple all over

How you do it
1 Stand up straight, feet apart, hands at sides, fingers pointing towards ground (9a).
2 Put right hand on waist and stretch left arm above head. Breathe out and bend body to the right (9b). Breathe in and straighten up.
3 Put left hand on waist and stretch right arm above head. Breathe out and bend body to the left. Breathe in and straighten up.
4 Repeat the whole exercise four times.

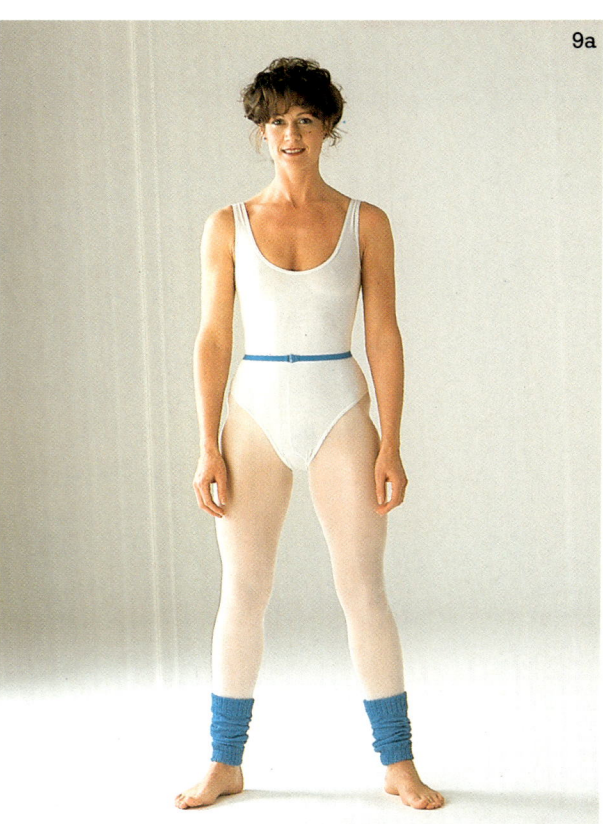

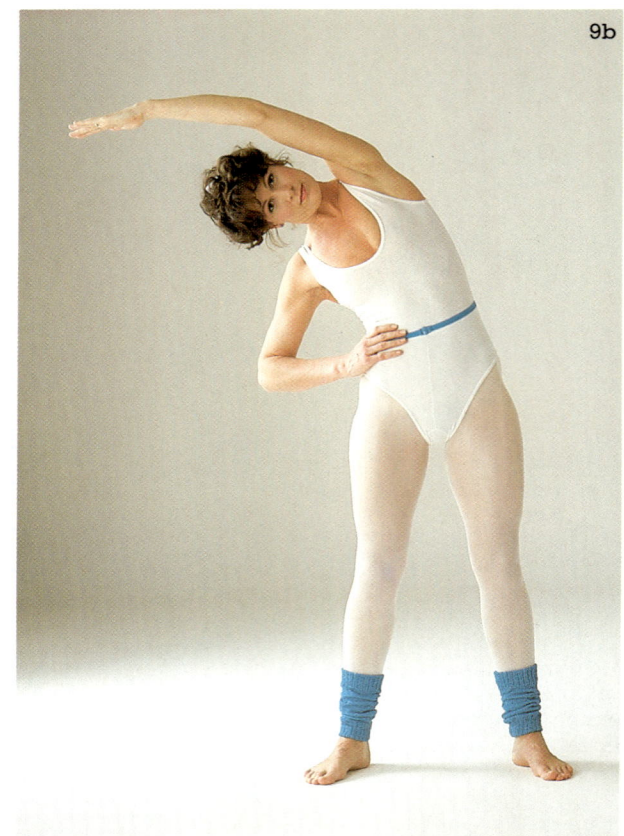

Exercise 10

What it does
Strengthens the thigh
muscles to cut flab and
sag

How you do it
1 Stand up straight, feet
together, arms stretched
out in front (10a).
2 Breathe out and bend
knees, keeping feet
together, heels on floor
and arms stretched out
(10b).
3 Breathe in, returning to
the standing position and
pulling in buttock
muscles as you rise.
4 Repeat the whole
exercise five times.

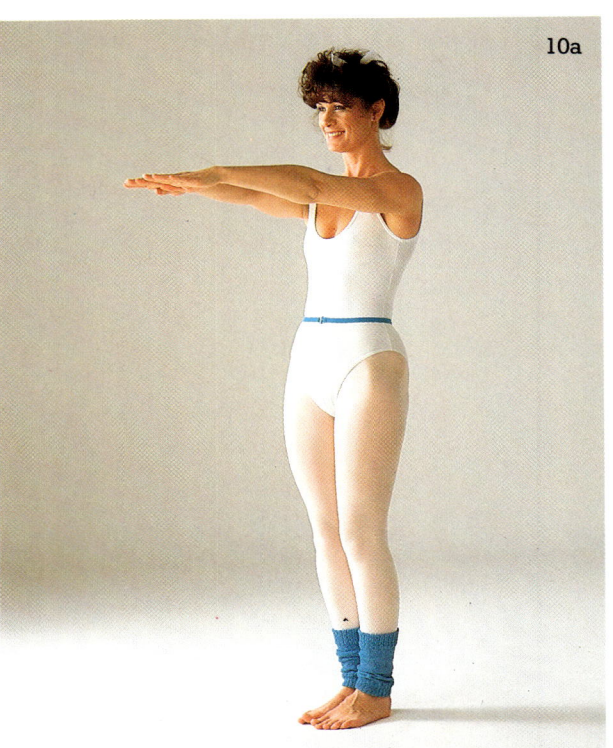
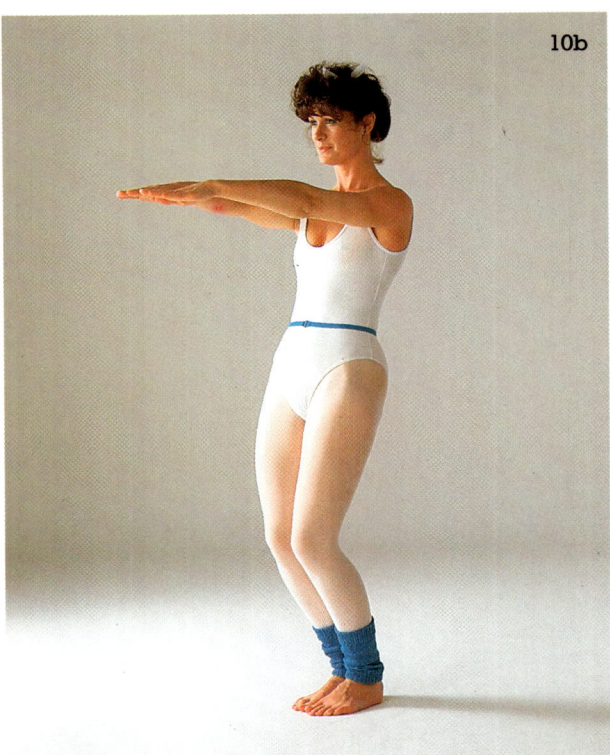

Exercise 11

What it does
Takes energetic toning
action on the stomach
and bottom

How you do it
1 Sit on the floor, back
straight, legs together
and stretched out in front
(11).
2 Raise arms in front to
shoulder level, keeping
them straight.
3 Floor-walk forward
briskly on your bottom
with a slight side-to-side
rolling motion. Extend
each leg in turn to its
fullest extent.
4 Floor-walk back to
your starting position by
reversing the movement.
5 Floor-walk across the
room until you reach the
wall, then reverse to
your original position.
Repeat this twice.

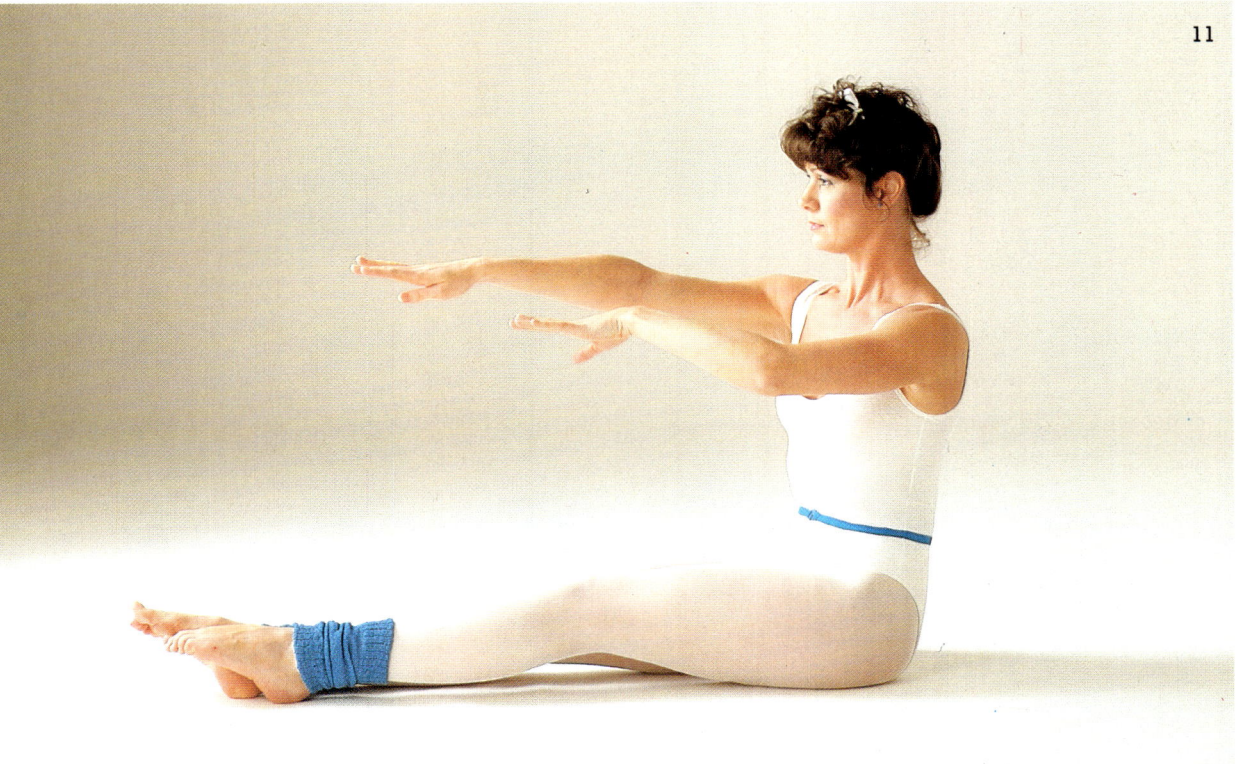

Exercise 12

What it does
Helps to trim and firm the bottom and rear of the thighs

How you do it
1 Lie flat on your back on the floor. Place arms by sides, palms of hands down.
2 Bend knees, keeping feet flat on floor, drawing heels directly under knees.
3 Breathe in as deeply as possible. Then breathe out, at the same time lifting bottom and pushing pubic bone towards the ceiling. Your weight should be on upper back, neck and feet and you'll feel your bottom and thighs tighten (12).
4 Hold position for 2 seconds. Breathe in and lower bottom to floor.
5 Repeat the whole exercise slowly four times.

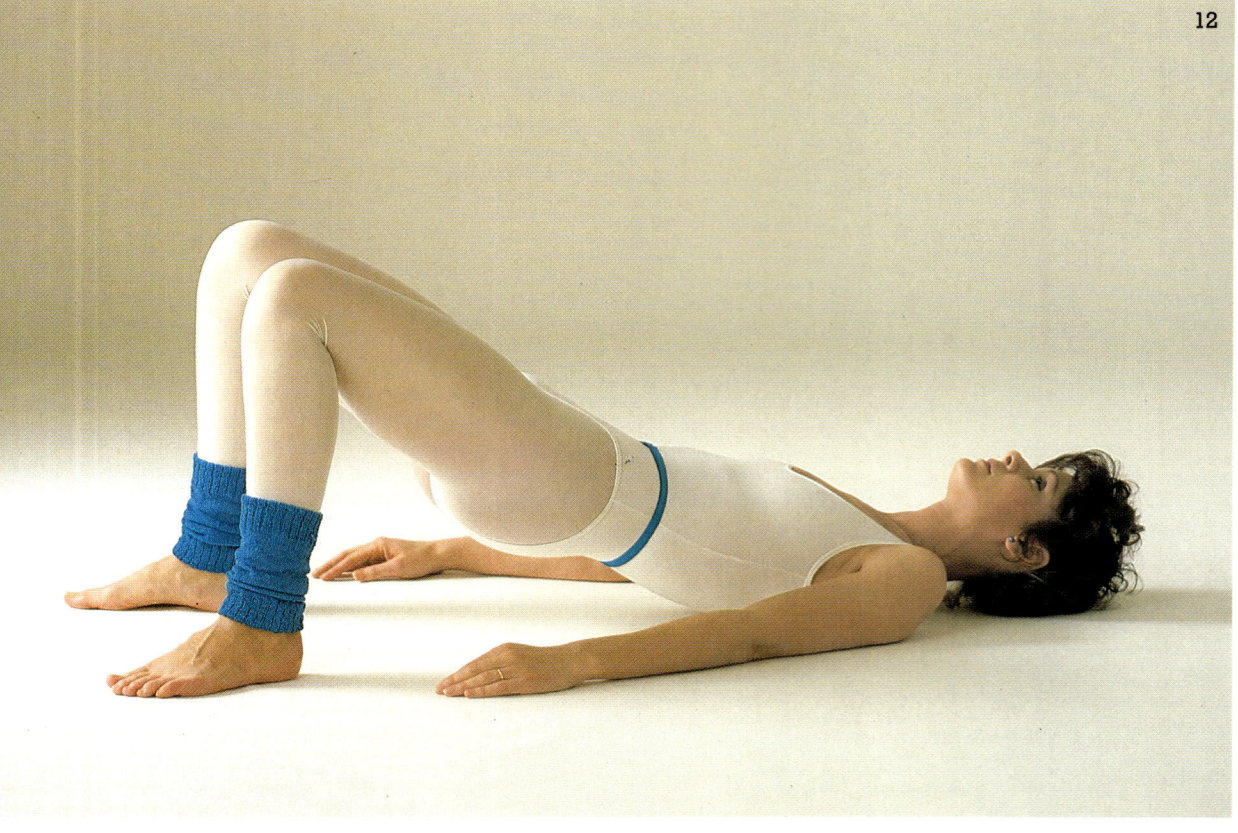

Exercise 13

What it does
Tones the waist and hips

How you do it
1 Lie flat on your back on the floor, arms stretched out horizontally on a line with shoulders.
2 Draw up knees to form a gentle inverted 'U', keeping feet flat on floor (13a).
3 Roll knees to the left, trying to touch floor with knees and allowing feet to turn on to their sides.
4 Return knees to the upright position, then roll to the right (13b).
5 Make sure you keep whole body above waist flat and motionless while doing this exercise.
6 Repeat the whole exercise 10 times.

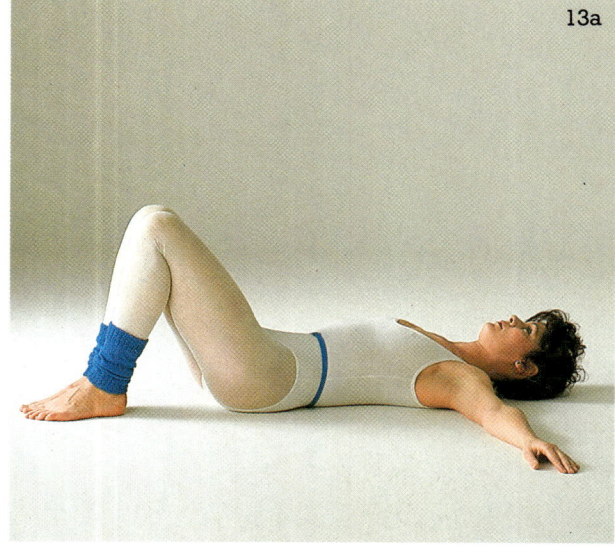

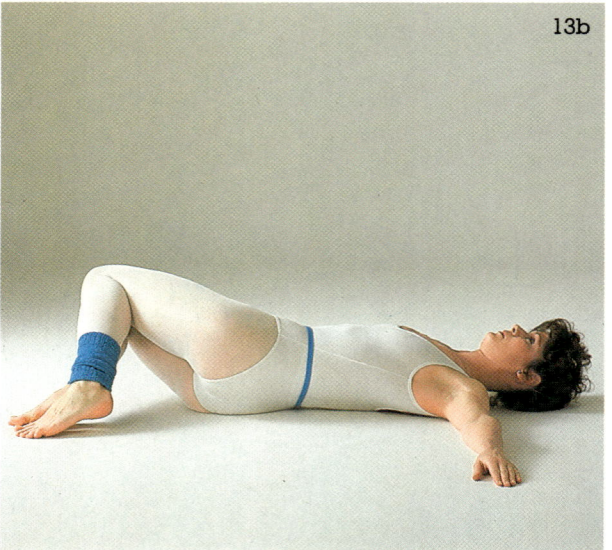

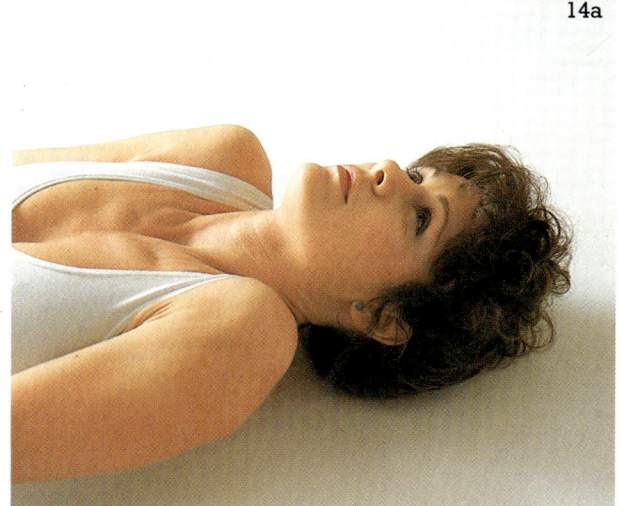

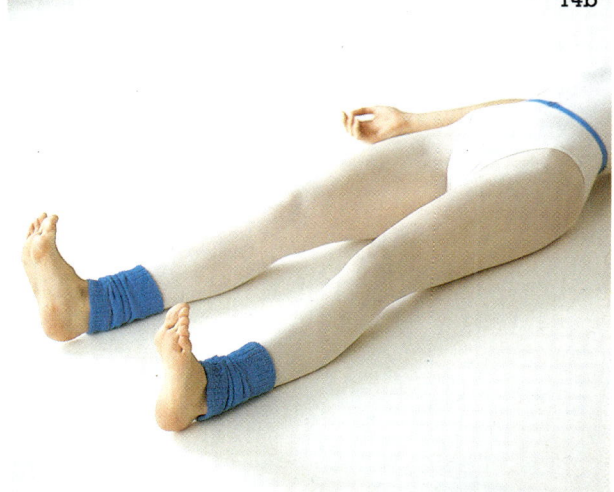

Relax

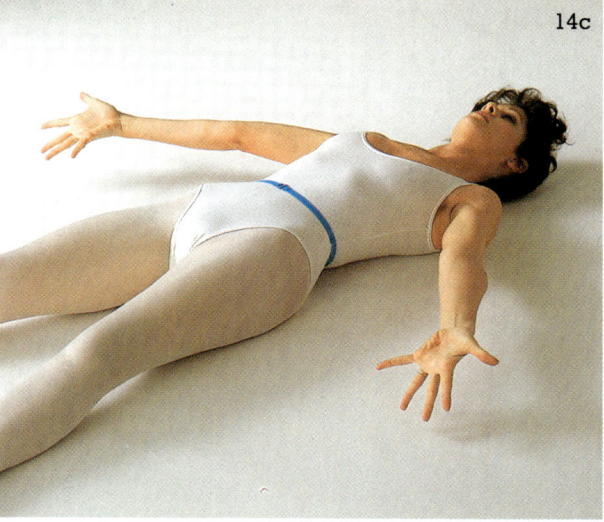

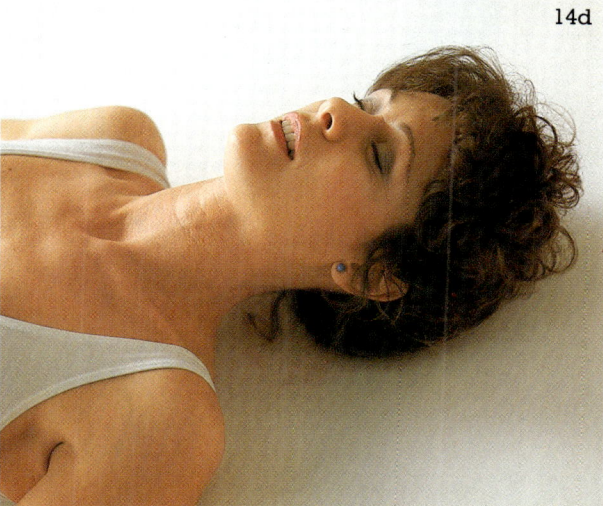

1 Lie flat on your back on the floor. Make sure you are lying in a straight line with head straight and chin tucked in.

2 Raise shoulders away from floor and up to ears, then relax them as you lower them back to floor (14a).

3 Raise bottom, press lower back into floor, clench buttocks, then relax as you lower them again.

4 Tense leg and feet muscles (14b), then relax them, allowing feet to flop outwards.

5 Stretch arms about 30 cm/12 inches from your body, stretching fingers outwards (14c), then relax arms and place palms facing upwards with fingers slightly curled in a relaxed position.

6 Tighten muscles in face, then relax (14d). Close eyes and breathe in and out very deeply for about five minutes (14e).

7 Roll over on your side and very slowly get to your feet.

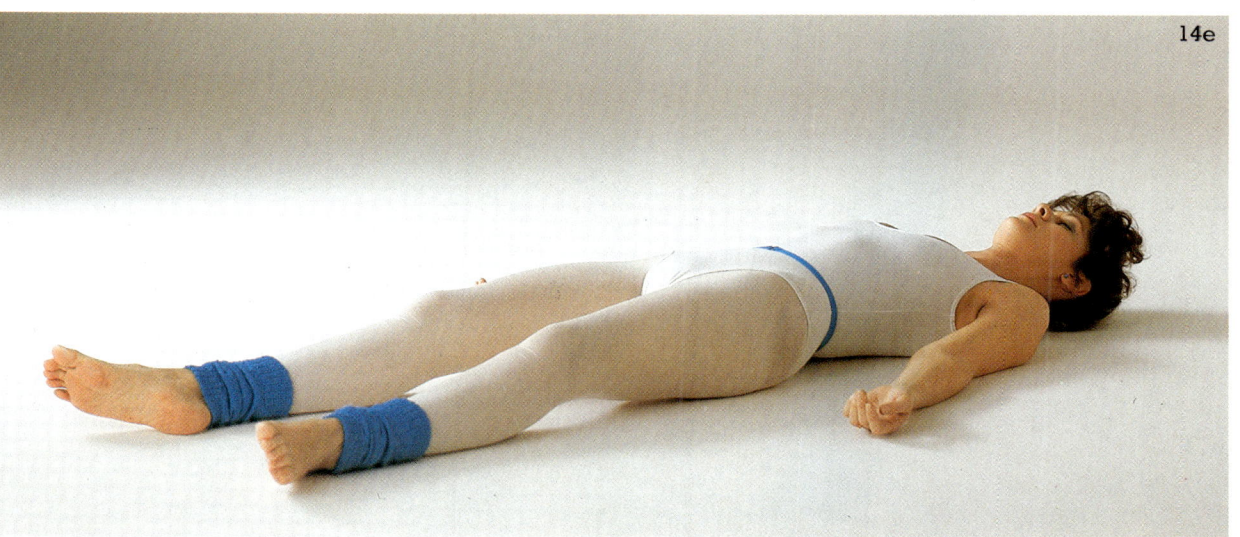

Beginner's Work-out 2

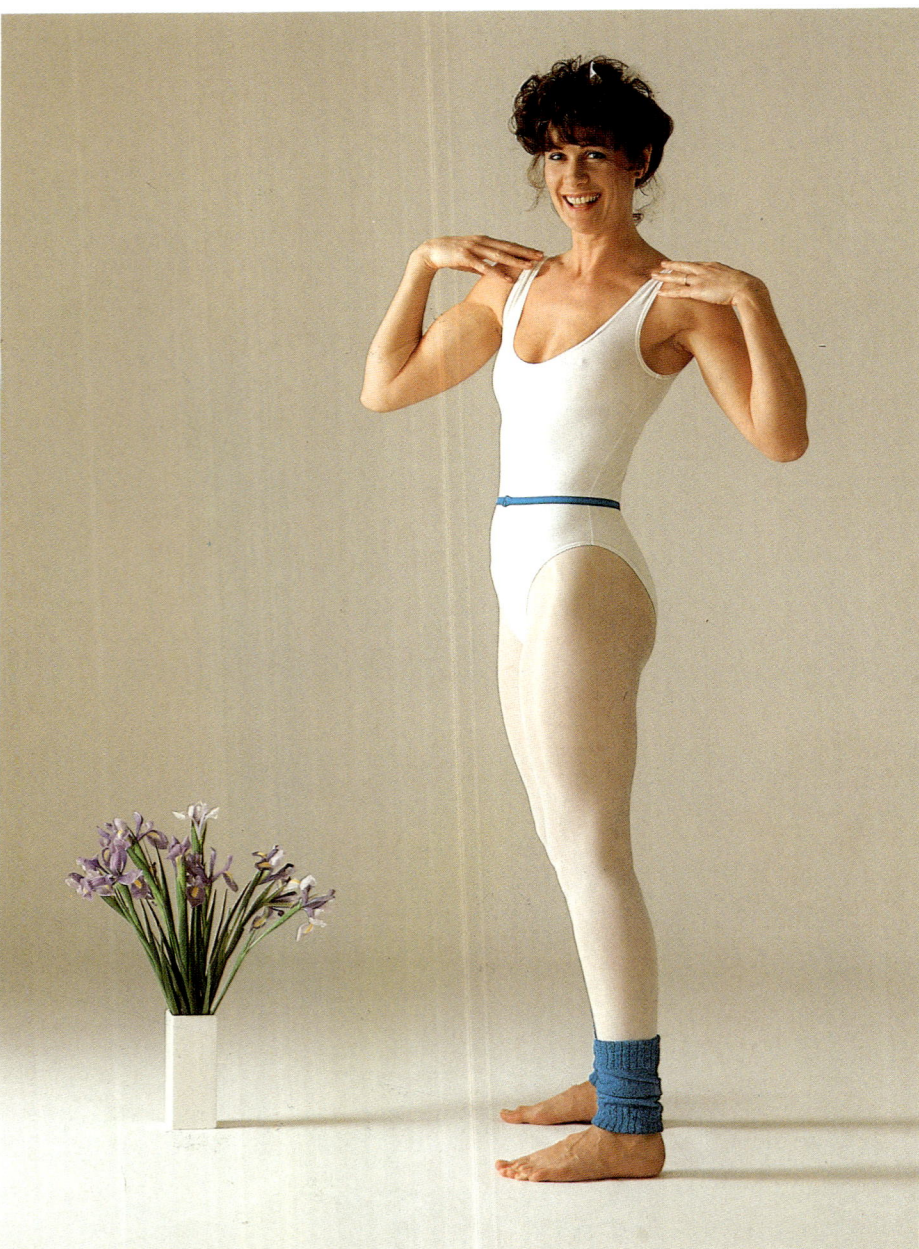

Allow 30 minutes for this session

When your body is working properly, you get so much *more* than just a better shape. Exercise helps the circulation, stimulates internal organs, improves your general health and makes you feel good, too. If you keep really fit you'll probably find you have far more stamina to do all sorts of jobs and chores. Stiff, heavy movements are instantly ageing – young is supple, light and flexible – so exercising will keep you looking youthful. If you're under 25 you may have a very good figure just by sheer luck: after 25, when the muscles start to slacken, you simply have to be prepared to work at it.

Exercise is vital if you are slimming since it ensures that your body muscles firm up as you shed weight. Dieting gets rid of surplus fat but could leave you saggy all over! And even if you have little or no weight to lose, properly toned muscles work to keep your whole figure in tip-top condition.

It is essential to start exercising gently, warming up slowly and easily. Never pick the hardest exercise you can find and work at it without doing some gentle tone-ups first. Don't exercise for too long, either. Just do as much as you comfortably can for your first few sessions; then, as your body gets used to the work-outs, you'll find them a little easier. If you have any health worries, please read the introduction to Beginner's Work-out 1.

These two beginners' programmes include exercises to improve the most common problem areas and are designed to give your body an all-over tone-up. Try to build one half-hour session into every day. Do not attempt to go on to the more difficult work-outs in this book until you have been doing one or both of these sessions regularly for at least two weeks.

Exercise 1

What it does
An all over stretch

How you do it
1 Lie flat on your back on the floor.
2 Stretch arms out behind head.
3 Stretch legs and point toes. Breathe in deeply.
4 Breathe out, stretching arms and legs as far as you can, pressing lower back into floor (1).
5 Repeat the whole exercise three times.

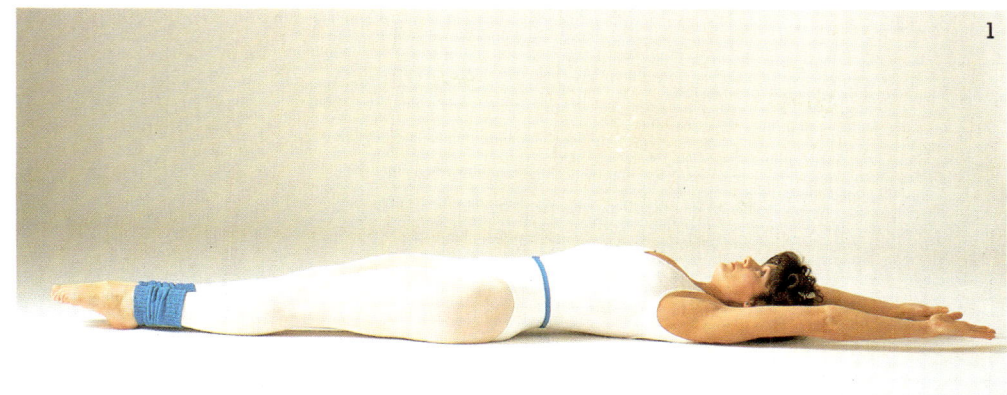

Exercise 2

What it does
Relaxes neck muscles

How you do it
1 Sit cross-legged on floor.
2 Keeping shoulders motionless, look over right shoulder, then over left (2a). Swivel your head as far as possible in each direction, with a clock's tick-tock rhythm.
3 Repeat five times on each side. Ignore any peculiar-sounding clicks and creaks; they'll gradually disappear as your neck relaxes and becomes more supple.
4 Now, to the same rhythm, drop head as far forwards as you can (2b), then lift and stretch back until you can see the ceiling (2c). Keep shoulders down throughout.
5 Repeat the exercise five times.
6 Now attempt the impossible: keeping head pointing forwards, try to touch right ear to right shoulder without letting shoulder rise (2d). Repeat with left ear to left shoulder. Repeat five times on each side.

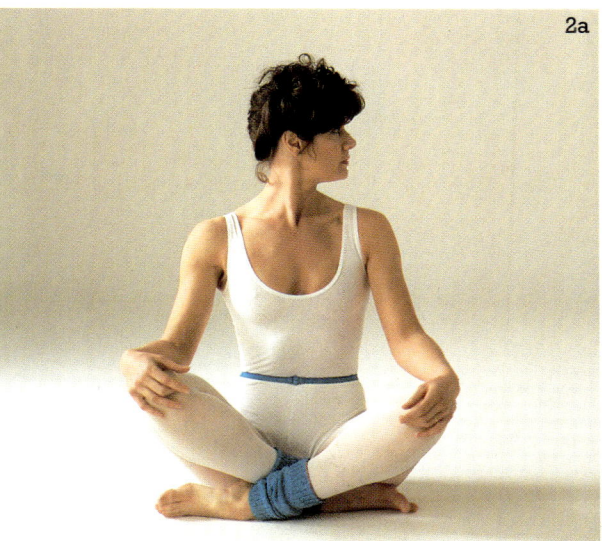

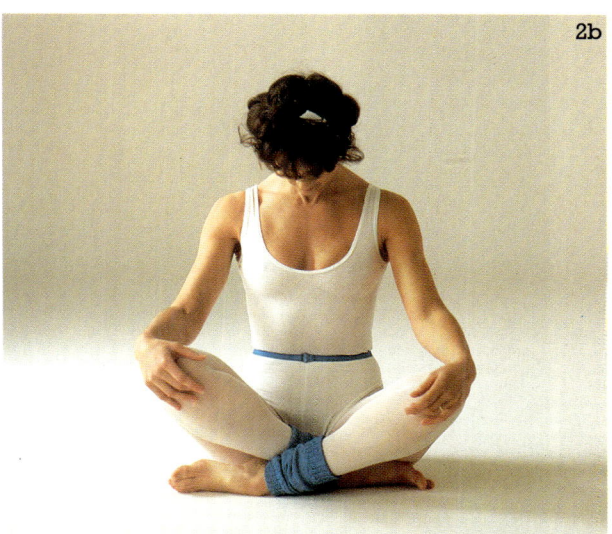

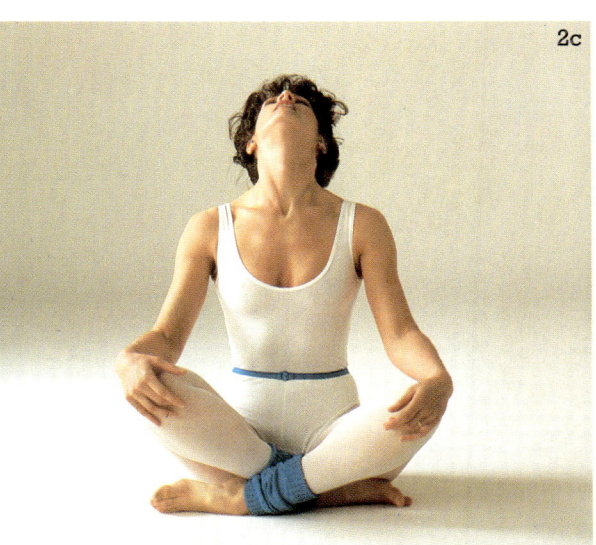

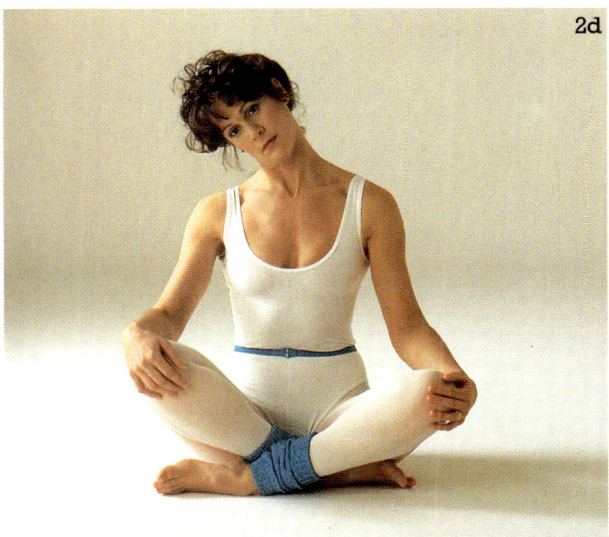

Exercise 3

What it does
Deals firmly with front-thigh sag

How you do it
1 Sit on floor, back supported against a wall, hips well back.
2 Place hands palms down on floor.
3 Tighten front thigh muscles as hard as you can and flex right foot, turning up toes and pulling them back towards you (3).
4 Breathe in, then breathe out and raise right leg 5–7.5 cm/2–3 inches in the air, keeping knees taut.
5 Breathe in and lower leg gently to ground.
6 Repeat the whole exercise five times, then repeat a further five times with left foot.

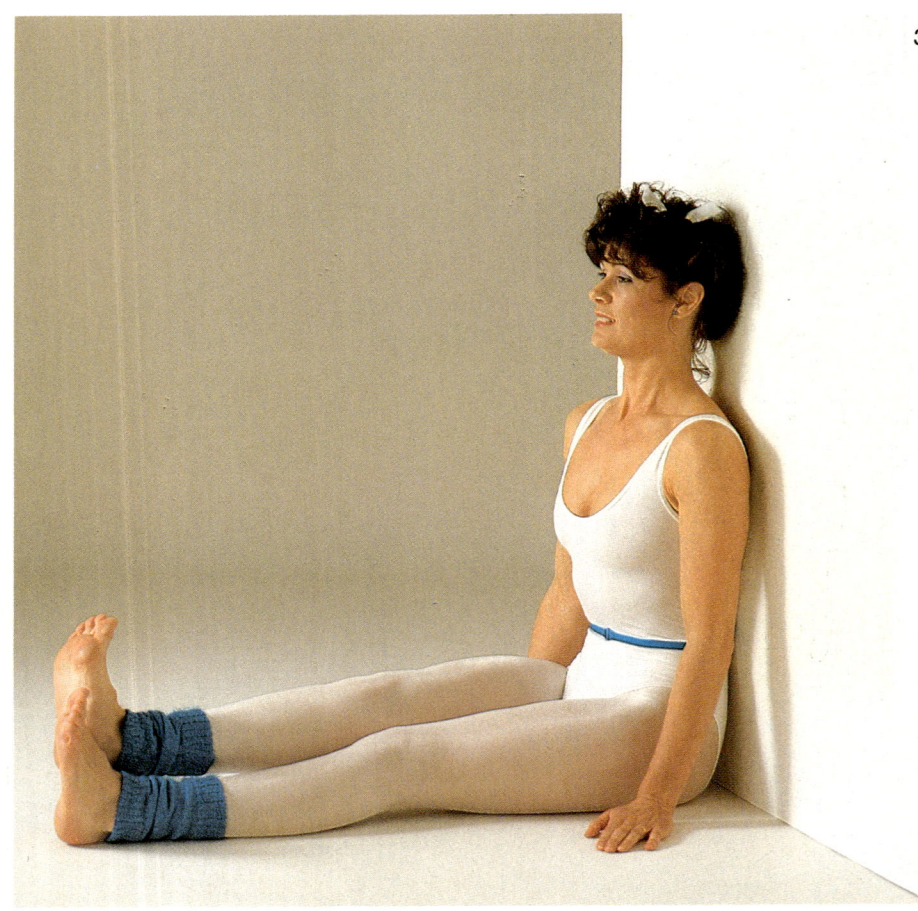

Exercise 5

What it does
Makes your waist, arms and shoulders beautifully supple

How you do it
1 Stand up straight, feet apart.
2 Bend forwards, allowing knees to bend a little, and swing arms to the left (5), then to the right.
3 Repeat 10 times.
4 Drop arms into centre again and slowly straighten up, keeping legs straight and bottom tucked under, with head coming up last.

Exercise 4

What it does
Helps slim the legs and limbers up the hips and bottom

How you do it
1 Stand up straight, feet apart.
2 Drop body forwards from hips, letting head flop down, and allowing knees to bend a little.
3 Push arms through legs as far as you can, making several small pushing movements (4).
4 Straighten up slowly from waist and return to starting position, arms at sides.
5 Repeat the whole exercise 10 times.

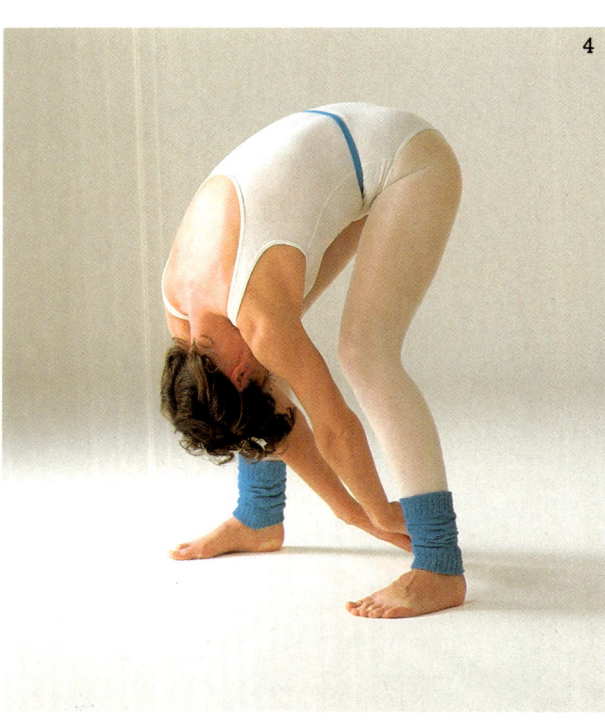

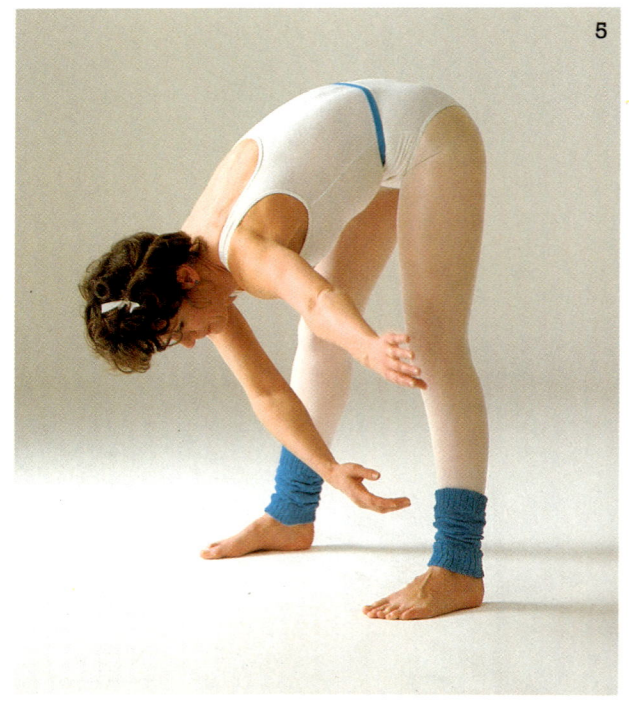

Exercise 6

What it does
Makes your waist trim
and taut

How you do it
1 Stand up straight, feet
slightly apart (6a).

2 Place hands on back of
head (6b) and make
several stretches, from
the waist to the left, then
to the right (6c).
3 Repeat the exercise 10
times, going a little
further each time.

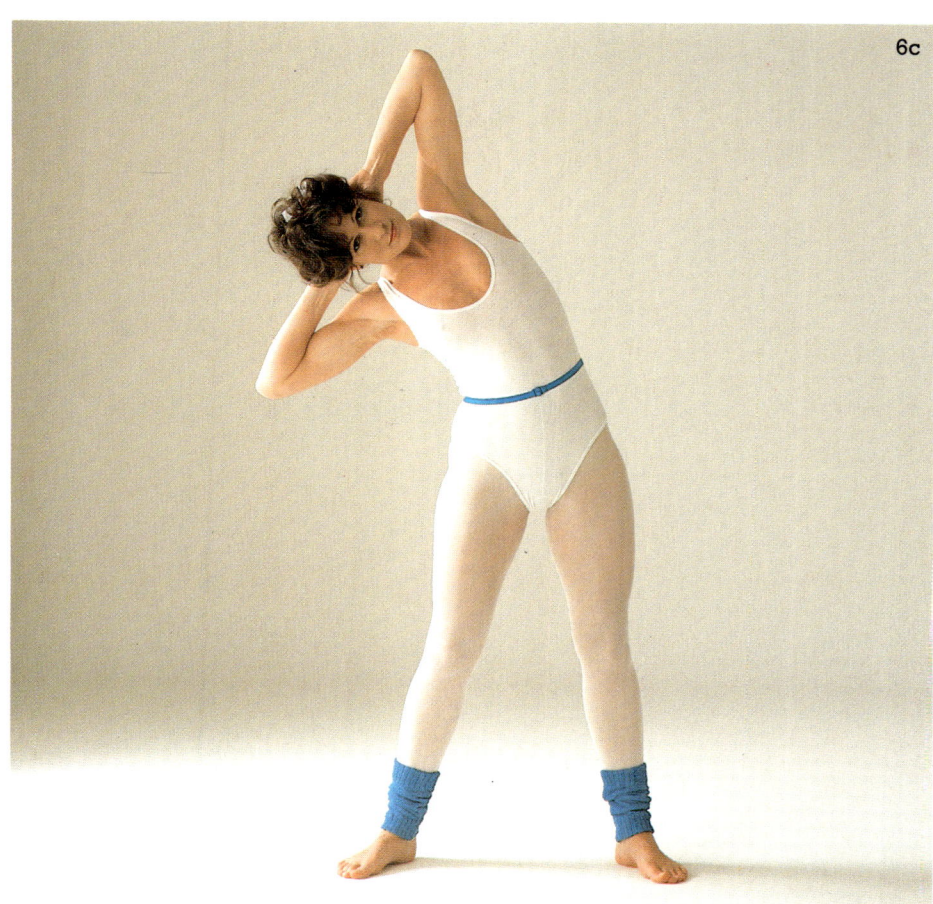

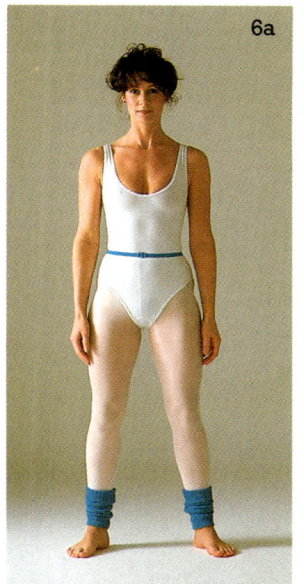

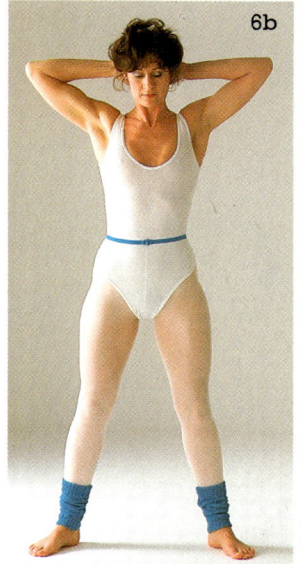

Exercise 7

What it does
Helps flatten the stomach

How you do it
1 Lie flat on your back
on the floor, with a chair
in front of you.
2 Raise one leg at a time
to rest on chair, bringing
knees right up to edge of
chair.
3 Holding on to chair, sit
up and bring head
towards knees (7).
4 Lie down again.
5 Repeat the exercise
five times.

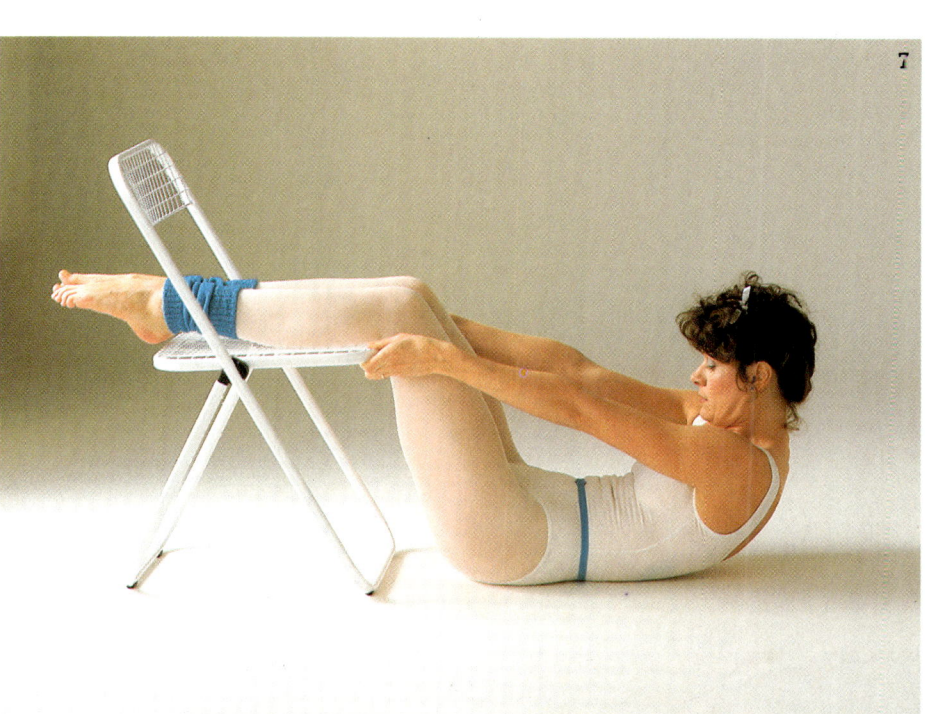

Exercise 8

What it does
Tones and firms the arms, bust and midriff

How you do it
1 Lie flat on stomach on floor, legs together and stretched out behind. Place hands under shoulders, palms down.
2 Push down on hands as you raise head and push upper torso backwards, until you are supporting yourself at full extent of arms. Keep shoulders down and try to keep hips on floor (8a).
3 Stretch back as far as you can and hold position for a few minutes, then slowly lower yourself to floor.
4 Repeat the exercise five times.
5 Raise to a kneeling position, slide arms alongside legs and tuck head and shoulders down to form a "ball" position. Hold for a few moments (8b).

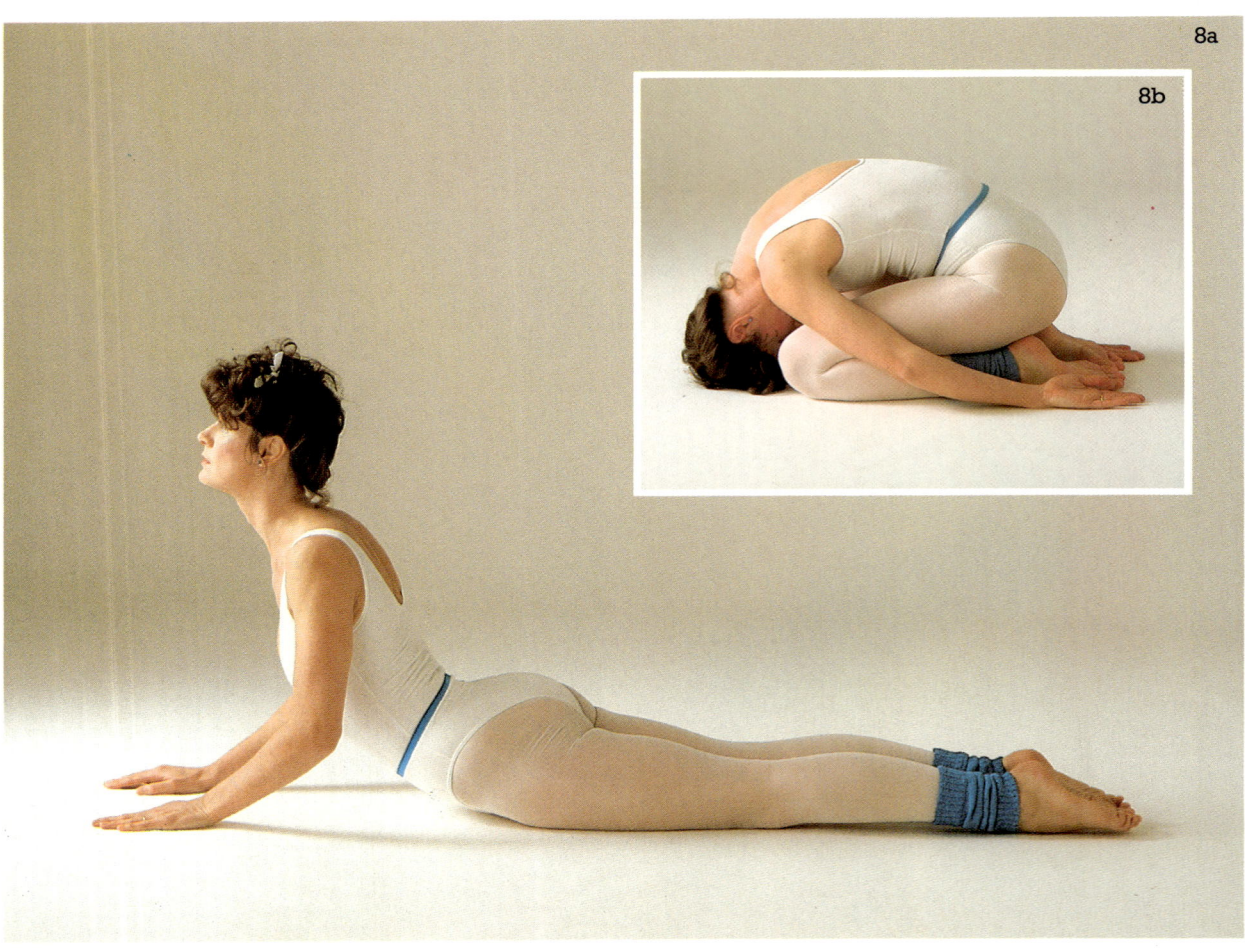

Exercise 9

What it does
Firms flabby, floppy upper arms

How you do it
1 Stand up straight, feet comfortably apart, weight evenly distributed and arms hugging sides, palms outwards (9a).
2 With a twist of the wrists, swing arms out and up and over head (9b) until backs of hands are facing each other and fingers touching as far as possible.
3 Stretch up as far as you can (9c), then swing arms down, so backs of hands touch sides of body.
4 Repeat the whole exercise 10 times.

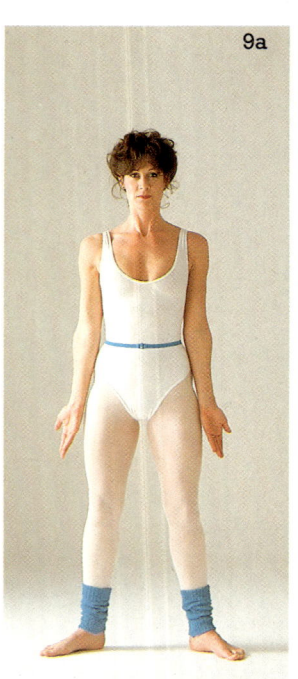
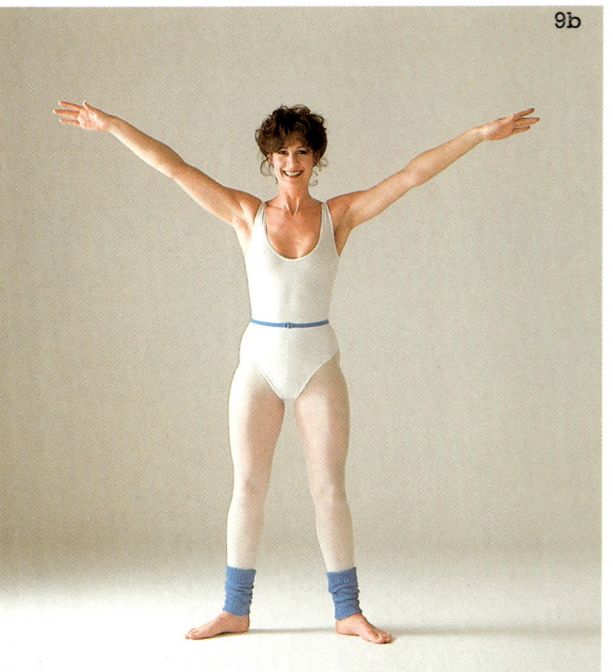
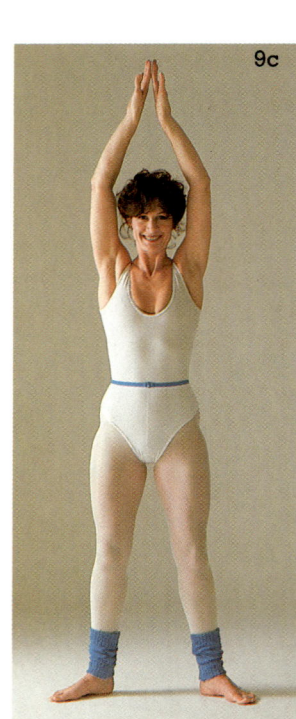

Exercise 10

What it does
A subtle but effective way of flattening the stomach

How you do it
1 Stand with feet slightly apart, knees slightly bent. Breathe in.
2 Keep one hand on your stomach, fingers outstretched, to check you are using stomach muscles and not simply lifting rib-cage. Keep your other hand in the small of your back (10).
3 As you breathe out, tuck bottom under, tilting pubic bone upwards in front and pulling stomach muscles in hard as you do so. Breathe in and release. Repeat several times.

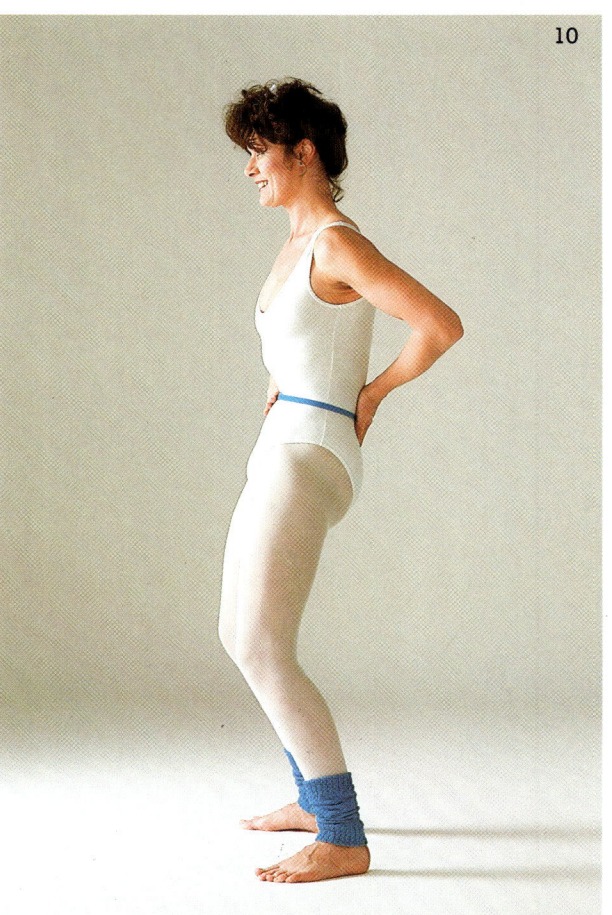

Relax

1 Lie flat on your back on the floor. Make sure you are lying in a straight line with chin tucked in.
2 Raise shoulders away from floor and up to ears then relax them as you lower them back to floor.
3 Raise bottom, press lower back into floor, clench buttocks, then relax as you lower them again.
4 Tense leg and feet muscles, then relax them, allowing feet to flop outwards.
5 Stretch arms about 30 cm/12 inches from your body, stretching fingers outwards, then relax arms and place palms facing upwards with fingers curled in a relaxed position.
6 Tighten muscles in face, then relax. Close eyes and breathe in and out very deeply for about five minutes (12).
7 Roll over on your side and very slowly get to your feet.

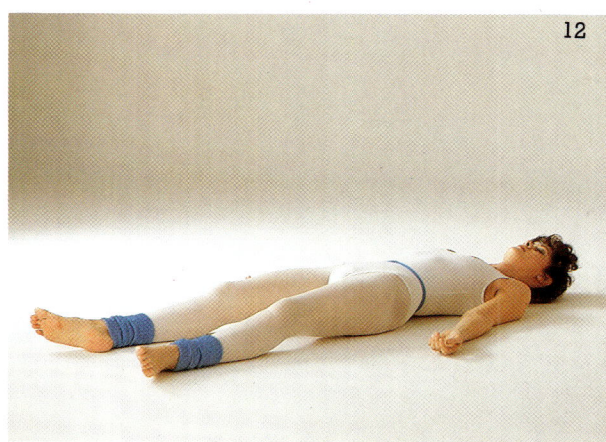

Exercise 11

What it does
An exercise to trim the waist

How you do it
1 Stand up straight, feet slightly apart. Raise arms and bend them in front at elbows so that fingers are just touching at shoulder level.
2 Keeping body straight, feet and pelvis facing forward, swing back with left elbow, fingers still touching, moving above waist only (11a).
3 Push back hard with three short, sharp movements.
4 Repeat the exercise to the right (11b), then repeat the exercise four times on each side.

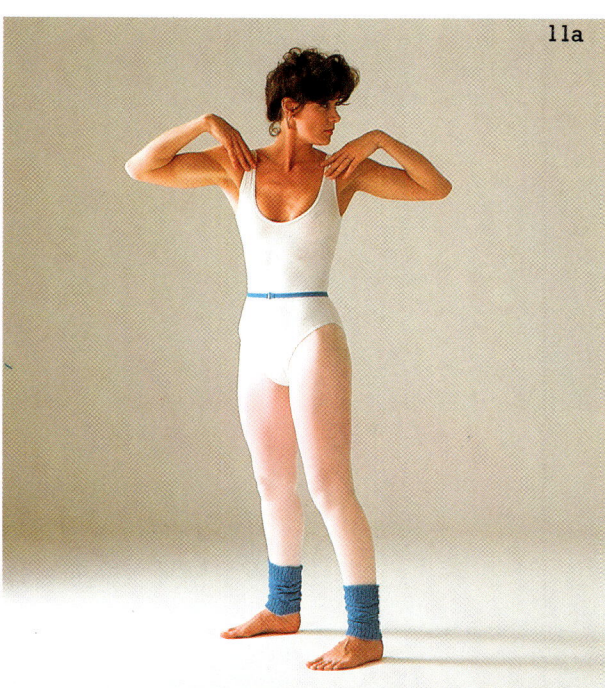

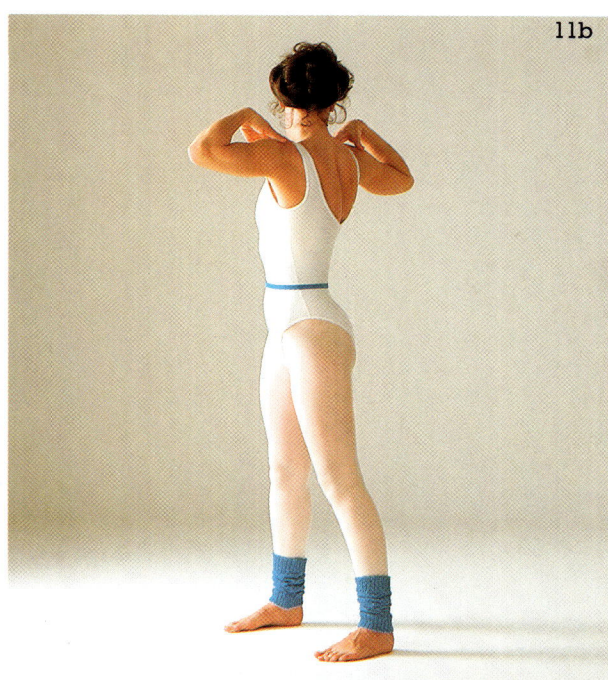

Allow 30 minutes for this session

Regular exercise will make you feel healthier in both mind and body. It can also help you improve your shape. Most women wish their whole shape was more streamlined, or think that certain parts could do with a lot of improvement . . . Whether the problem centres on a droopy pear-shape, plump waistline or flabby tum, the first step is to get down to your correct weight. Then, while you are losing every last ounce of flab, take steps to tone up the slack muscles that can blur your bodyline.

Thick thighs are probably the most stubborn-to-trim zone. But don't get down-hearted or settle for anything less than the sleekest hip-to-knee line that's humanly possible for you: the solution is to *concentrate* on exercising this area each day.

Your waist is probably the most responsive-to-exercise part of your anatomy. Work every day at a waist-improver exercise and within weeks this area should be firmer, tighter and trimmer.

Saggy bottom? The muscles in that area haven't been worked enough. As well as the bottom-firming routines that you'll find in this section, there's a simple exercise you can do any time during the day when you have a few minutes to spare . . . Sit on a hard chair and clench your buttock muscles as you briskly bounce up, lifting your bottom off the chair. Sit down and relax. Do this as often as you can manage.

Fat on and around the upper arms accumulates very easily, but neither fat nor flab is inevitable. Here, as everywhere else on the body, firm shapeliness depends on two things: correct weight and good muscle tone. And even if you've rather neglected yourself in both areas, it's never too late to work for a really magical improvement – we show you how!

Strenuous exercises aren't for people with health problems, though. If you are in doubt, consult with your doctor before attempting any work-out. This session takes half an hour. If you are used to exercising at least once a week, you could easily manage two half-hour sessions in one day. If you've been exercising less frequently take it very easy on your first day and gradually build up your sessions.

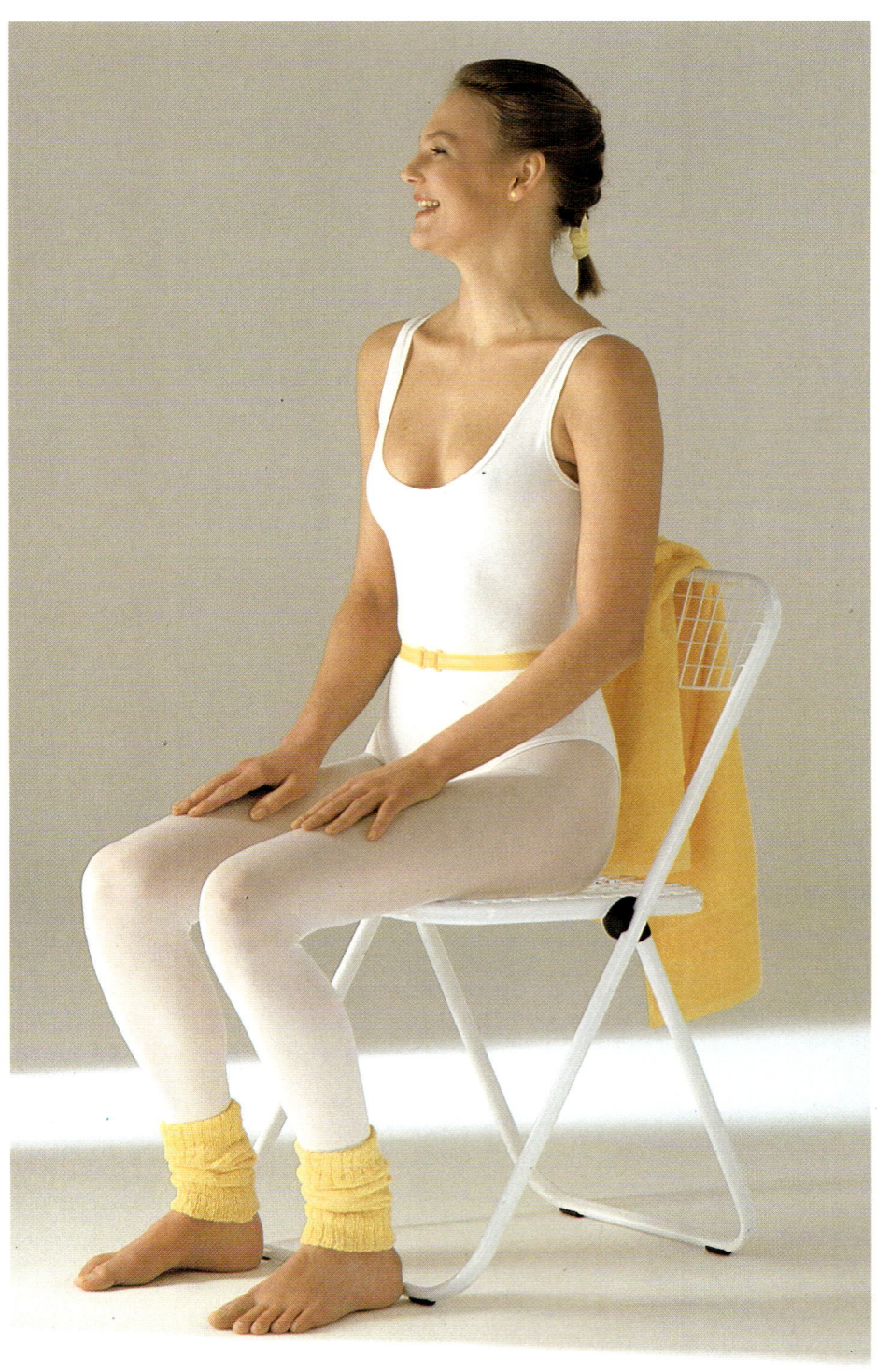

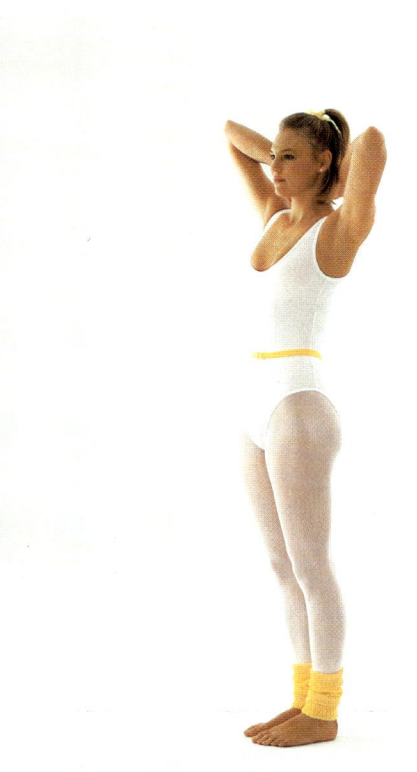

1a

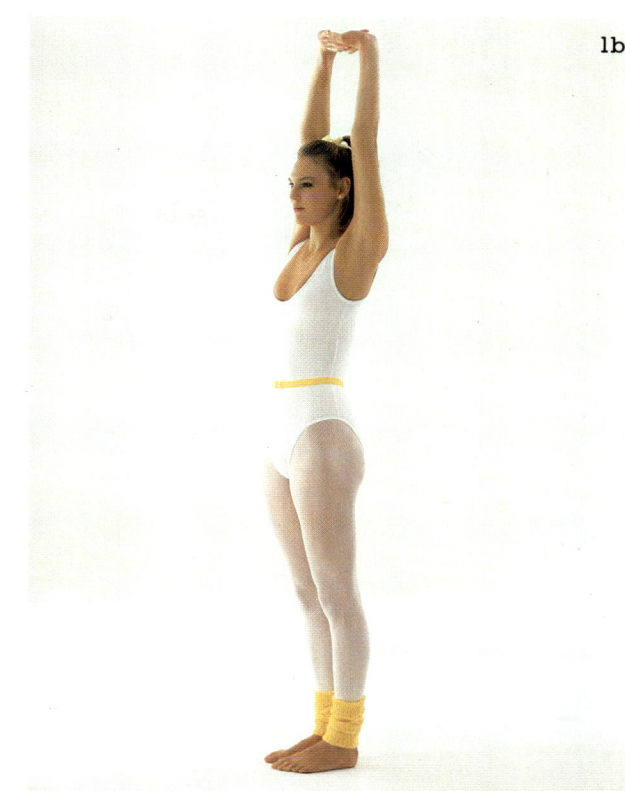

1b

Exercise 1

What it does
Stretches and tones the
whole body

How you do it
1 Stand up straight, feet
together, arms by sides.
2 Raise arms and let
hands drop behind head,
linking fingers (1a).
3 Stretch arms upwards
as far as you can and hold
for a count of five (1b).
4 Drop hands behind
head again, then return
to original position.
6 Repeat the whole
exercise five times.

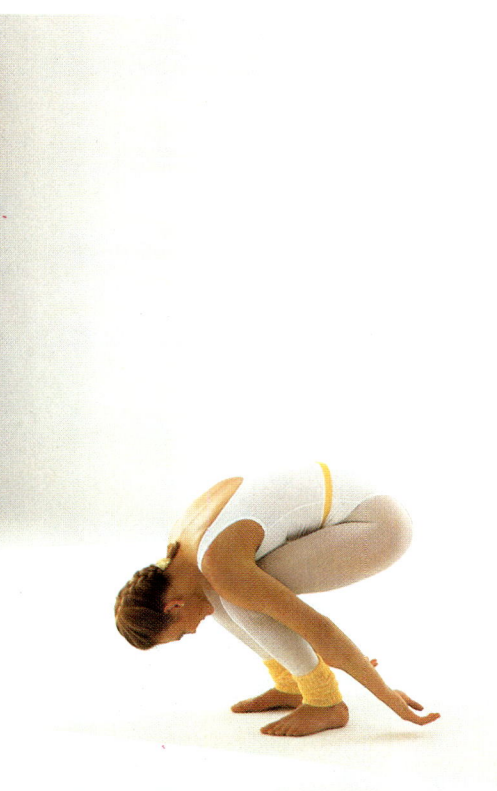

2a

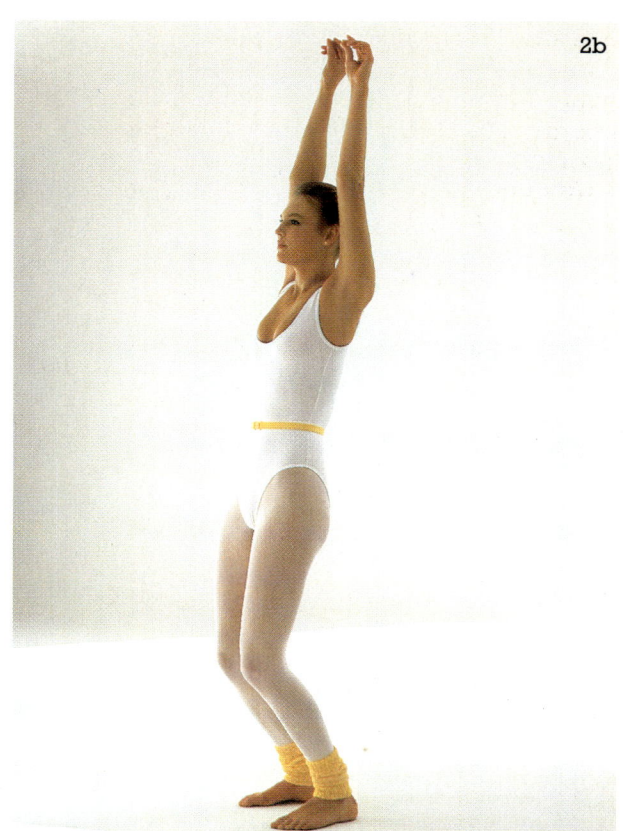

2b

Exercise 2

What it does
Acts as a general warm-
up

How you do it
1 Stand up straight, feet
apart, stomach held in
and bottom tucked under.
2 Stretch arms above
head, then drop body
forwards from waist,
swinging arms down and
back behind you,
bending knees as you go
(2a).
3 Now swing arms, body
and head up and back,
keeping knees bent (2b).
4 Repeat the whole
exercise five times.

Exercise 3

What it does
Limbers up your spine

How you do it
1 Bend forwards from hips and stretch arms out in front of you, keeping knees straight. Look up and hold position for a count of 10 (3a).
2 Flop down to floor, bending from hips, allowing knees to bend. Grasp your ankles and pull head as low as you can (3b). Hold position for a count of five, straightening knees a little until you feel a stretch in legs.
3 Straighten up and repeat the whole exercise twice.

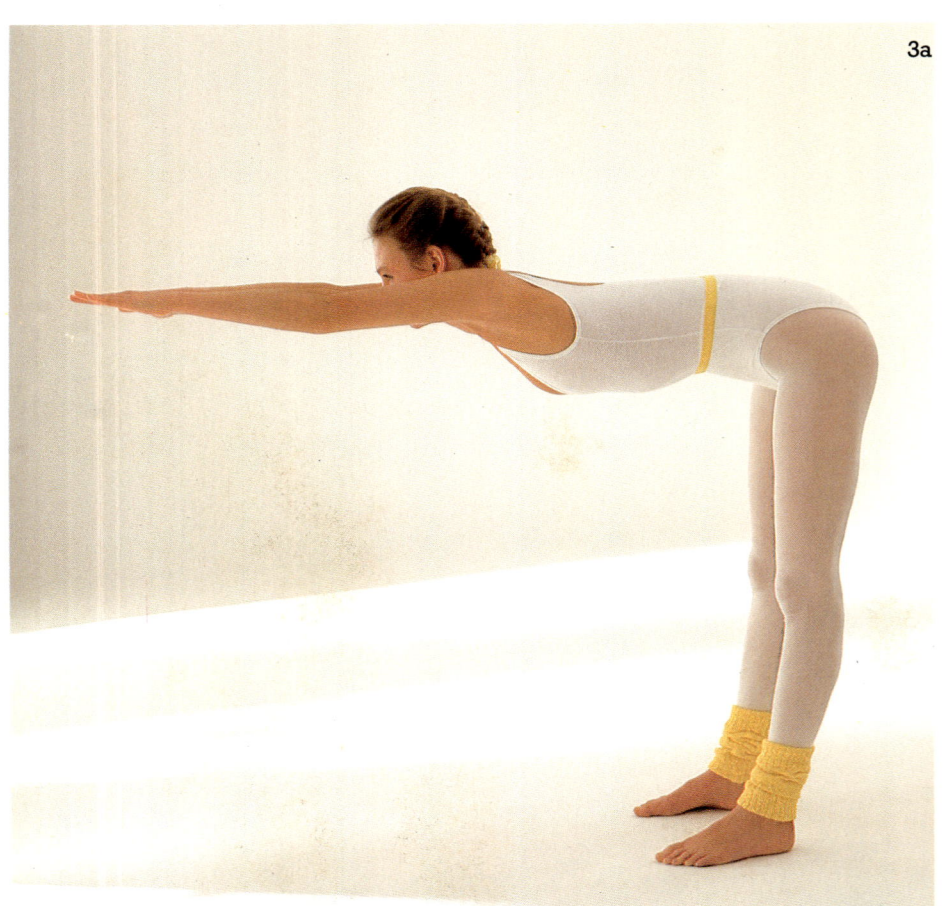

3a

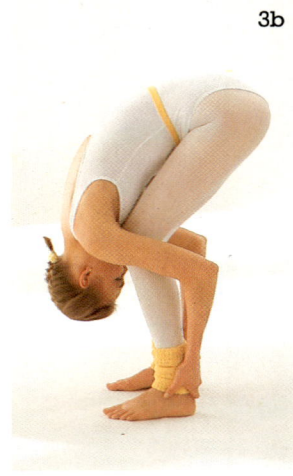

3b

Exercise 4

What it does
Excellent for the waist

How you do it
1 Stand up straight, feet apart, arms by sides.
2 Put right hand on hip and bend to the left, sliding left hand down left leg as far as you can. Stretch sideways from waist, without bending forward (4a).
3 Straighten up, then put left hand on left hip and bend to the right.
4 Repeat these two bends 10 times.
5 Bend to the left, but this time let right arm reach over head (4b). Then pull to the right, letting left arm reach over head. Repeat 10 times.

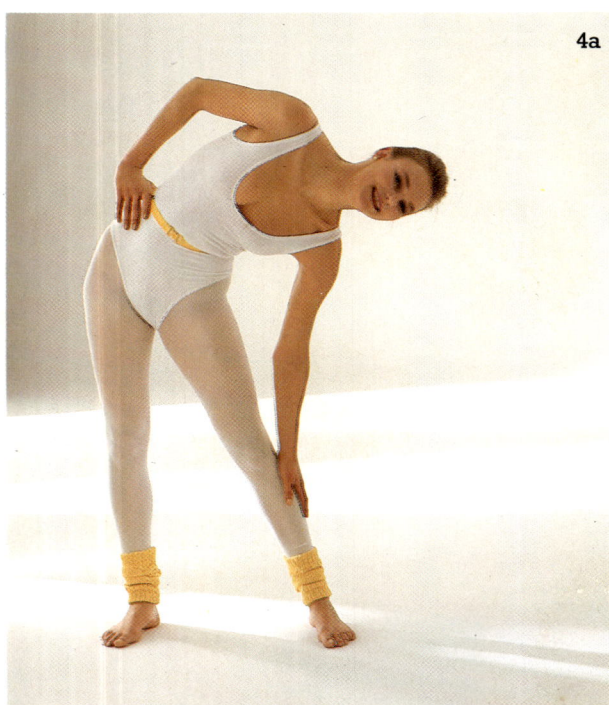

4a

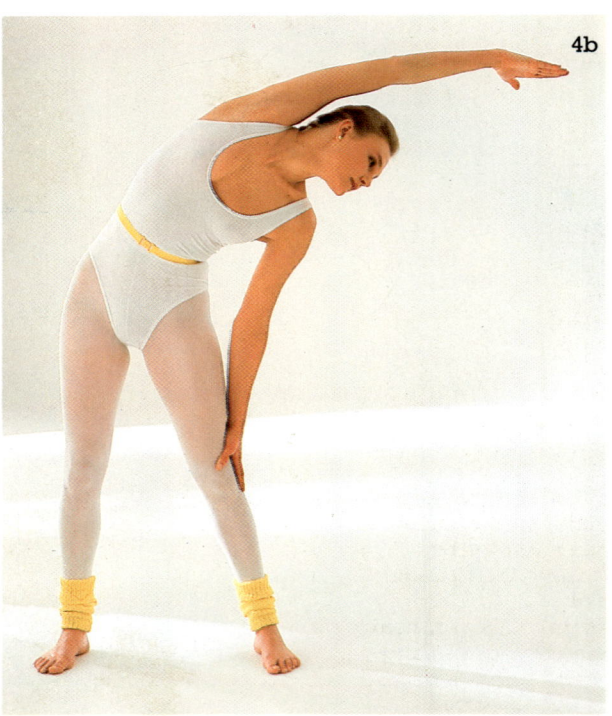

4b

Exercise 5

What it does
Relieves wrinkle-inducing tension in the neck and shoulders

How you do it
1 Sit cross-legged on the floor.
2 Breathe in and turn head to the right.
3 Breathe out and turn head to the left (5a).
4 Breathe in and lift head backwards (5b).
5 Breathe out and lower head forwards (5c).
6 Repeat the whole exercise 15 times.

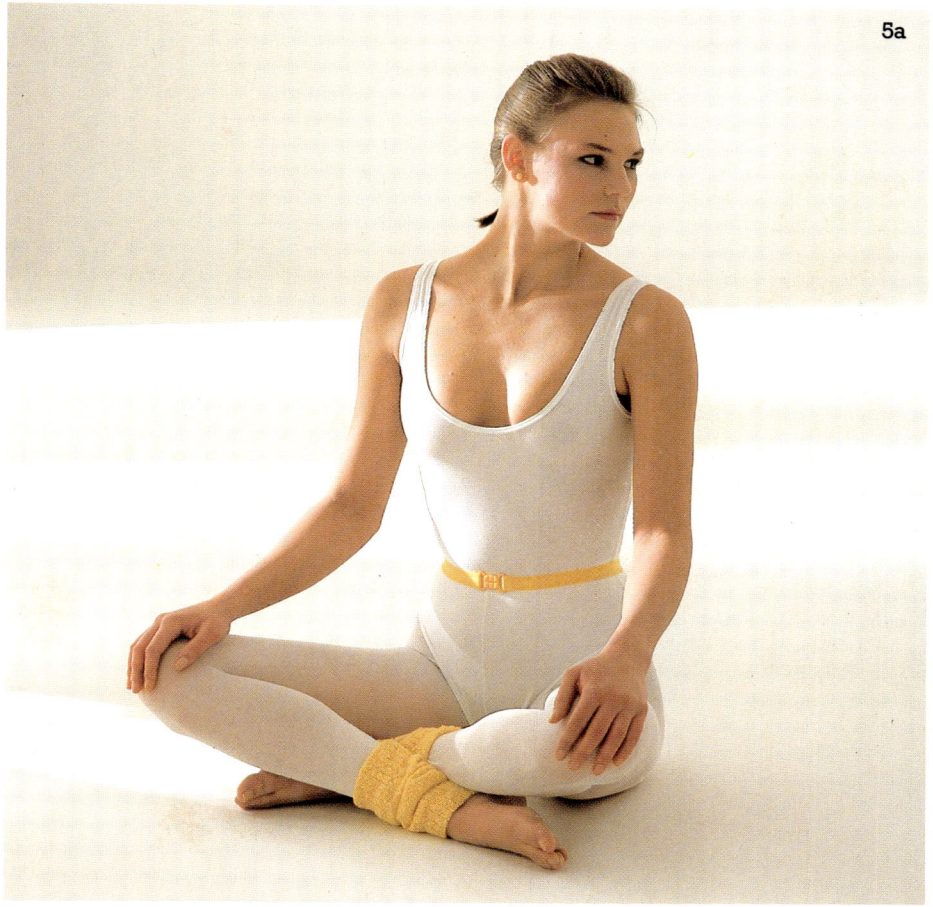
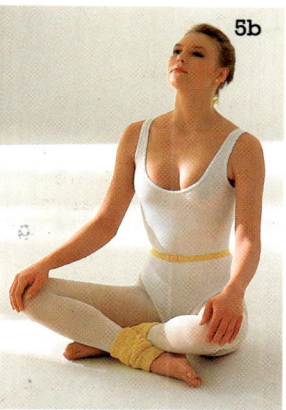
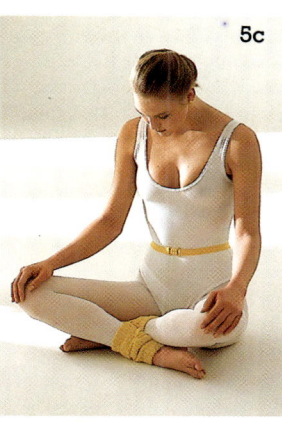

Exercise 6

What it does
Firms the thighs

How you do it
1 Sit on the floor, legs stretched straight out in front of you, back straight and palms of hands down on floor by sides (6a).
2 Cross right leg over left leg, bending knee and placing right foot on floor close to left knee (6b).
3 Now raise left leg, hold for a few seconds (6c) and lower to the floor again. Repeat five times.
4 Sit with legs stretched straight out in front of you and cross left leg over right leg, bending knee and placing left foot on floor close to right knee.
5 Raise right leg, hold for a few minutes and lower to the floor again. Repeat five times.

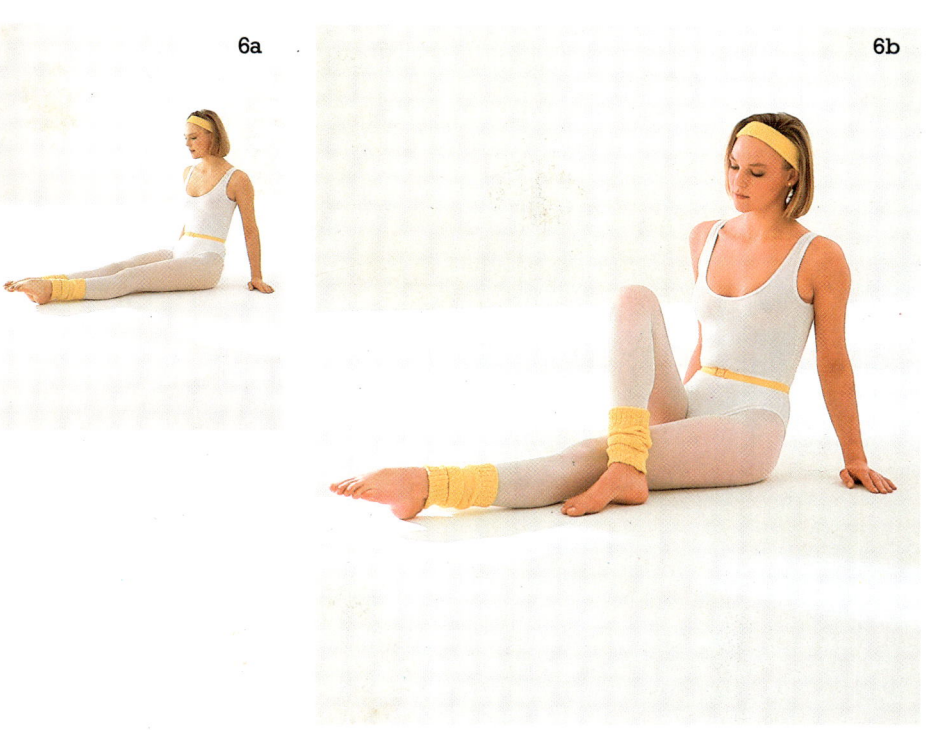
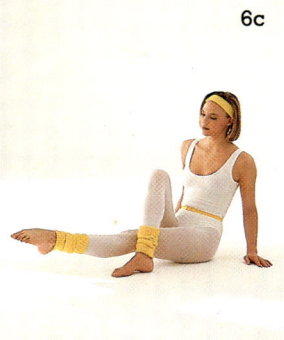

Exercise 7

What it does
Trims the waist and stretches the spine

How you do it
1 Kneel down on floor, resting hands on floor directly below shoulders and keeping back parallel to floor.
2 Draw right knee up beneath you and touch chest, dropping head down towards knee (7a).
3 Stretch back and up, straightening knee, to reach out as far as and as high as possible while pulling up and back with head and shoulders (7b).
4 Relax and return to kneeling position. Repeat with left leg.
5 Repeat the whole exercise 10 times.

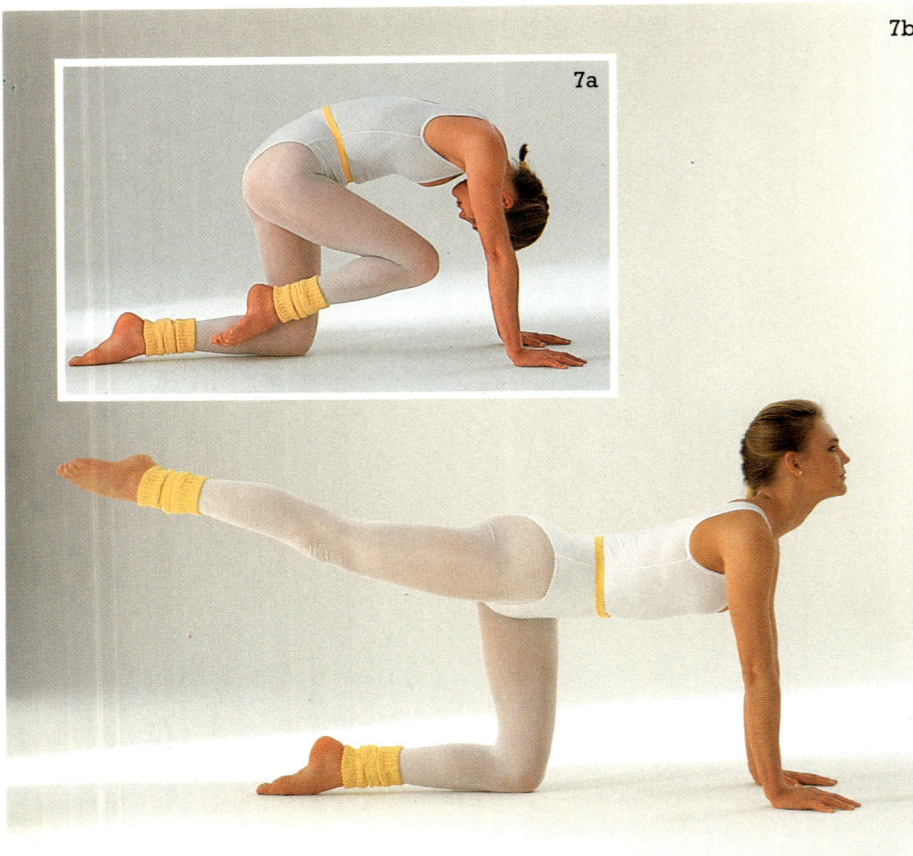

Exercise 8

What it does
Helps to lift the bustline

How you do it
1 Stand up straight, feet together, stomach held in, bottom tucked under.
2 Raise arms to chin level and grasp wrists. Holding them firmly, push against wrists until you feel pectoral muscles jump (8).
3 Relax, then repeat the exercise 10 times.

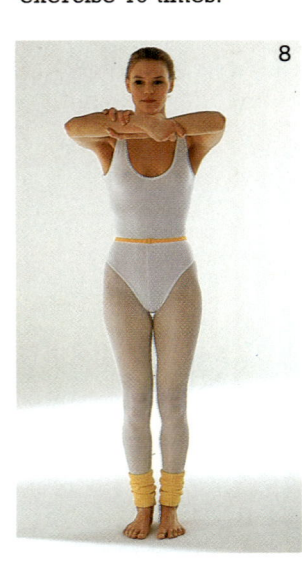

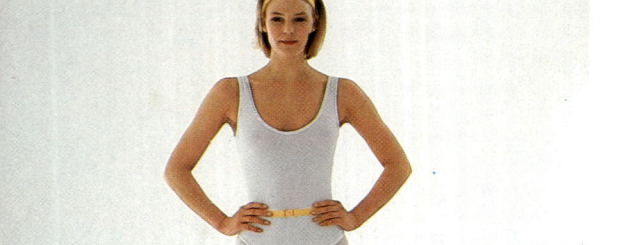

Exercise 9

What it does
Fights bottom droop and thigh sag

How you do it
1 Stand up straight, feet apart, tummy held in, hands on hips (9a).
2 Keeping body straight, bend right knee and lunge sideways over it, keeping left leg straight. Do not let right knee or foot roll inwards (9b).
3 Return to starting position, then bend left knee and lunge sideways over it, keeping right leg straight. Do not let left knee or foot roll inwards.
4 Repeat 10 times.

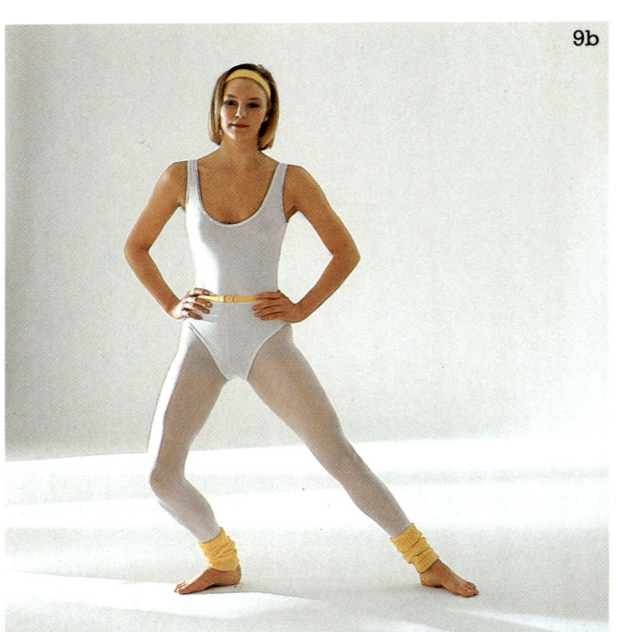

Exercise 10

What it does
Helps to trim the ankles and calves

How you do it
1 Stand on a large book, heels hanging over edge. Steady yourself with the back of a chair if necessary.
2 With feet together, rise up on tiptoe (10a), then lower gradually, pushing heels down as far as possible (10b).
3 Repeat the same movements, standing first with toes turned out, then with toes together and heels out.
4 Repeat the whole exercise five times.

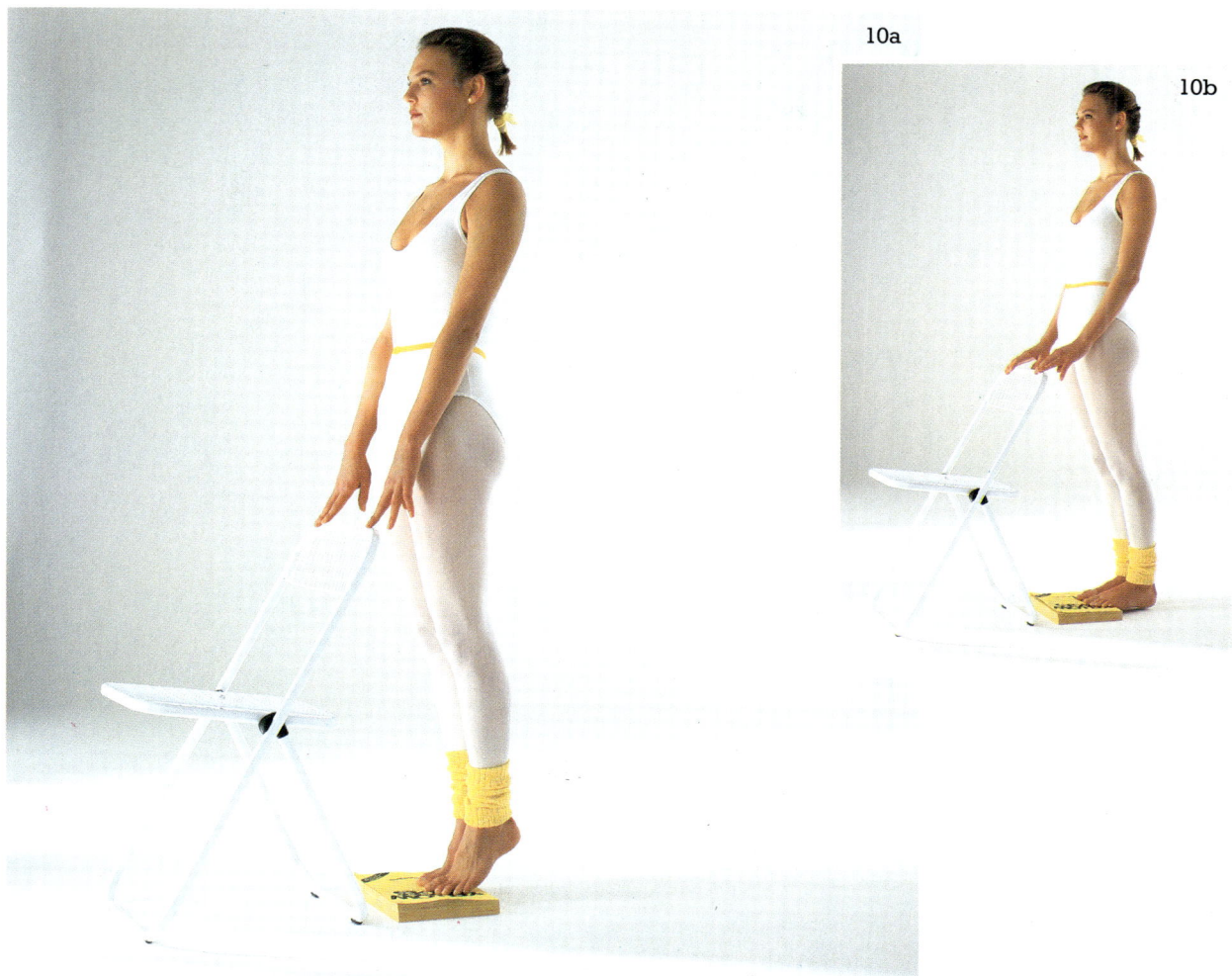

10a

10b

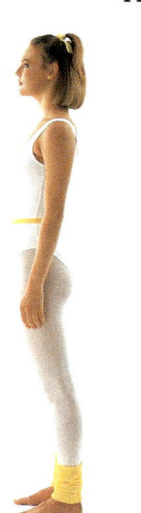

11a

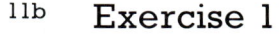

11b

Exercise 11

What it does
Helps firm upper-arm flab

How you do it
1 Stand up straight, feet apart, hands at sides, fingers pointing towards ground (11a).
2 Raise arms in front to shoulder level (11b), then raise them above head, fingers pointing upwards (11c).
3 Pull shoulder-blades back hard and circle arms behind (11d), bringing them down to sides.
4 Repeat the whole exercise 10 times.

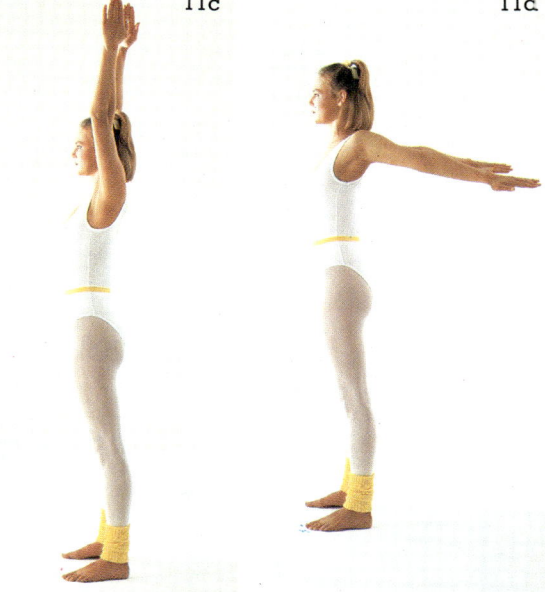

11c

11d

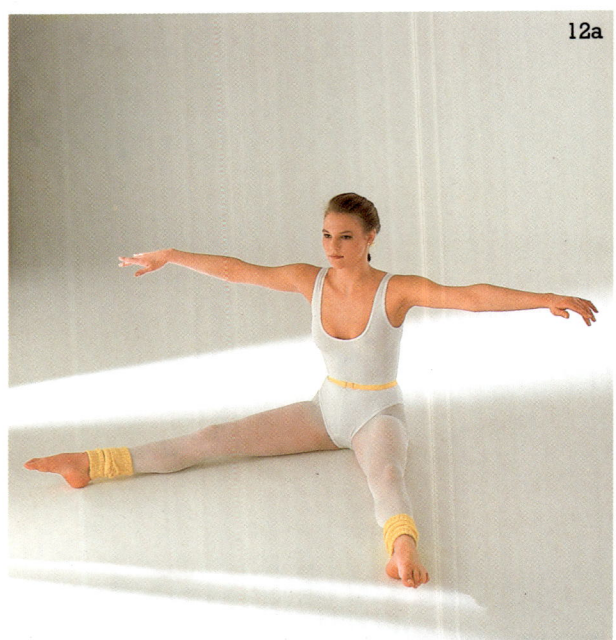

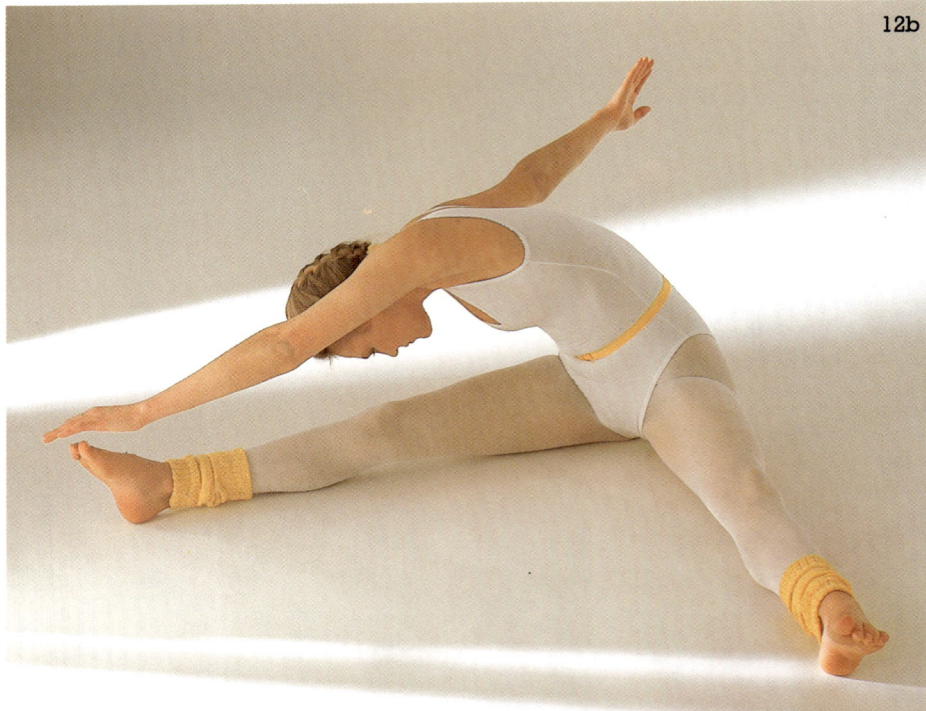

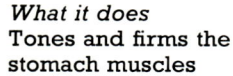

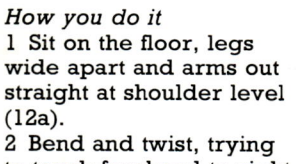

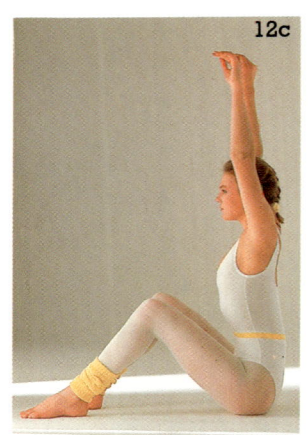

Exercise 12

What it does
Tones and firms the stomach muscles

How you do it
1 Sit on the floor, legs wide apart and arms out straight at shoulder level (12a).
2 Bend and twist, trying to touch forehead to right knee. At the same time slide left hand down right leg as far as you can, holding right arm out behind (12b).
3 Return to starting position and repeat with forehead and left leg.
4 Repeat the whole exercise five times on each side.
5 Now bring legs together and bend knees, back straight, feet flat on floor. Stretch arms up over head (12c). Carefully lower yourself to floor, uncurling spine one vertebra at a time. Allow arms to pull forwards as you uncurl (12d).
6 Relax for a few minutes (12e).

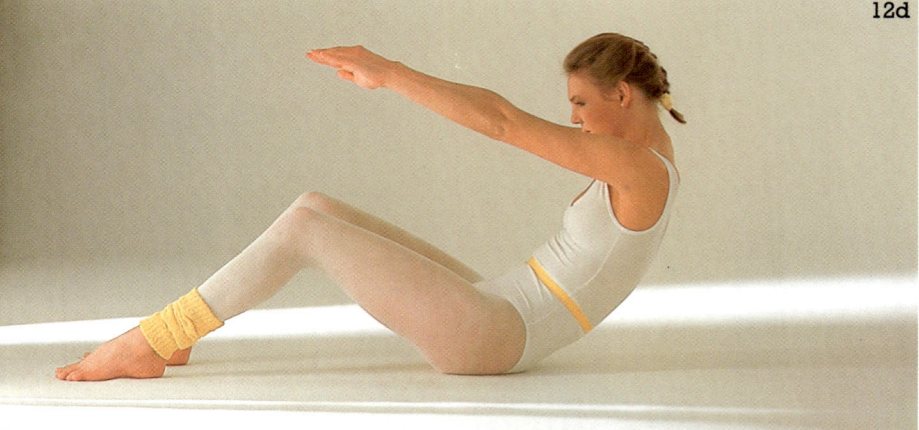

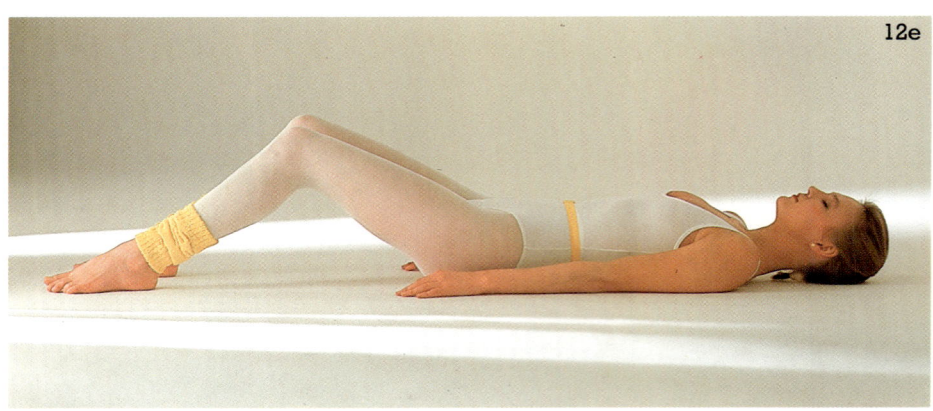

Exercise 13

What it does
An all-over toner that works on legs, stomach and arms

How you do it
1 Kneel on floor, arms straight down from shoulders, palms of hands against floor (13a).
2 Turn toes inwards and move trunk forwards as you raise body as high as possible.
3 Straighten legs and arms, bringing head between arms.
4 Raise yourself on tiptoe (13b), then lower feet until soles are flat on the floor (13c). Raise yourself on tiptoe and lower once more.
5 Lower knees to floor and sit back on heels.
6 Repeat the whole exercise five times.

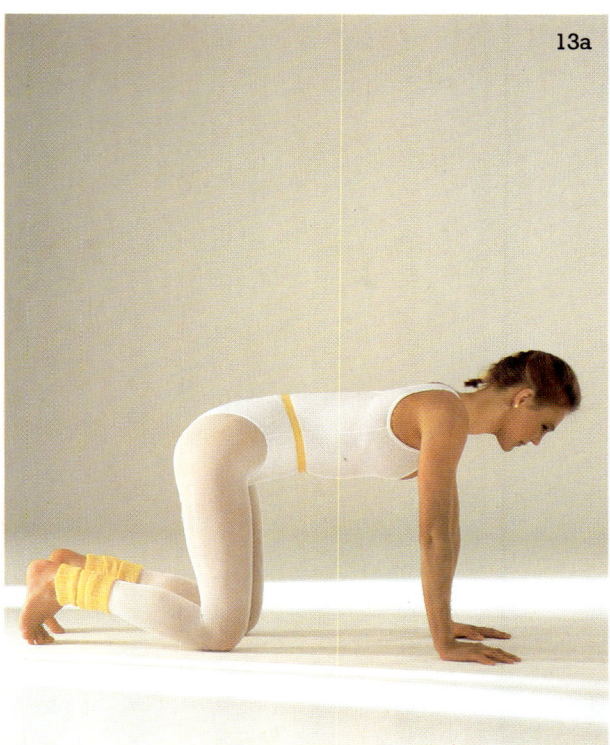

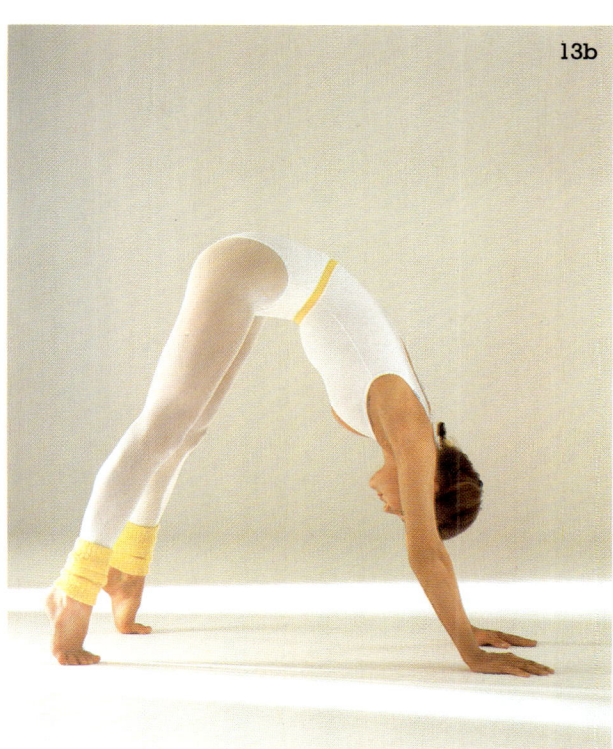

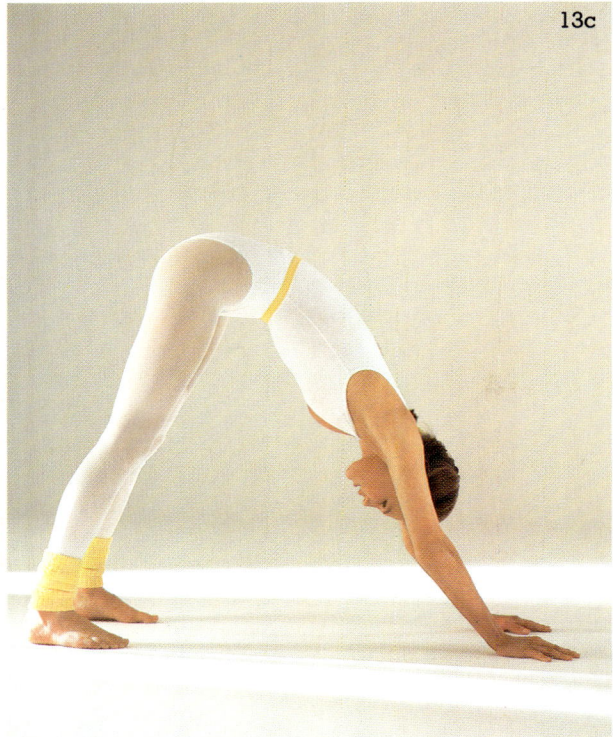

Relax

1 Lie flat on your back on the floor. Make sure you are lying in a straight line with head straight and chin tucked in (14).
2 Raise shoulders away from floor and up to ears, then relax them as you lower them back to floor.
3 Raise bottom, press lower back into floor, clench buttocks, then relax as you lower them again.
4 Tense leg and feet muscles, then relax them allowing feet to flop outwards.
5 Stretch arms about 30 cm/12 inches from your body, stretching fingers outwards, then relax arms and place palms facing upwards with your fingers slightly curled in a relaxed position.

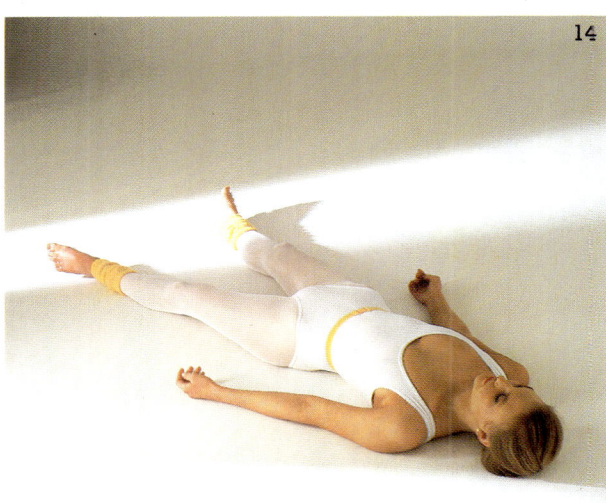

6 Tighten muscles in face, then relax. Close eyes and breathe in and out very deeply for about five minutes.
7 Roll over on your side, slowly get to your feet.

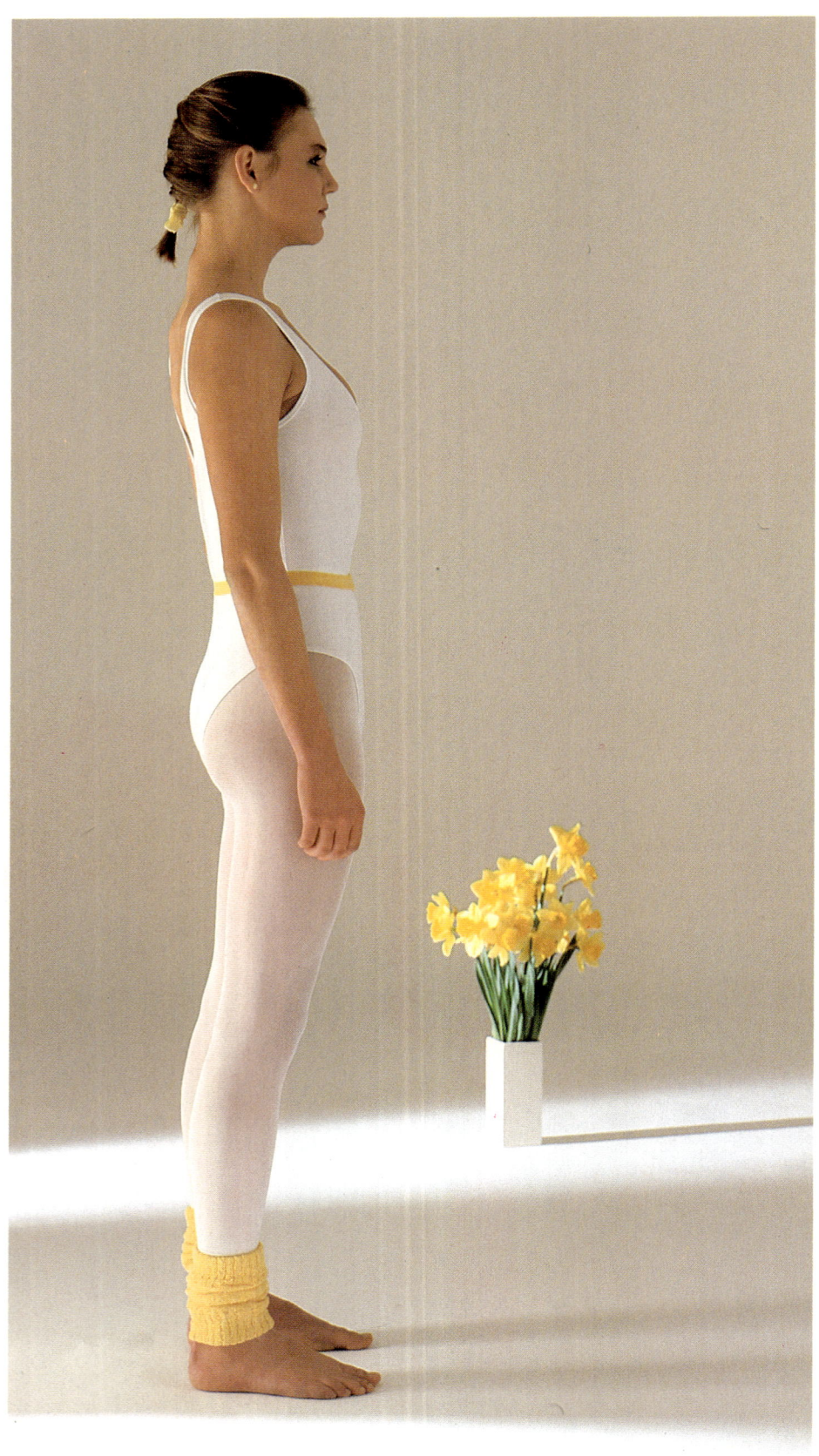

It is possible to look pounds thinner by simply improving your posture. Before you start this work-out, think about how you hold yourself. Do you habitually tend to slump or stoop? If so, however successfully you are losing weight, you won't look in pretty shape because you are allowing the muscles that keep flesh firm to become slack and droopy. You must retrain yourself to move tall.

Not like a soldier, with shoulders thrust back. This encourages stiffness and tension. Try to walk and move from the centre of your body. Imagine you are suspended by a thread from the top of your head and you will find yourself moving as a dancer does, with your head and spine in natural alignment. This way of moving makes you look more graceful and feel healthier and better psychologically. If you have got into the habit of stooping, you will have to keep reminding yourself. It is easy to slip back into bad habits.

Many facial lines which get embedded at too early an age may also be due to bad posture. Badly held neck and shoulders can create massive tension, reinforce frown-lines, even lead to headaches.

If you stretch up, you will immediately look as if you've shed pounds, even if your slimming campaign still has some way to go. But note that the following exercise session is only for a person with no health problems. You can concentrate on doing Work-out 2 and repeating the whole session whenever you want, or you could combine this work-out with Work-out 1 to make an hour-long session.

Remember, though, it is not how *long* you exercise in one session that matters: it's how *well* you do the exercise that counts. Placid exercises without a pull on the muscles are no use. You must be prepared to work at them until you feel some tension. If you can't, you aren't doing them properly! If you get tired after half an hour or even ten minutes, it is better to take a break, then continue your exercises later. When you are tired you're much less likely to put a lot of effort into making sure you do the exercises really well, and that's what is most important. Finish every exercise session with a period of relaxation; it is important to rest for a few minutes after strenuous exercise.

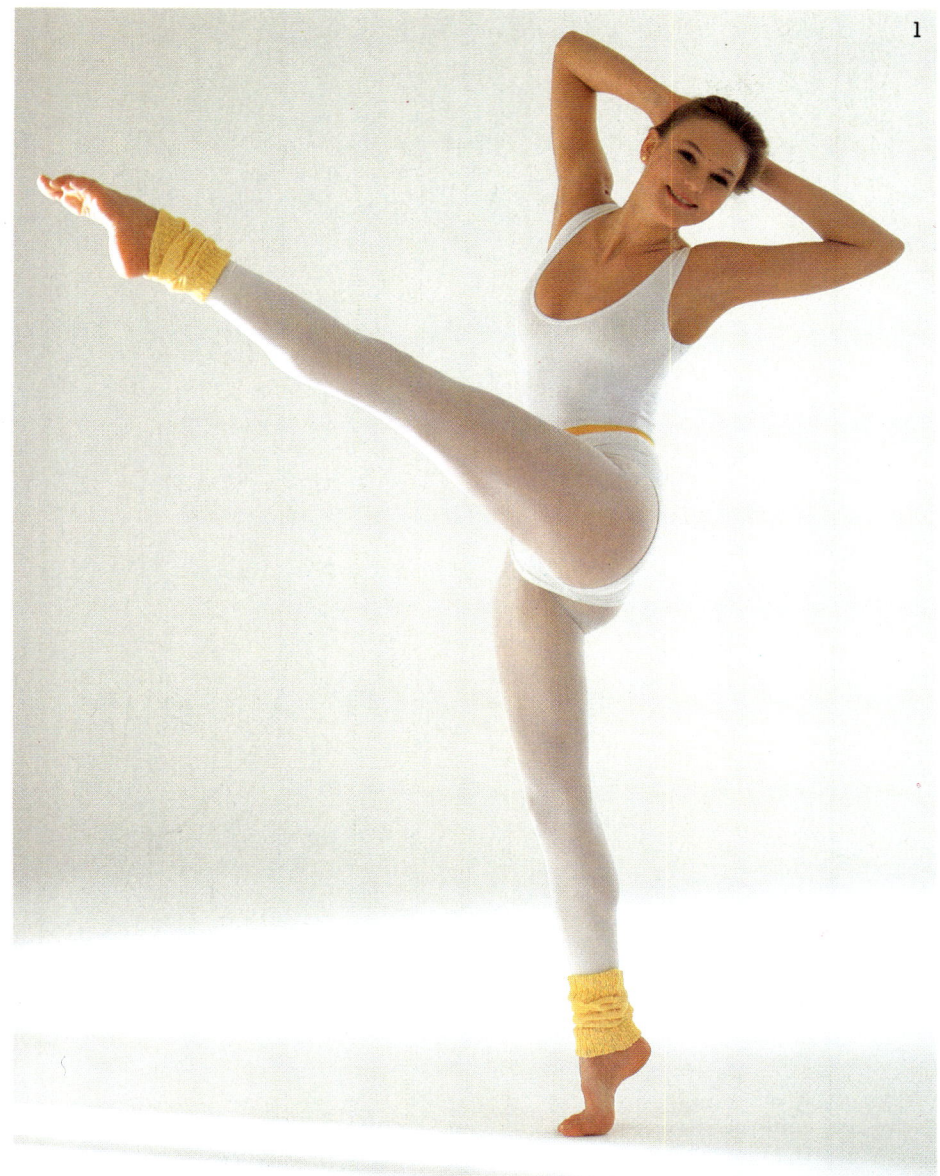

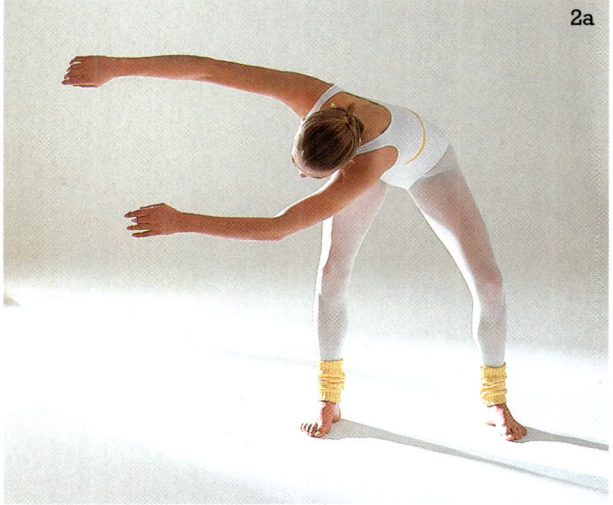

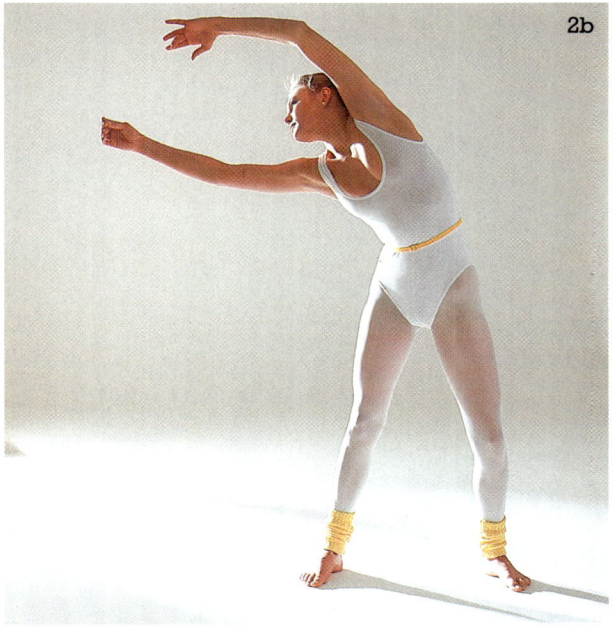

Exercise 1

What it does
A warm-up that stretches and tones the whole body

How you do it
1 Stand up straight, feet very slightly apart, hands clasped lightly at back of head, elbows back and shoulders down.
2 Try to push the crown of your head through your hands.
3 Keeping stretched spine upright, walk around the room three times in a series of slow, deliberate goose-steps, or strides with the leg raised high (1).

Exercise 2

What it does
An all-over warm-up to get you moving

How you do it
1 Stand, feet apart, knees flexed and ready to bend, arms loose at sides.
2 Swing arms rhythmically from left to right, building up momentum and letting each knee bend as the arms swing towards it. Develop the arm swings until you are reaching up and out as far as possible on each side and dropping forwards and down to the front (2a).

3 Take the whole movement up and over in a big circle, reaching out above your head and stretching out and down in front as you continue the circle right round (2b). Take the circles as high as you can, reaching up on tiptoe and leaning back slightly at the topmost point.
4 Relax back to the side-to-side swings as you reverse the movement in the opposite direction.

Exercise 3

What it does
A tough treatment to firm the thighs

How you do it
1 Find a really firm support such as the back of a chair or the stair banisters.
2 Hold on for support with one hand and place other hand at waist. Rise up on tiptoe, keeping back straight and bottom tucked well in.
3 Still with back straight, bend knees until you're squatting on your haunches, still on tiptoe (3a).
4 Rise just a few cm/inches, holding basic position, and stick bottom out.
5 Still holding same position, tuck bottom under (3b).
6 Repeat the whole exercise five times.

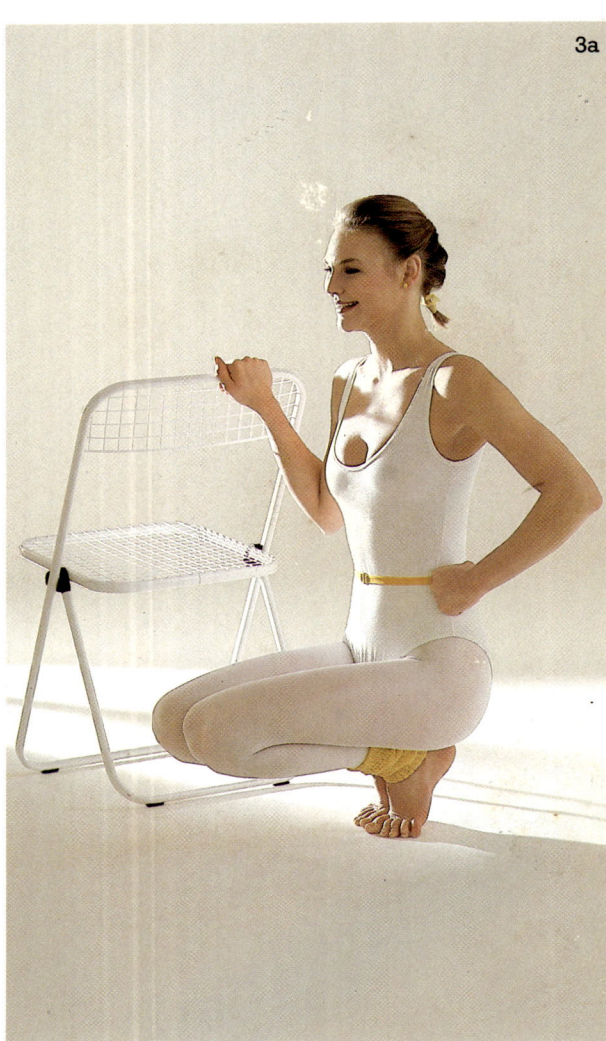
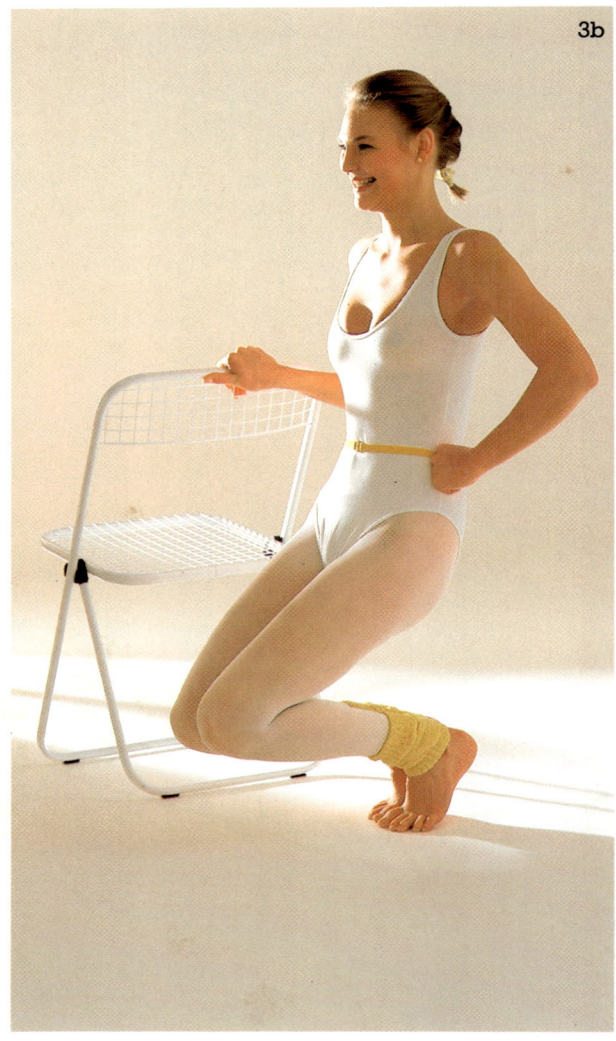

Exercise 4

What it does
This exercise tones the hips and the waist

How you do it
1 Stand up straight with legs together. Raise arms at sides to shoulder height, keeping them straight (4a).
2 Keeping shoulders and arms still, and legs straight, swing hips from side to side 20 times (4b).

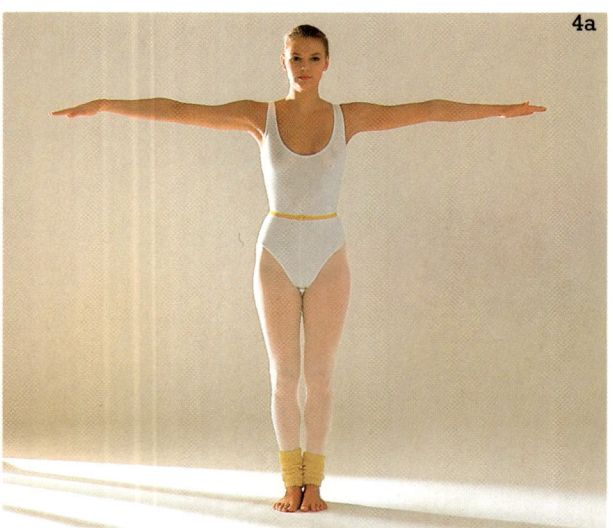
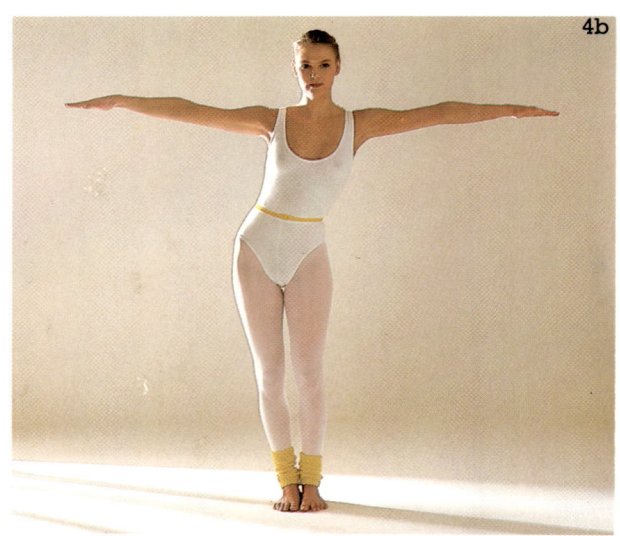

Exercise 5

What it does
Firms flabby upper arms
and relaxes tired
shoulders

How you do it
1 Lie on your back, arms
by sides, legs together.
2 Raise arms up and
back over head (5a),
stretching as much as
possible (5b), then circle
them out to the sides (5c)
and back to starting
position. Do the whole
exercise in an easy,
continuous movement.
3 Repeat the exercise 10
times.

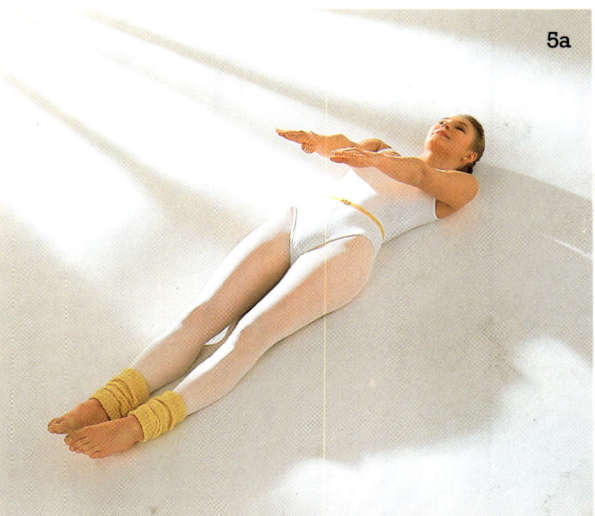

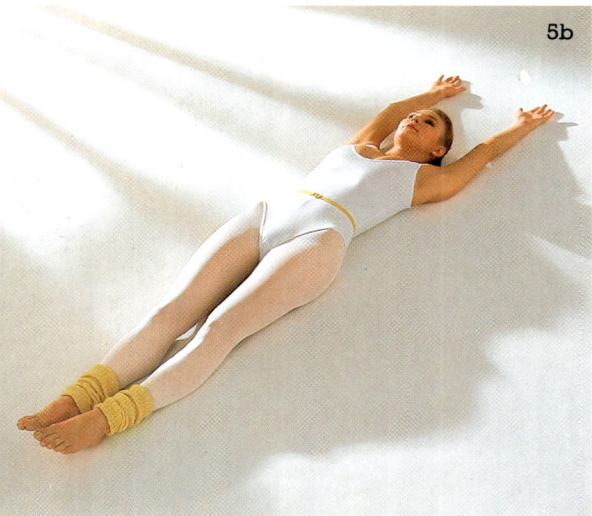

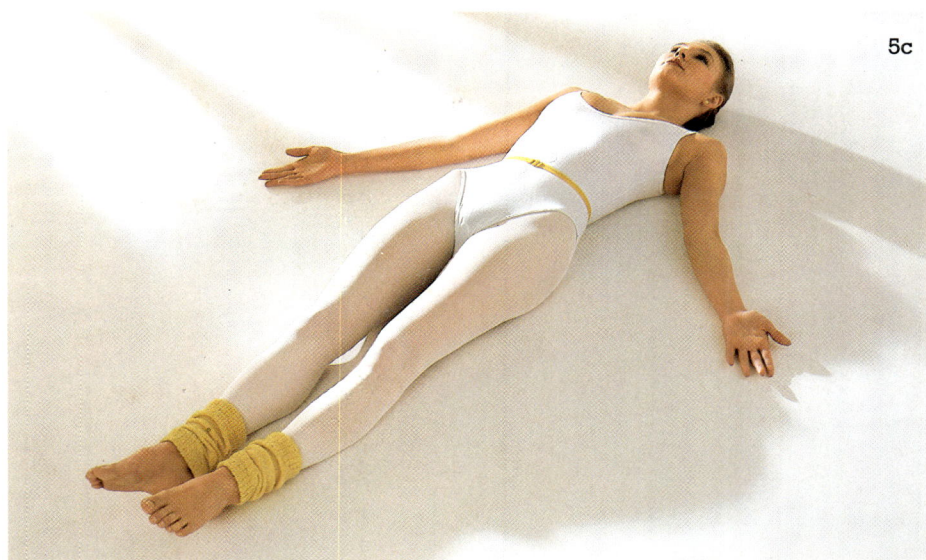

Exercise 6

What it does
Firms the stomach
muscles

How you do it
1 Lie on your back, arms
by sides, legs together
and stretched out in front
(6a).
2 Raise head and
shoulders, lifting hands
off floor, until you can
see your heels (6b).
Don't try to rise any
higher than this.
3 Lower smoothly to
floor and repeat the
exercise five times.

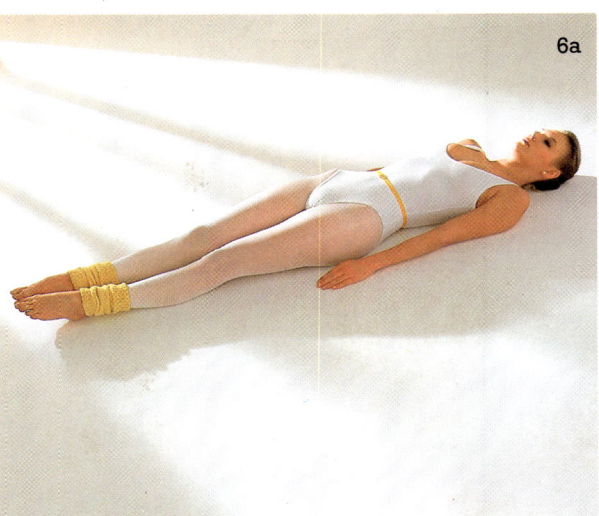

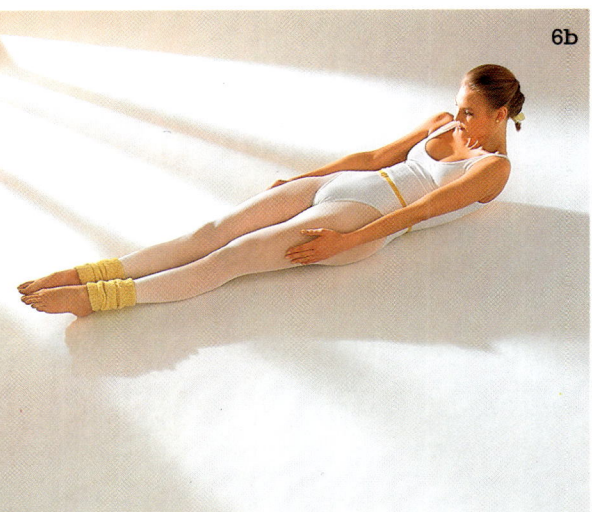

Exercise 7

What it does
Tones the hips and legs and fights thigh flab

How you do it
1 Lie on right side, supporting head with right arm, legs straight (7a).
2 Raise both legs off floor, keeping them straight (7b). Then lower.
3 Keeping body in a straight line, raise left leg into the air and swing it forwards to touch floor with foot as near to shoulder level as you can (7c).
4 Raise leg straight into the air (7d) and return to starting position.
5 Raise both legs off floor, keeping them straight. Hold position for a minute, then lower to floor.
6 Roll over on to left side and repeat the exercise.
7 Repeat the whole exercise twice.

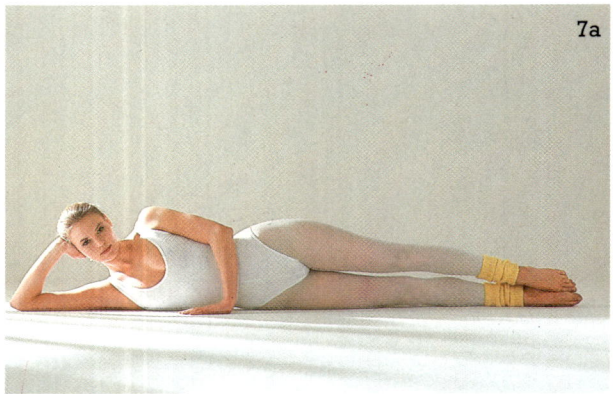
7a

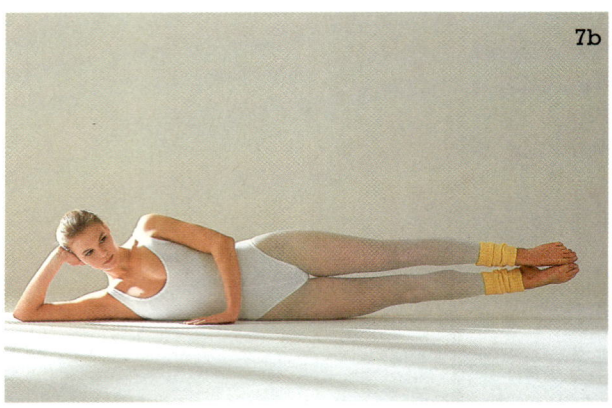
7b

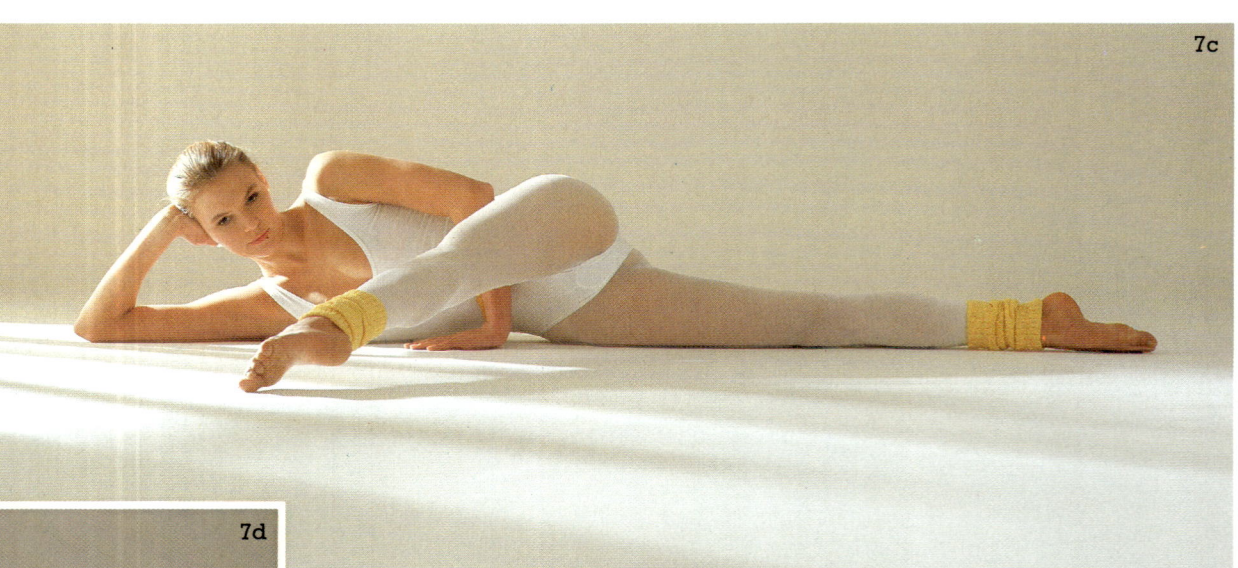
7c

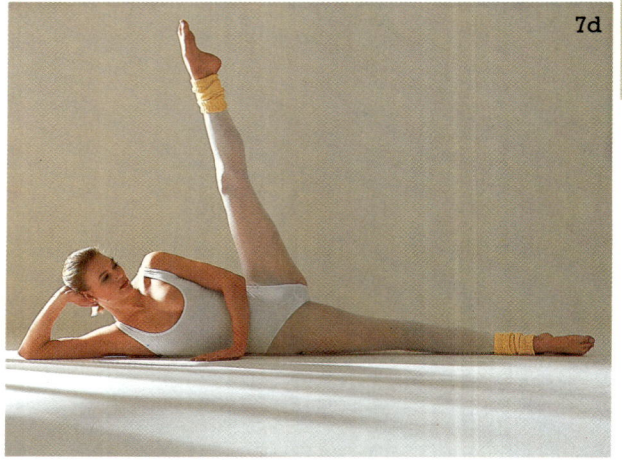
7d

Exercise 8

What it does
Firms the buttocks and gives your bottom a lift

How you do it
1 Kneel on the floor, holding on to a firm table or chair.
2 Leaning on the table or chair, and keeping body upright, extend left leg straight behind you, pushing knee away from body (8).
3 Return to kneeling position, then extend right leg.
4 Return to kneeling position and repeat the exercise five times.

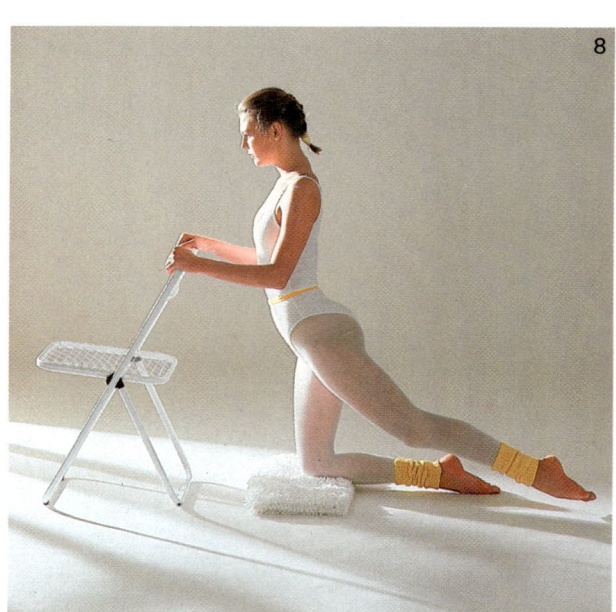
8

Exercise 9

What it does
Trims the waist and midriff and tones the arms

How you do it
1 Sit on floor, right foot back, left foot tucked under right thigh, back straight, arms by sides.
2 Push your left hip down into the floor as you slowly raise arms above head, stretching top half of body up as far as you can.
3 Bend body to the right as you swing arms down in the same direction (9).
4 Swing arms up above head again, then lower them to sides. Repeat four times.
5 Relax for a moment. Sit with left foot back, right foot tucked under left thigh, then repeat the movement, this time bending towards the left. Repeat four times.

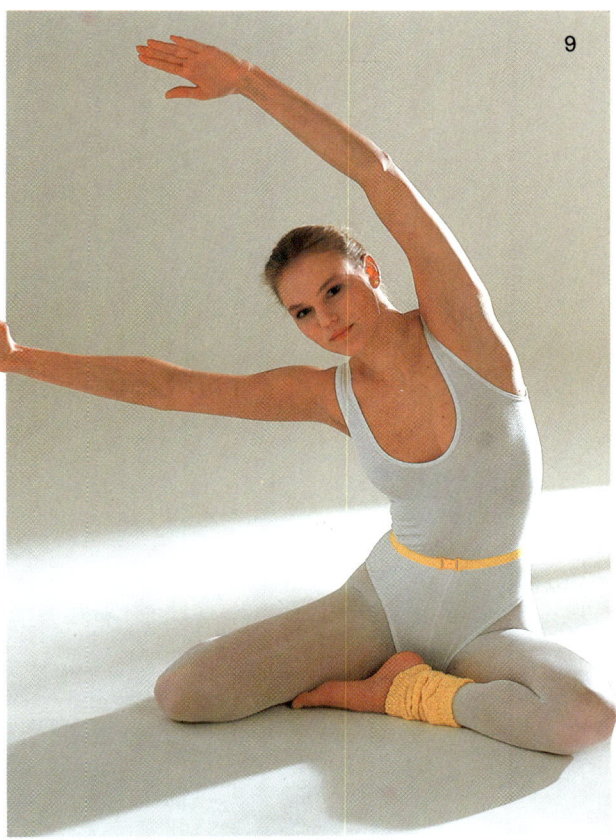

Exercise 10

What it does
Flattens the stomach

How you do it
1 Lie on your back with legs bent and feet flat on floor.
2 Breathe in. As you breathe out, push lower back into floor and lift your head and chest, reaching forward for knees (10).
3 Lower yourself gently to floor as you return leg to starting position.
4 Repeat the whole exercise five times.

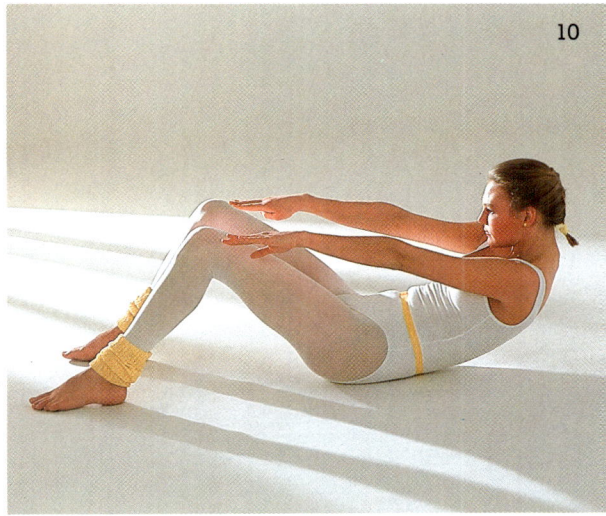

Exercise 11

What it does
Tones up the legs to make them shapelier

How you do it
1 Stand up straight, feet apart, arms by sides.
2 Breathe out, bend knees with arms relaxed in front (11a).
3 Breathe in, stretch arms above head, straighten the legs and rise up on tiptoe (11b).
4 Repeat the exercise eight times.

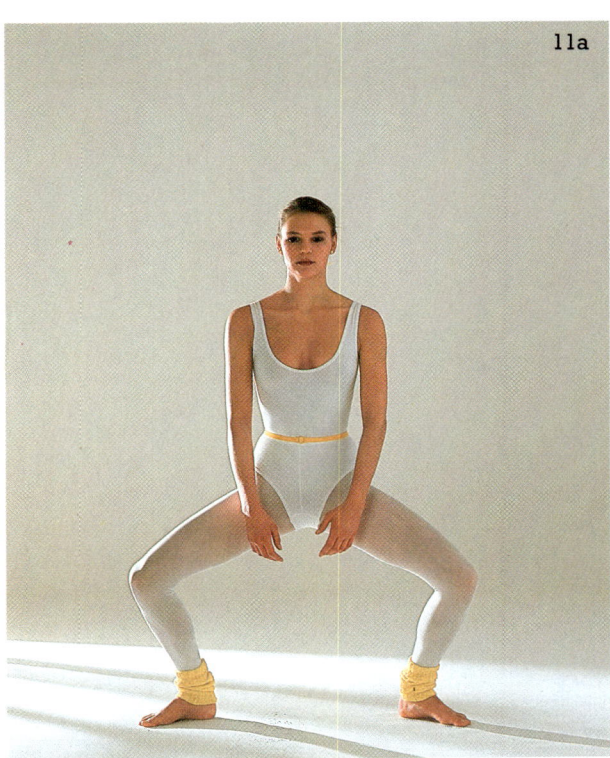

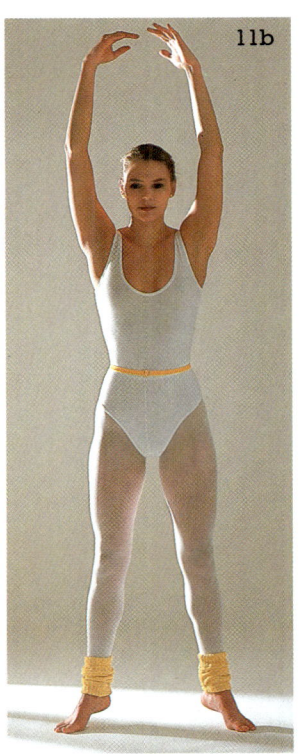

Exercise 12

What it does
Helps lift the bustline

How you do it
1 Stand up straight and place palms of hands together in front of you at bust level (12a).
2 Press hard against your hands in sharp, short pushes. Push 10 times.
3 Repeat the exercise at forehead level (12b), stomach level and then, with fingers pointing downwards (12c).

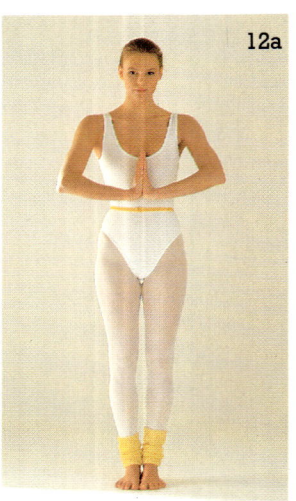
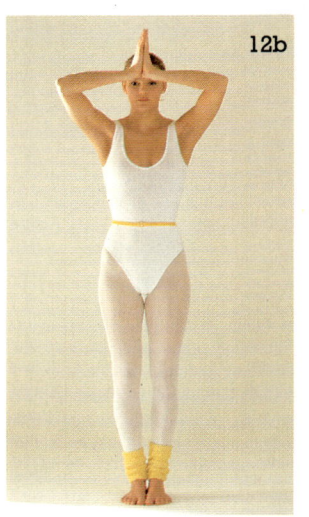
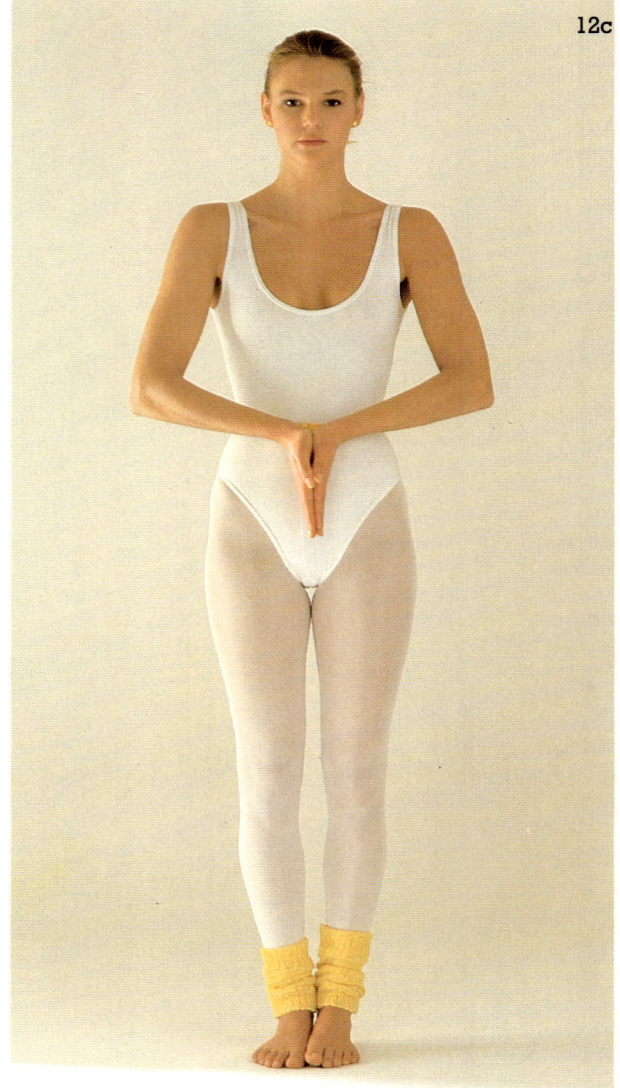

Exercise 13

What it does
Firms up the bottom

How you do it
1 Lie flat on your stomach, face and shoulders on floor, arms by sides, palms of hands down.
2 Bend knees and lift bent left leg off floor from hipbone (13). Lower again to floor.
3 Repeat with bent right leg. Repeat exercise six times.

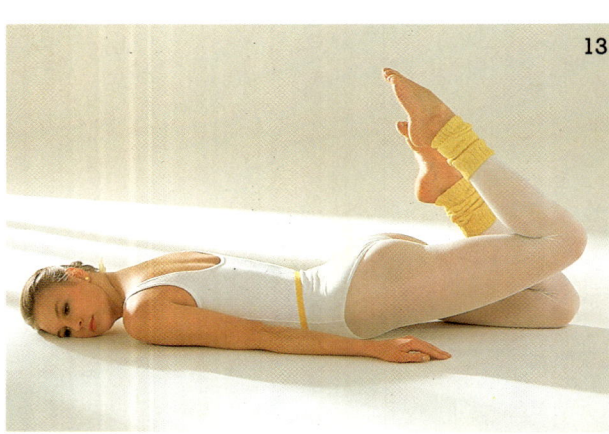

Exercise 14

What it does
Tones the top of the thighs by exercising both inner and outer thigh muscles

How you do it
1 Lie flat on your back and place feet against outside of a chair's legs.
2 Keeping legs straight, push in hard with short, rhythmic pushes, as if trying to bring feet together. Repeat pushes 10 times (14a).
3 Place feet against inside of chair's legs. Keeping legs straight, push out hard with short, rhythmic pushes. Repeat pushes 10 times (14b).

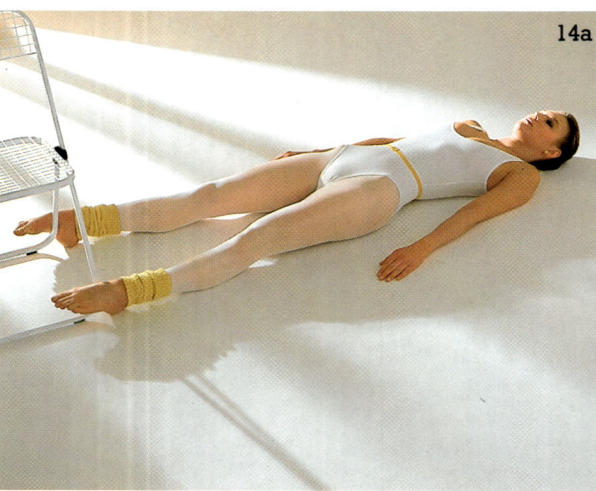
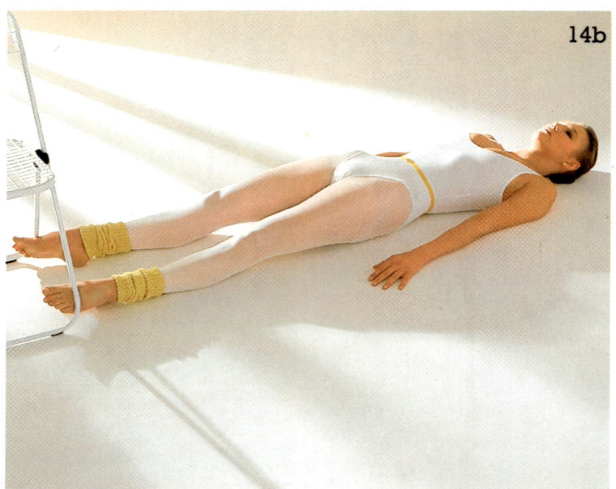

Exercise 15

What it does
Tones up buttocks, stomach, thigh and calf muscles

How you do it
1 Lie on your back, hands, palms down under pelvis. Bend knees towards chest (15a).
2 Straighten legs, stretching legs and feet upwards strongly (15b).
3 Keeping both legs straight, lower left leg towards floor on left side (15c). Raise leg to upright position again. Repeat with the right leg, lowering towards floor on right side.
4 Repeat the whole exercise 10 times.

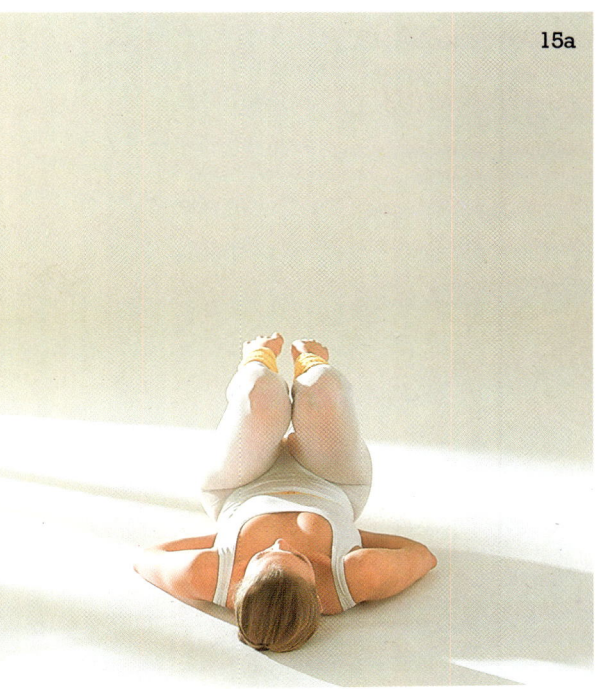

15a

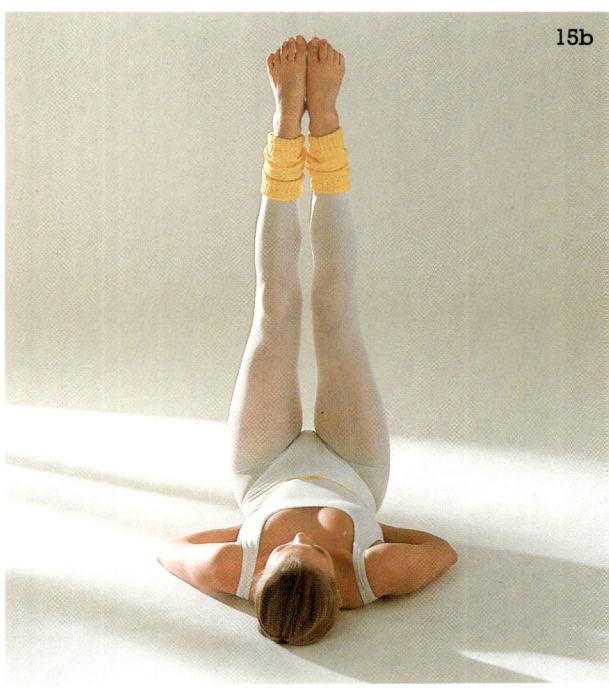

15b

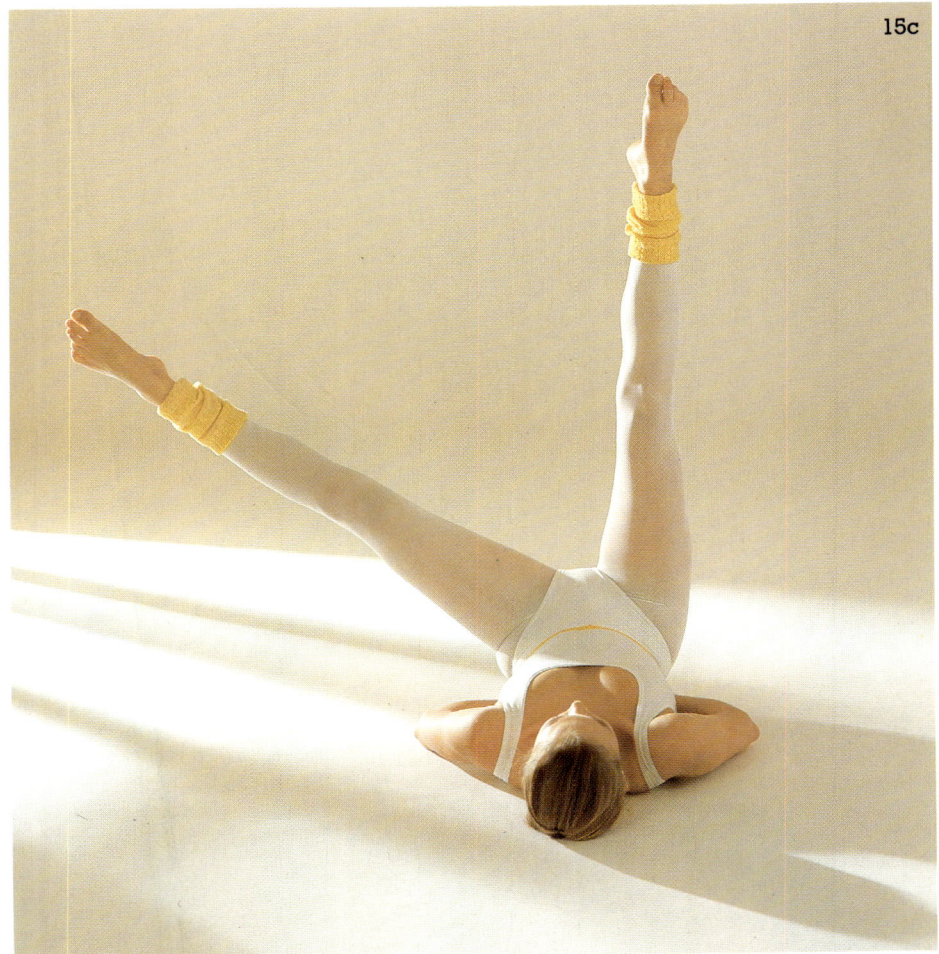

15c

Relax

1 Lie flat on your back on the floor. Make sure you are lying in a straight line with head straight and chin tucked in.
2 Raise shoulders away from floor and up to ears, then relax them as you lower them back to floor.
3 Raise bottom, press lower back into floor, clench buttocks, then relax as you lower them again.
4 Tense leg and feet muscles then relax them, allowing feet to flop outwards.
5 Stretch arms about 30 cm/12 inches from your body, stretching fingers outwards, then relax arms and place palms upwards with fingers slightly curled in a relaxed position.
6 Tighten muscles in face, then relax. Close eyes and breathe in and out very deeply for about five minutes (16).
7 Roll over on your side and very slowly get to your feet.

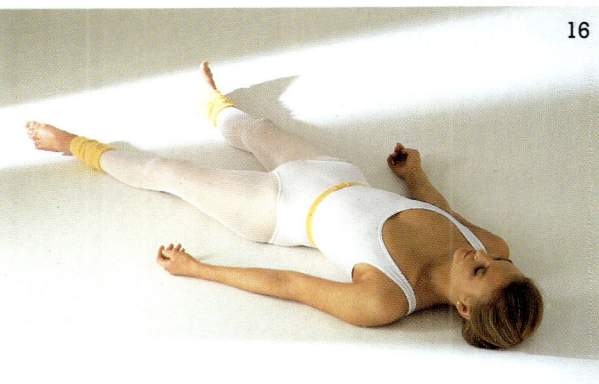

16

Expert Work-out

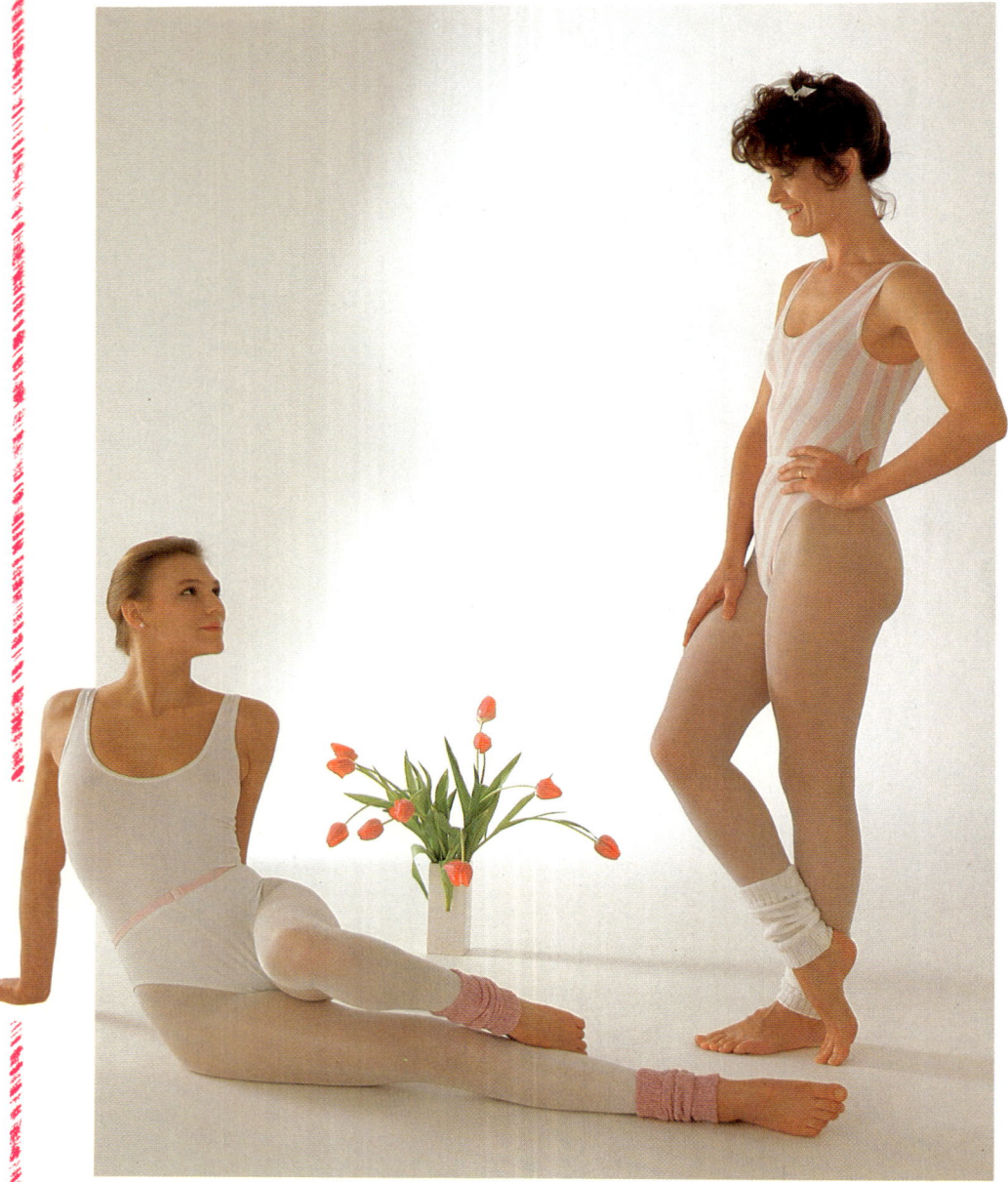

RIGHT **WRONG**

Note

It is not the speed with which you exercise that counts but rather the care you take to work the right muscles. The girl wearing the white leotard uses the correct positions and illustrates how you will gain maximum benefit from the exercises. The girl in the pink-striped leotard shows how and where you can go wrong.

Time required for this session depends upon the number of exercises selected

Done correctly, daily work-outs can refirm and reshape your figure, banish flab and make you look and feel so much livelier.

However, you may be faithfully doing your 'daily dozen' yet nothing much seems to happen. It could be that you just need to persevere, as muscles can take up to six months or more to get back into trim. But it could also be that you aren't exercising correctly. Many women gain only 25 per cent of the value of exercises because they do them badly.

The brutal truth is that you can stretch, bend and twist all you like but, unless you work your muscles the right way, you are wasting a lot of your time.

One thing to remember is that fat always seems to cling in the places where you least want it. If your waist or thighs are your biggest problem areas, you will have to get *right* down to your target weight before the flab finally disappears. In the meantime, exercises done the right way will achieve real benefits in flattening bulges and firming flabby areas. Limbering up for a few minutes before you start is essential to flex muscles and get your body ready for sterner exercises, otherwise you will be tense and muscles may be strained. Start off with the general warm-up that follows, then select the exercises for the areas you'd particularly like to improve. Devote your first session or two to learning how to do one or two exercises really well. Then work your way up, adding more exercises until you have a daily exercise programme that suits the time you have available. To start with, break your exercises into half-hour sessions – the warm-up will take about 15 minutes.

The slimmer you are, the more quickly you will obtain results from exercise. The younger you are, the easier it will be, too. But everyone can benefit from an exercise session done really well. If you are over 45 you may find the results of your efforts aren't immediately obvious, but keep working on your problem areas and they will eventually improve.

Exercises should be done rhythmically without jerkiness (music helps here) and no exercise should be rushed through – take a second or two to relax between each movement.

As we always remind you, exercises are for healthy people; check any fitness doubts with your doctor.

Warm-up stretch 1

How you do it
1 Stand up straight, feet firmly on floor.
2 Raise left leg and place foot on inside of right leg.
3 Stretch arms above head, palms together (1), and rise on tiptoe. Keep knee well back.
4 Stretch arms up as far as you can and hold position for a count of 10.
5 Return to starting position, then repeat the exercise standing on left leg. If you have trouble balancing at first, this exercise can be done with your back to a wall.

Warm-up stretch 3

How you do it
1 Stand on left leg and put right leg against a wall or on top of a firm chair, foot parallel to ground (3a).
2 Bend at waist towards raised leg, hands on hips. Repeat five times (3b).
3 Turn and repeat the exercise with other leg.

Warm-up stretch 4

How you do it
1 Stand with feet apart. Bend slowly forwards from hips, allowing knees to bend as necessary.
2 Touch floor in front of feet with palms of hands, straightening knees a little as you hold (4).
3 Hold position and stretch for a count of 25.

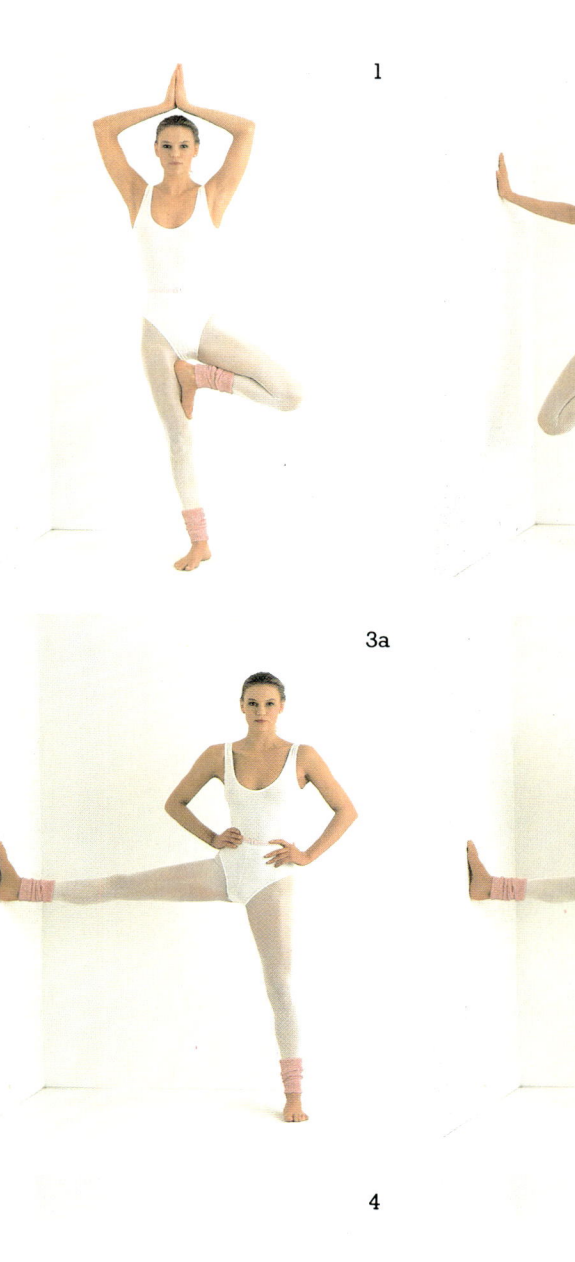

1

2

3a

3b

4

5

Warm-up stretch 2

How you do it
1 Stand in front of a wall, right arm outstretched, fingers touching wall.
2 Keeping right foot firmly on floor, bend left leg backwards, holding foot with left hand.
3 Pull heel towards buttocks and hold for a count of 30 (2).
4 Repeat exercise with other leg.

Warm-up stretch 5

How you do it
1 Stand up straight facing a wall and raise left leg so left foot is flat against wall.
2 Keeping right leg straight, foot flat on floor, grasp left ankle with both hands and bend forwards from hips until you feel the pull in your raised leg. Hold position for a count of 20 (5).
3 Repeat the exercise with other leg.

Warm-up stretch 6

How you do it
1 Sit on the floor and bend legs in front of you with feet together.
2 Hold your toes and bend forwards from hips keeping back straight.
3 Pull feet in towards body for a few seconds, pressing knees down towards floor (6).
4 Return to starting position and repeat the whole exercise.

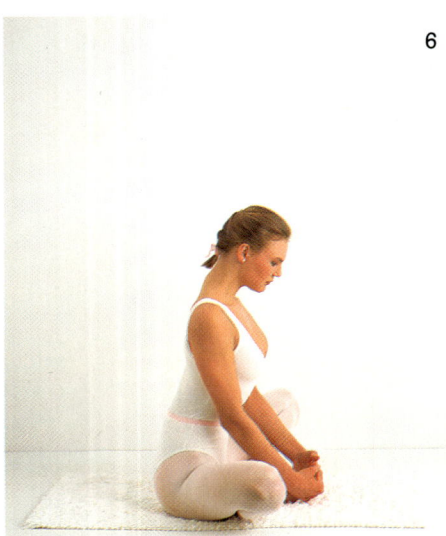

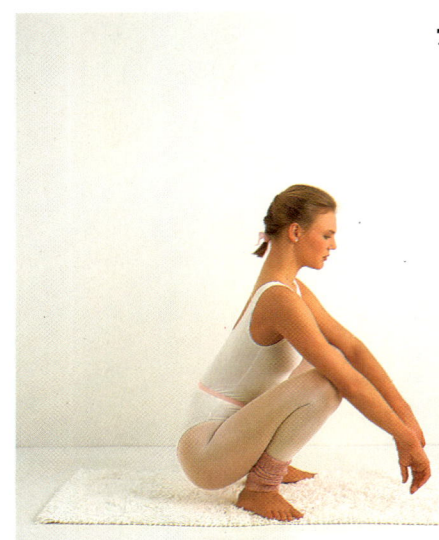

Warm-up stretch 7

How you do it
1 Stand up straight, feet slightly apart.
2 Squat down on haunches, feet flat on floor and toes pointed out at 15°.
3 Relax arms between feet (7).
4 Return to starting position and repeat slowly 2–3 times.

Warm-up stretch 8

How you do it
1 Sit on the floor, hands behind you, palms down, fingers facing backwards.
2 Bend right leg so that heel is just outside right hip.
3 Bend left leg so that sole of left foot is flat against upper right leg. Push chest forward and straighten back, making sure heel is well in to body and knees are flat on floor (8).
4 Return to starting position and repeat the exercise, starting with left leg.

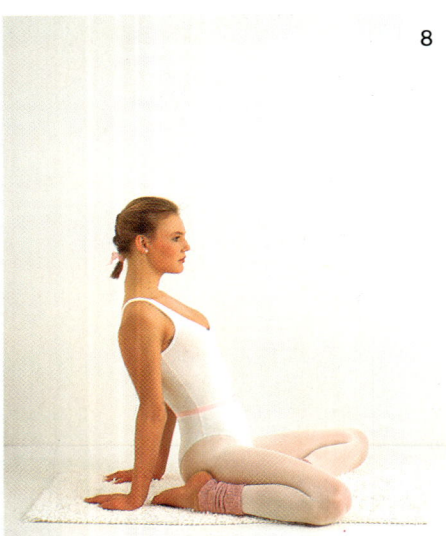

Warm-up stretch 9

How you do it
1 Stand up straight, feet together, arms by sides.
2 Jump so that feet are apart and arms raised to shoulder level (9).
3 Jump back to starting position.
4 Repeat the exercise 20 to 30 times.

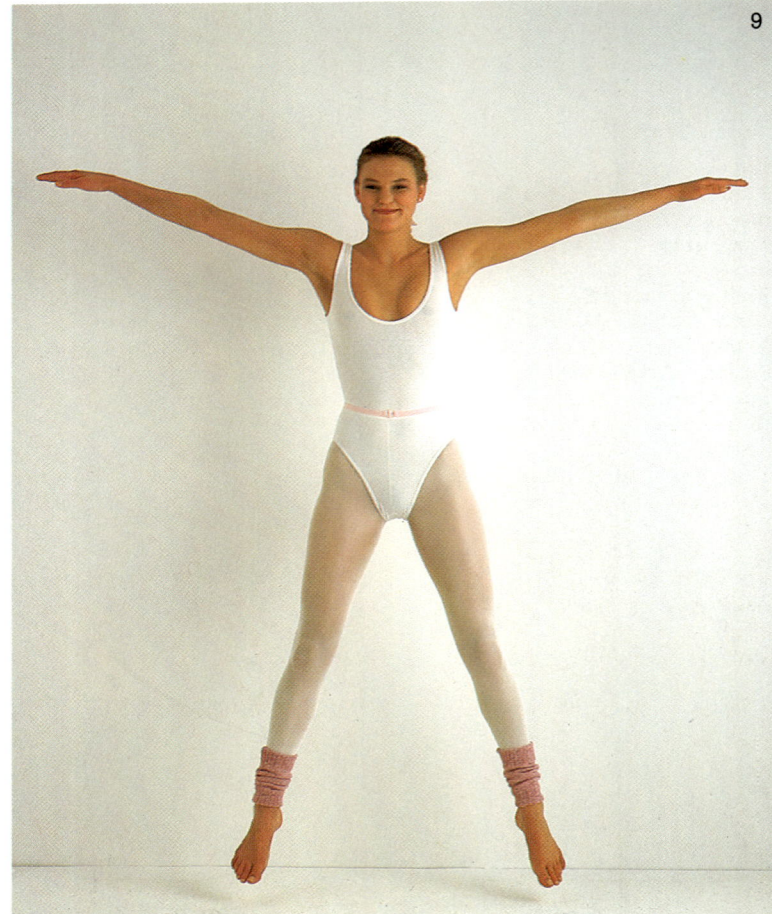

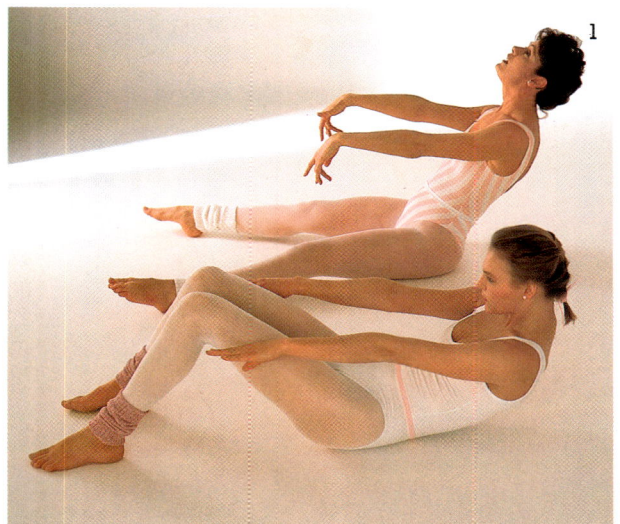

Exercise 2

What it does
Tones calves and thighs for neater looking legs

How you do it
1 Lie on your back. Bring legs up and over, lifting hips off floor and supporting weight with hands and elbows. Make big, slow cycling movements in the air, stretching each leg up as far as you can and pointing toes (2).

It's wrong if . . .
You do the exercise without supporting your back. Then the whole of the weight of the legs and lower body is balanced on the delicate vertebrae of upper shoulders and neck.

Exercise 3

What it does
Trims the waist, firms buttocks and hips

How you do it
1 Sit on the floor, leaning back slightly and supporting yourself with outstretched arms, hands on floor, palms down, a little behind your back.
2 With a rolling motion, swing right knee up and over left leg, allowing body to turn at waist and hips only, and try to touch floor on opposite side of leg with knee (3).
3 Roll back to starting position and repeat several times with a rhythmic, rocking motion.
4 Repeat the exercise using left knee.

It's wrong if . . .
Upper part of body is curled over, hands are too near hips, waist and hips do not turn with movement of knee, stomach is allowed to bulge.

Exercise 1

What it does
Firms the stomach, midriff and thighs

How you do it
1 Lie flat on your back on the floor, legs slightly apart, knees slightly bent.
2 Sit up, gradually curving arms up in front, letting head curl up towards them and curving spine as if trying to bring each vertebra in turn off floor (1).

It's wrong if . . .
Back hollows instead of curving, head does not 'lead' but is held back, arms are kept to the sides or legs are straight

3 Straighten and stretch legs as you reach sitting position, pull in stomach, lift midriff and sit up straight.
4 Reverse the movement, allowing knees to lift and bend as spine curls back down to floor until you are lying down flat again.

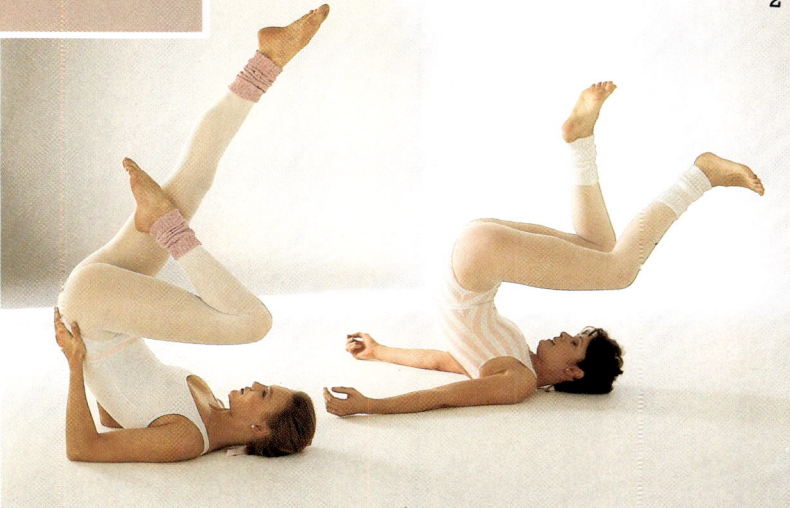

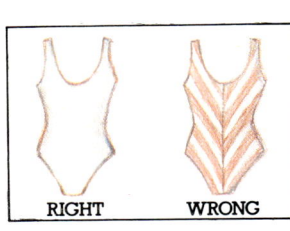

RIGHT   WRONG

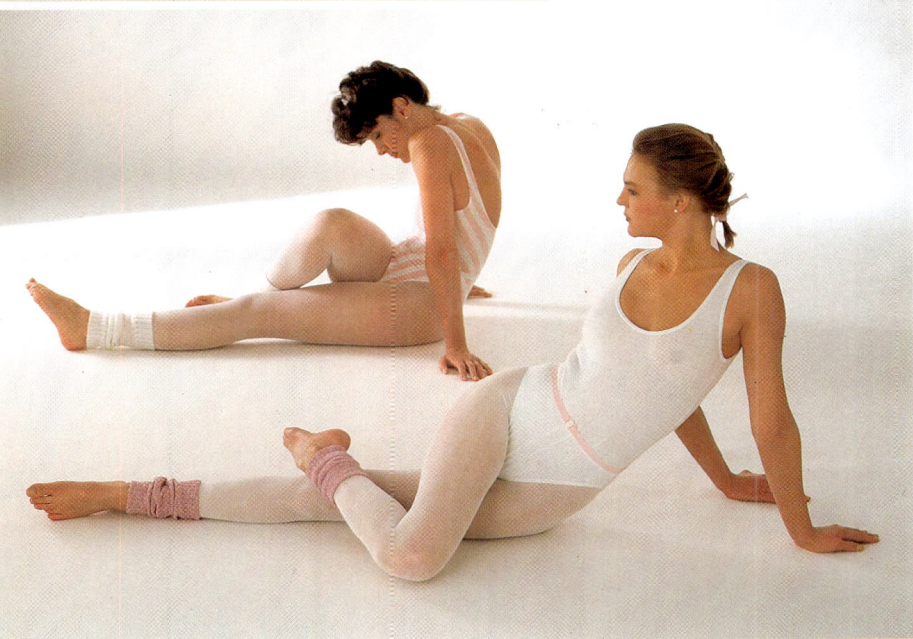

Exercise 4

What it does
This is stern treatment for the stomach, waist and thighs

How you do it
1 Lie on your back on the floor, legs raised at right angle to body and slightly bent at knees, arms stretched out behind head (4a).

It's wrong if . . .
Back is not hard down on floor. Legs should be well up and elbows relaxed.

2 Pressing lower back into floor, tilt pelvis and raise upper part of body. Grasp legs (4b).

It's wrong if . . .
Top part of body isn't curled forward.

3 Lower arms and legs, relax, then repeat the whole exercise.

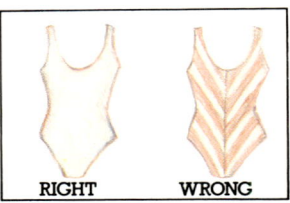

RIGHT   WRONG

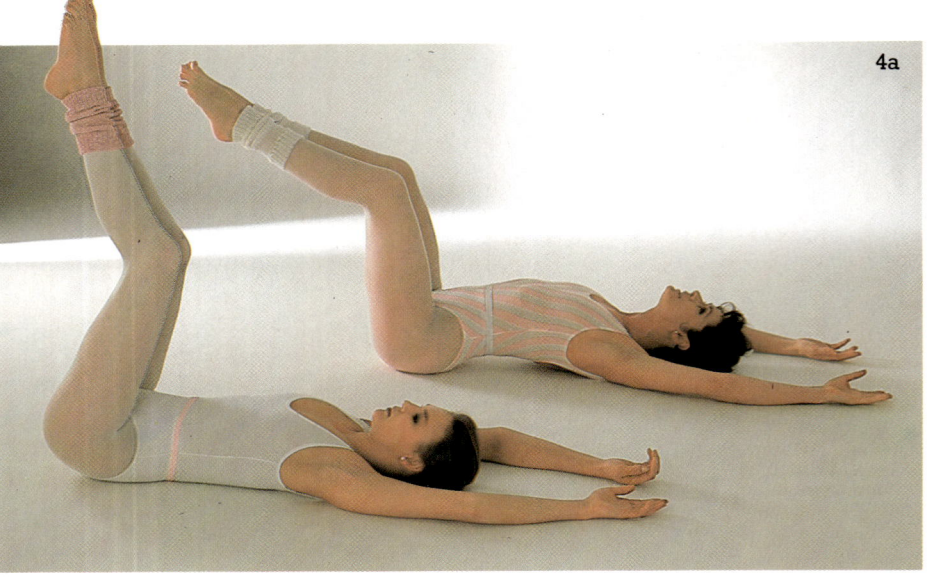

4a

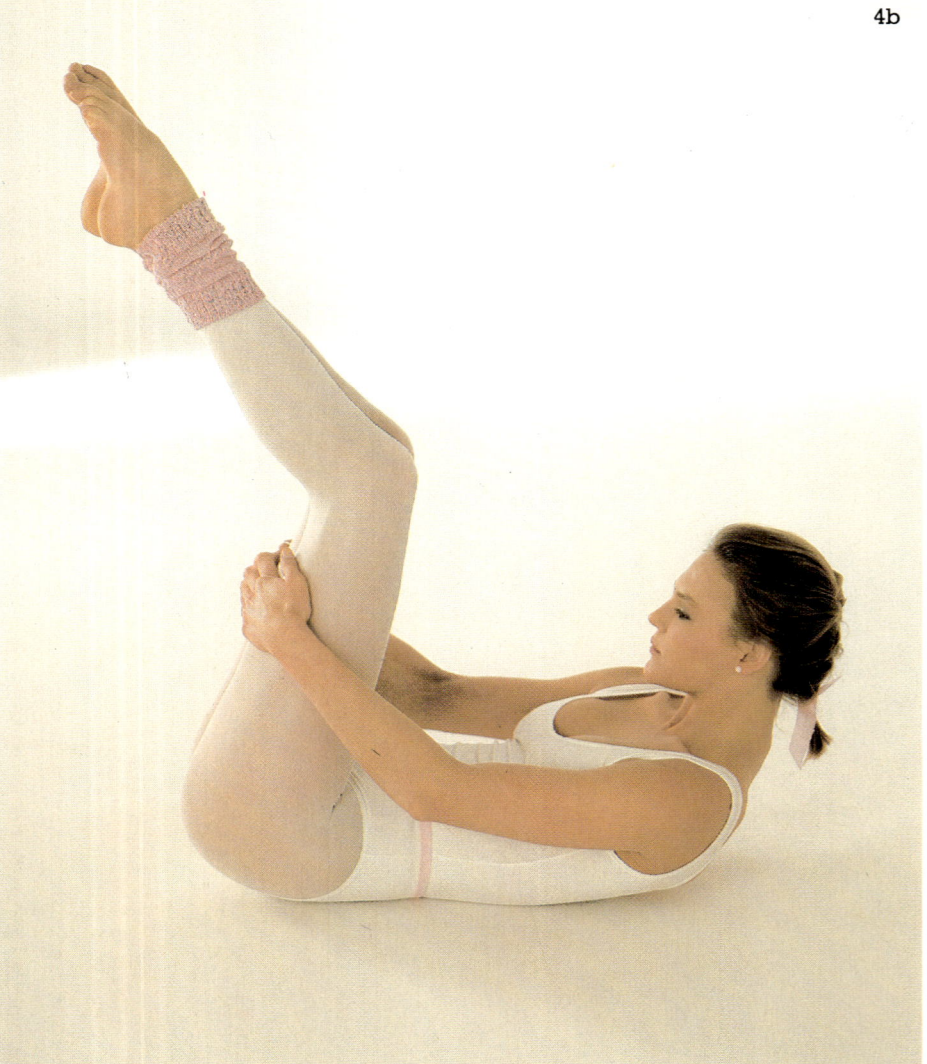

4b

Exercise 5

What it does
Firms the thighs

How you do it
1 Kneel on a carpet, knees slightly apart, and lean backwards as far as you can, keeping upper body rounded forwards. You'll feel a pull on thigh muscles (5a).

It's wrong if . . .
Back is arched, not rounded.

2 Without moving upper body, thrust pelvis forwards from hips and push forwards until thighs and body are upright.

It's wrong if . . .
Pelvis doesn't come right forward. Imagine you're pushing it forward with a click.

3 Follow through with upper body, raise arms (5b) and bring body upright, stretching towards ceiling (5c). Aim to get pelvis and thighs completely forward before moving upper body – that's the part of you that must do the work.

It's wrong if . . .
Your body is not completely straight as you stretch to the ceiling.

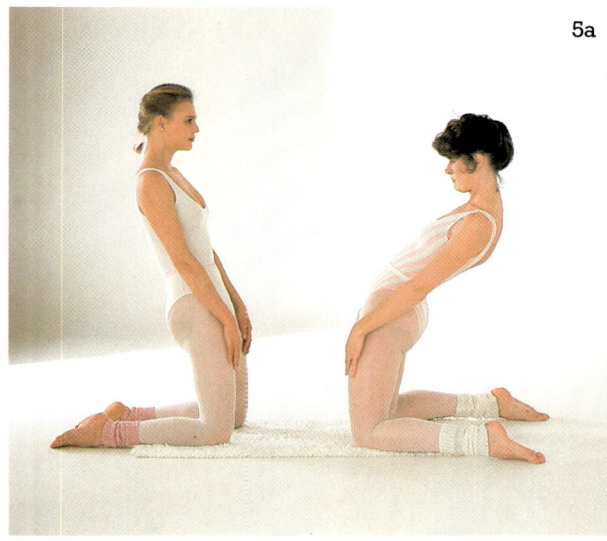

5a

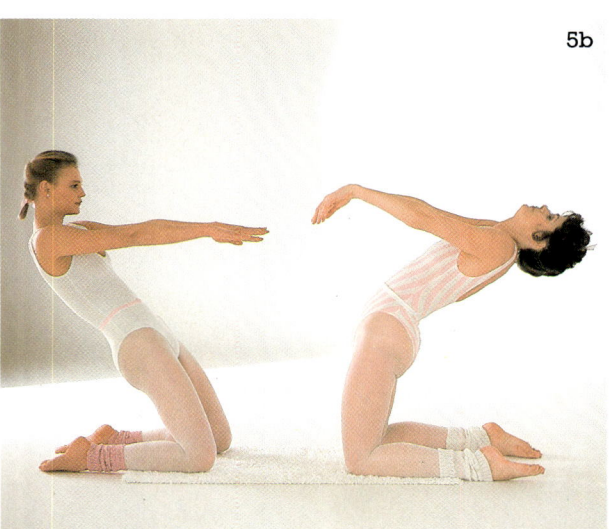

5b

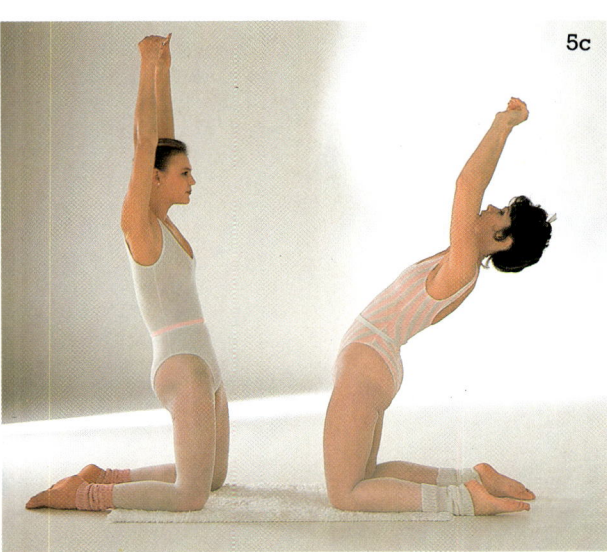

5c

Exercise 6

What it does
Firms and trims the waist

How you do it
1 Stand up straight, legs apart, and stretch up as far as you can (6a).

It's wrong if . . .
You are not standing straight nor stretching arms from waist upwards.

2 Keeping legs straight, swing left arm over head and slide right arm down right leg. Stretch over as far as you can, so that you feel a pull on waist. Keep hips centred (6b).

It's wrong if . . .
Hips aren't in line and left hip is sticking out.

3 Swing back upright, then stretch over the other side.

It's wrong if . . .
Arms aren't coming really low. Don't lean forward or back. If possible, do this exercise sideways on to a mirror so that you can check that legs, body and arms are in line.

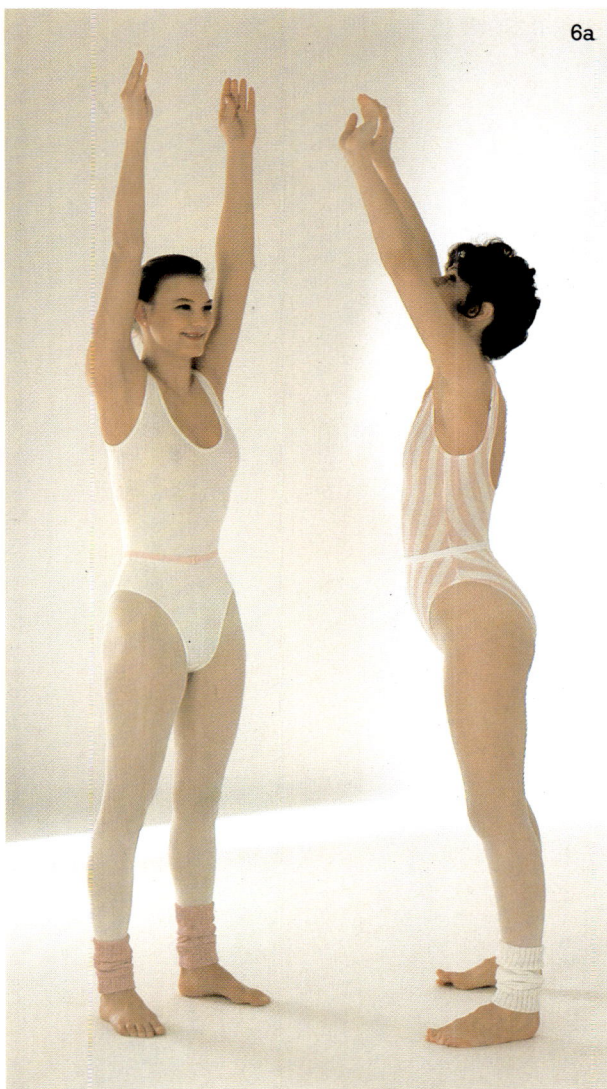

6a

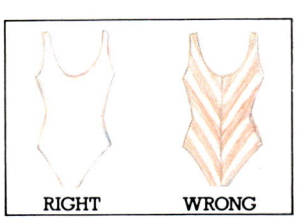

RIGHT   WRONG

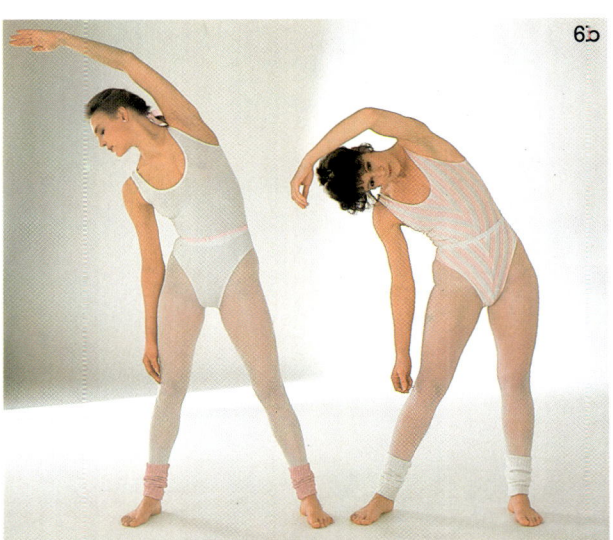

6b

Exercise 7

What it does
Firms the legs from top
to toe

How you do it
1 Stand up straight, feet
apart, hands resting on
top of hips, bottom
tucked in, pelvis centred
(7a).

It's wrong if . . .
You are turtle-topped.
Straighten neck, lift
head up from
shoulders, keep
midriff and chest held
high.

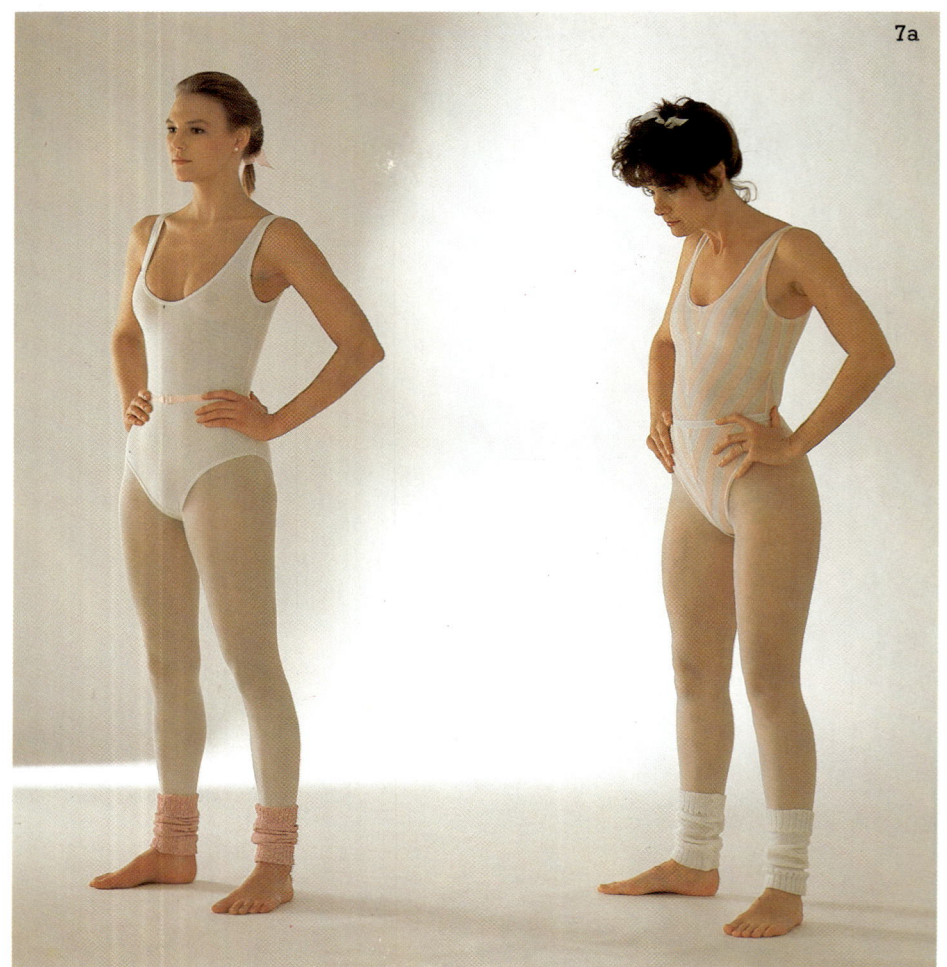

7a

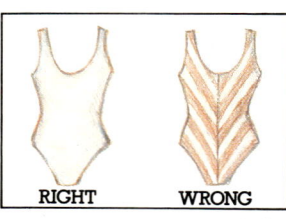

RIGHT WRONG

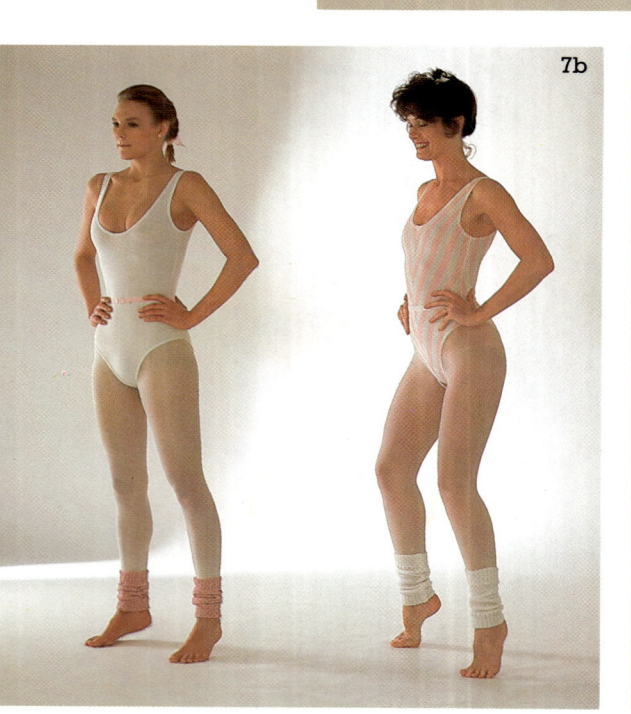

7b

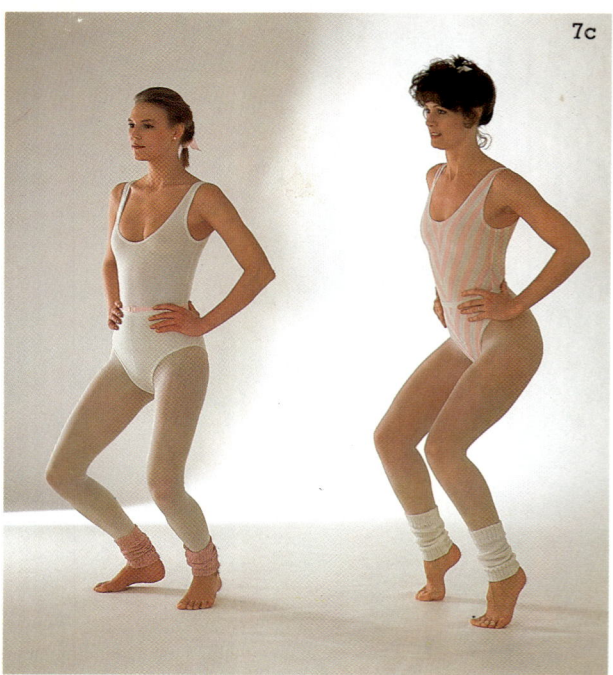

7c

2 Rise up on tiptoe, head
still held high, chest up,
bottom tucked in (7b).
You'll feel your calf
muscles working. If they
cramp slightly, don't
give in . . . relax to
starting position for a
moment before
continuing with the
exercise.

It's wrong if . . .
You start to wobble.
Grip hipbones firmly
for steadying effect.

3 Bend knees, directly in
line with angle of feet
(7c). It is vital that knees
keep to exact line of feet,
splayed out over them.
Top half of body should
be absolutely upright.
Don't bend forward from
waist.

It's wrong if . . .
You go down knock-
kneed or in a wide
apart squat. Keep
bottom tucked under.

4 Stand up straight again, feet together. Keep left hand resting on left hip, stretch out right arm until fingertips just touch a wall or chair (7d). This helps you keep upright and maintain your balance during the next movement.

5 Swing left leg forward and raise to a comfortable level. Point toes, keeping leg straight (7e). You'll feel the front thigh muscle working.

It's wrong if . . .
Your body is swaying, bending, or even leaning towards the wall. You should be moving from below waist only.

6 Swing left leg back, stretching leg and keeping it straight, pointing toes (7f). You'll feel the back of the thigh tighten.

It's wrong if . . .
Your body sways forwards to 'balance' the movement. Keep standing absolutely straight.

7 Reverse position and repeat the exercise with right leg.
8 Swing leg out to side. Keep leg and foot really stretched and knee facing forwards (7g). You'll feel the outside thigh muscle working.

It's wrong if . . .
You lean towards wall, taking the weight of your top half on the supporting hand.

9 Turn round and repeat side-swing with other leg.
10 Repeat the whole exercise three times, working up to six times a session.

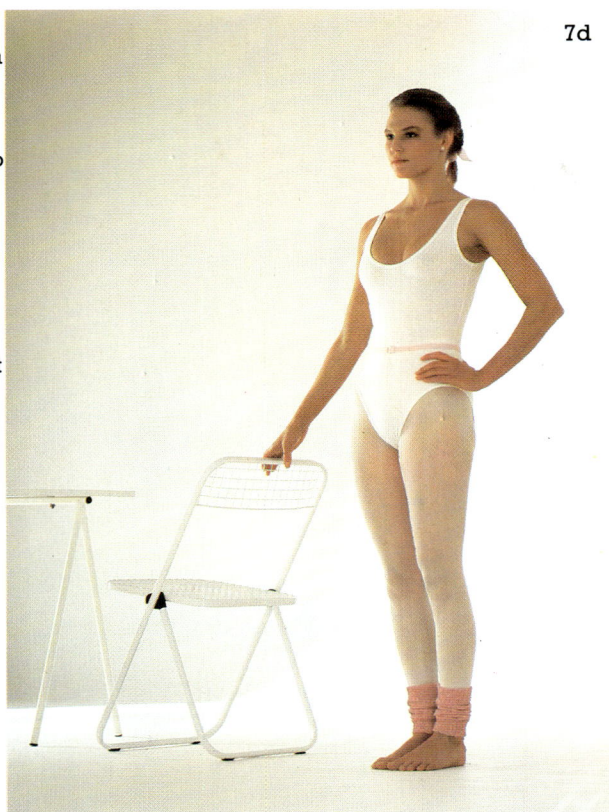

7d

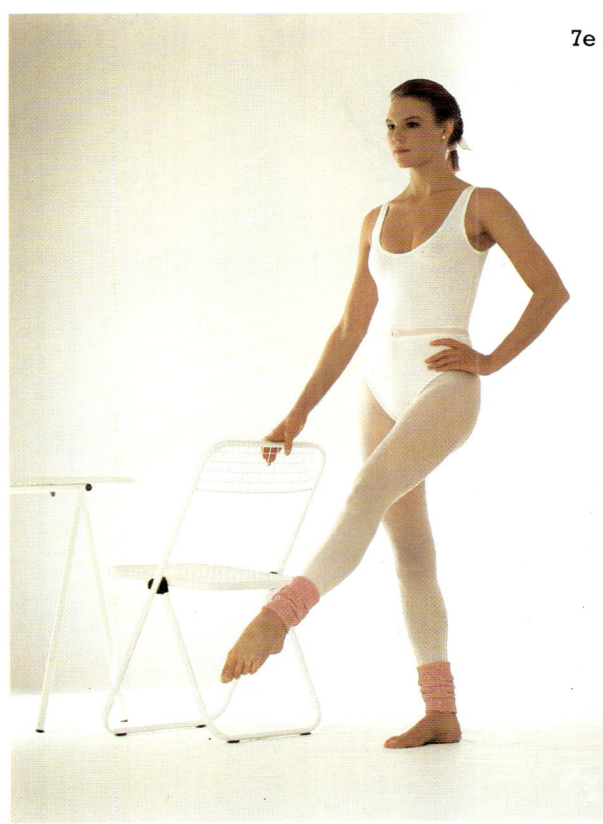

7e

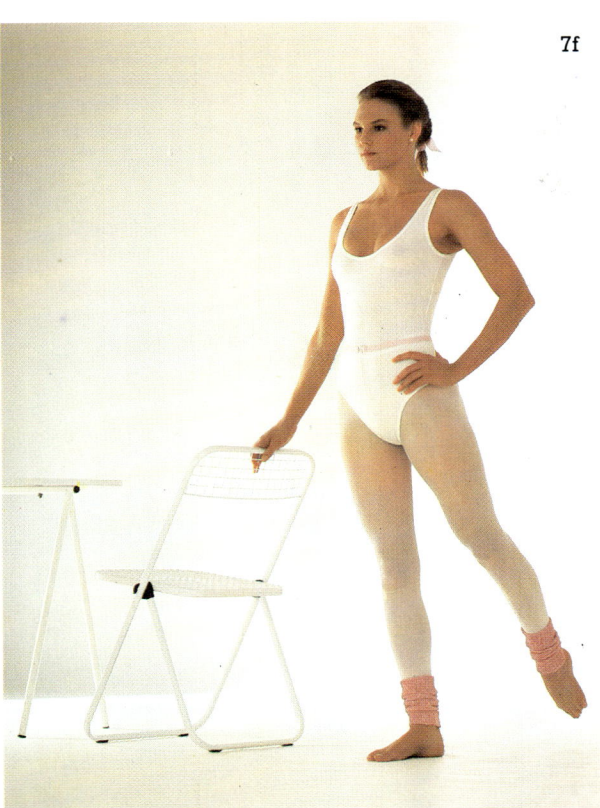

7f

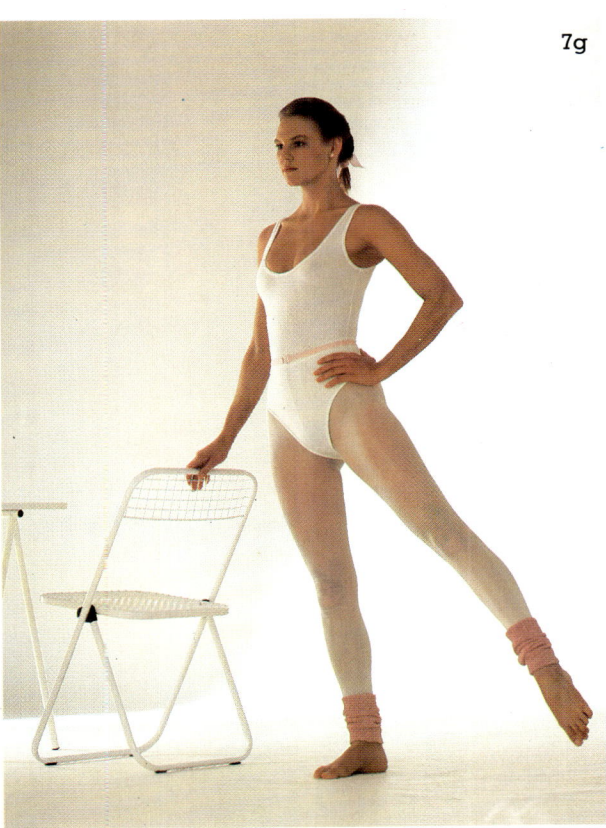

7g

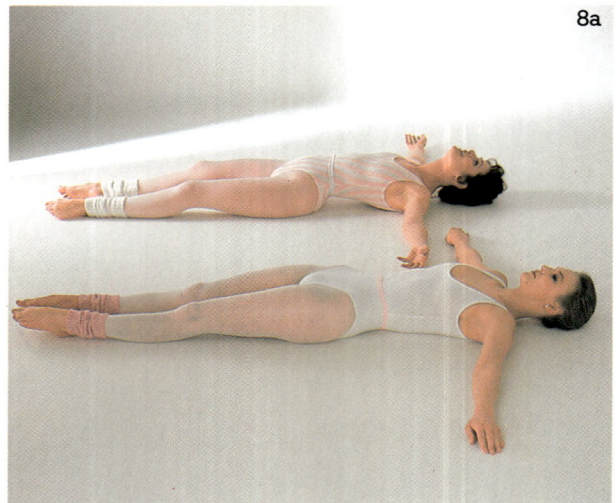

8a

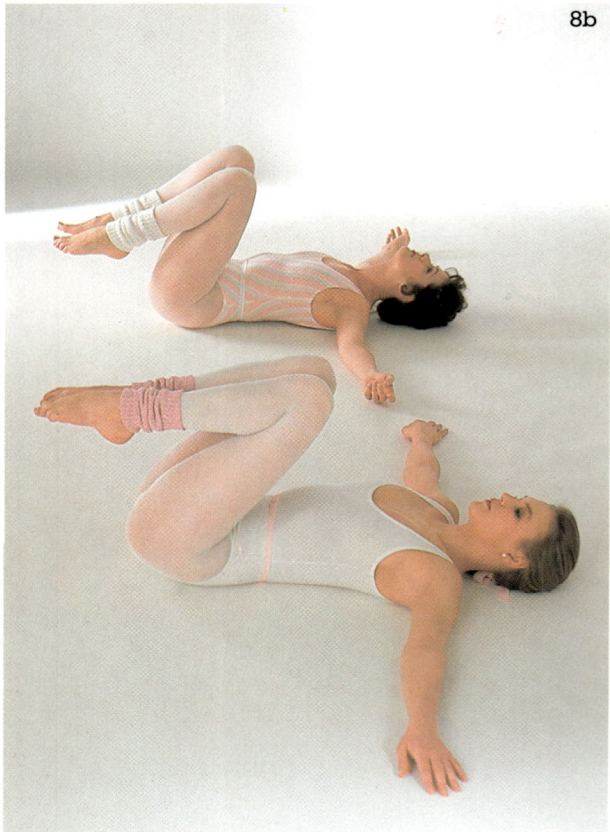

8b

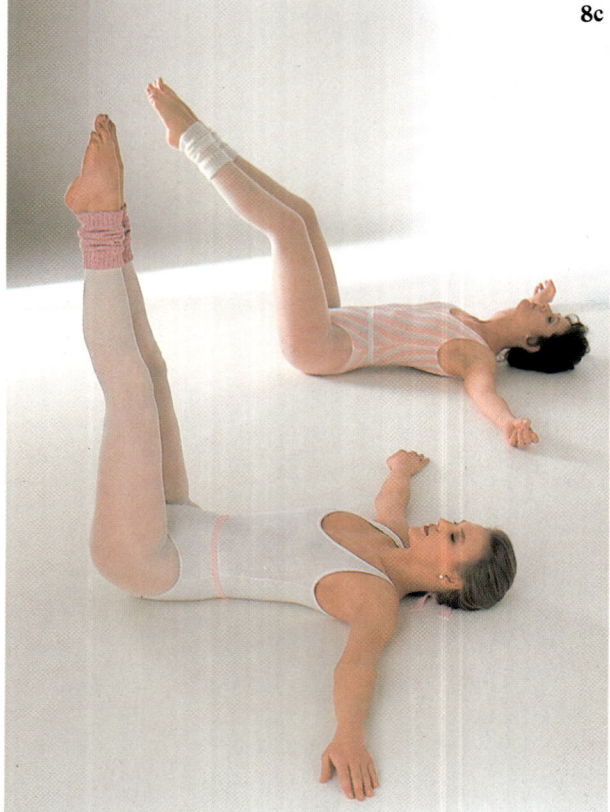

8c

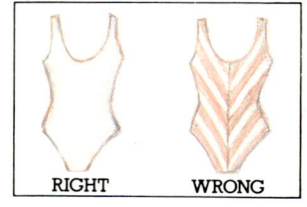

RIGHT   WRONG

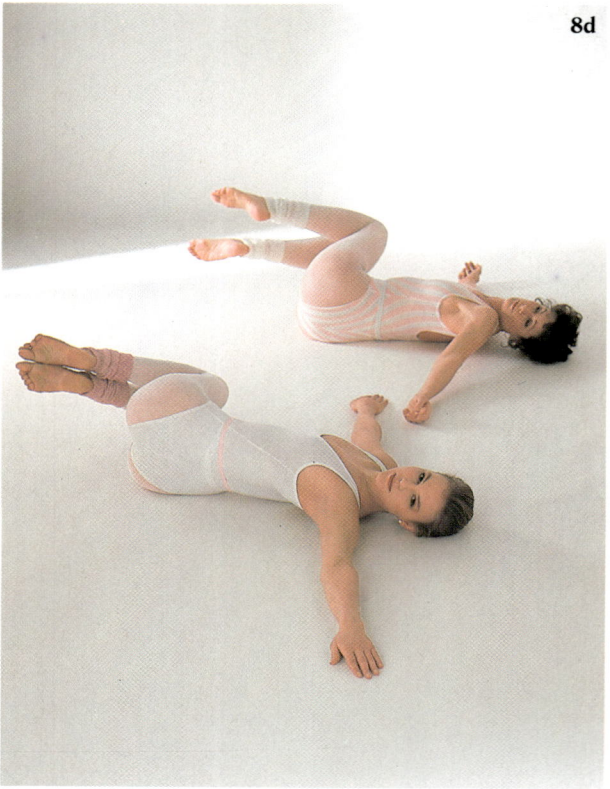

8d

Exercise 8

What it does
Firms the stomach and trims the waist

How you do it
1 Lie down flat on your back, legs stretched out in front and toes pointed. Press back of waist firmly into floor and pull stomach down. Keep arms outstretched at shoulder level, fingers and palms flat on floor, chin tucked in (8a).

It's wrong if . . .
Back is hollowed. Make each vertebra touch the ground.

2 Bring knees up to chest, keeping toes relaxed (8b).

It's wrong if . . .
Knees separate. Try holding a piece of paper between them to keep them touching. Are you breathing in and out normally? If you are holding your breath this will keep your top half raised.

3 Straighten legs so that they are at right angles to body, toes pointing gently towards ceiling (8c).

It's wrong if . . .
Knees are bent. If back is arched, press spine back down to floor.

4 Slowly bend knees and return legs to floor, to starting position.
5 Relax for a minute. Think about your stomach. It has cross-muscles as well as the main long one. These are oblique, rather like the side panel of a girdle, and are very important they're the muscles that pull in your waist.

6 Bring knees up to chest, swing over towards right elbow, head turning to left. If you can't quite make it, don't worry. Your basic body proportions determine how near you can get. You'll feel a sharp twist at the side of waist as the muscles shorten with the movement (8d).

It's wrong if . . .
You move shoulders and arms. They should still be flat on the floor, arms outstretched.

7 Bring knees over to touch left elbow, then back to centre.
8 Straighten legs in air (8e).
9 Spread legs in big V-shape, pointing toes outwards, following the line and angle of leg (8f).

It's wrong if . . .
Back is arched and knees are bent. Legs should be stretched and straightened, shoulders pulled back and flat on floor.

10 Bring one leg in front of the other, then repeat with opposite leg, to perform a scissor movement in the air. Do not bend knees – keep legs straight and stretched throughout (8g).

It's wrong if . . .
Leg's aren't still at right angles to body – or as near as you can manage. It is tempting to lower them a little at this point but try hard not to.

11 Do scissor movements for as long as you can manage, then bend knees towards chest and lower legs to floor. Lie flat and relax.

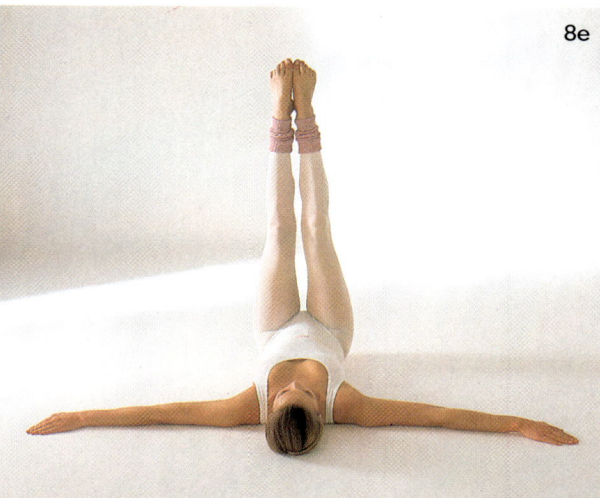

8e

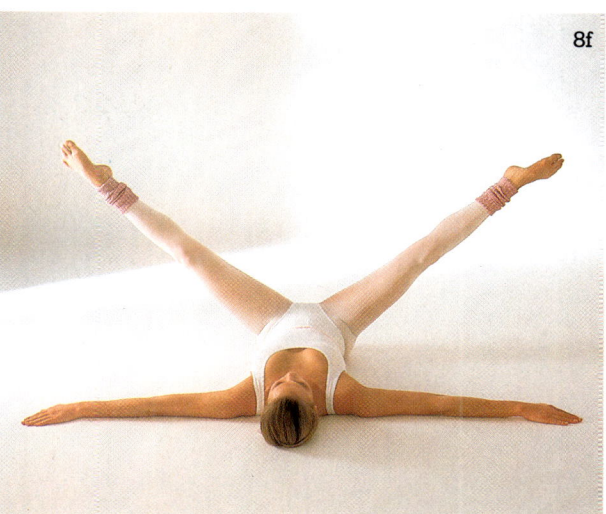

8f

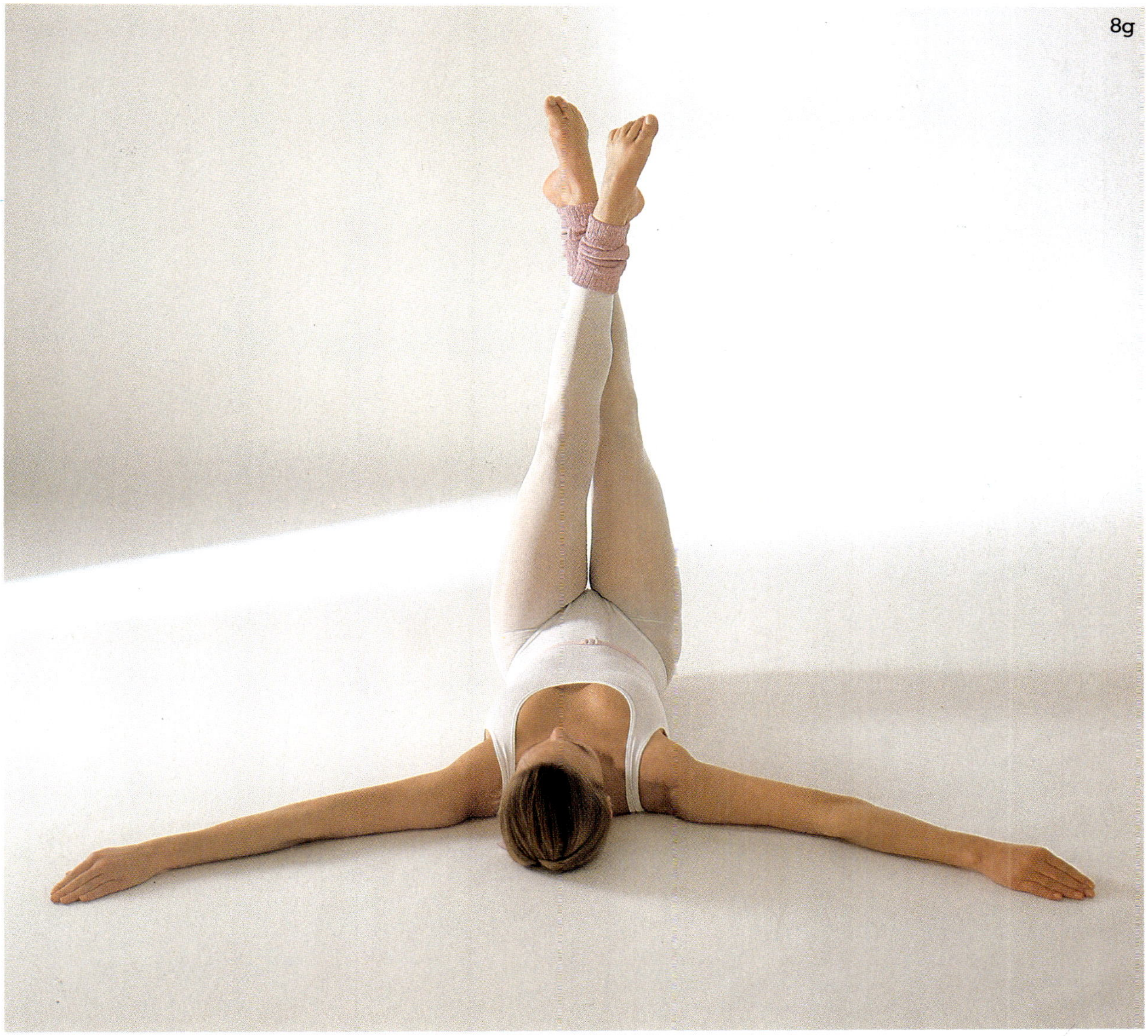

8g

Exercise 9

What it does
Takes care of upper arm flab

How you do it
1 Stand up straight, feet slightly apart, head held straight. Place hands on shoulders (9a).
2 Keeping hands on shoulders, bring elbows down and forward to touch each other.
3 Now bring joined elbows upwards to face level (9b).

It's wrong if . . .
You allow elbows to separate as you raise arms. Keep fingers touching shoulders.

4 Let elbows continue upwards, then move them outwards to complete a circular movement.

It's wrong if . . .
You don't keep elbows as high as possible. Open them as wide as you can each time.

5 Repeat the whole exercise five to eight times in a continuous movement.

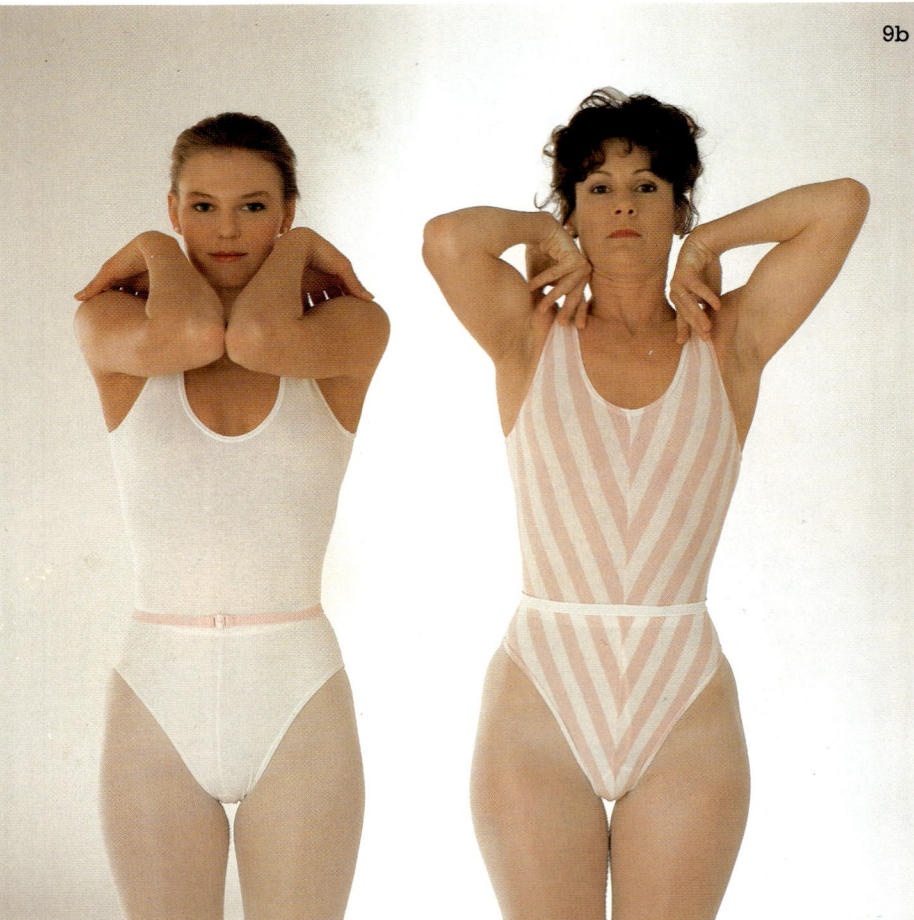

9b

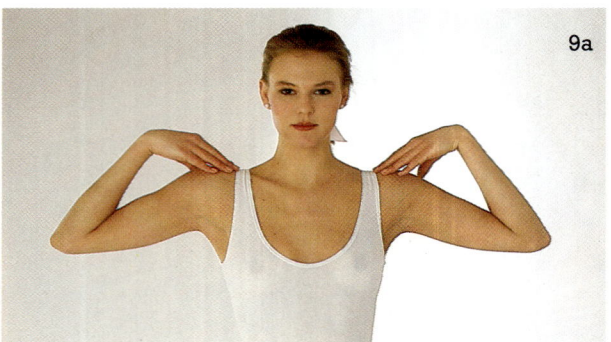

9a

Exercise 10

What it does
Firms the buttocks

How you do it
1 Kneel on a carpet, holding on to edge of a firm table.
2 Extend left leg diagonally behind you, left knee slightly bent (10a).
3 Lean over extended leg.
4 Now roll left hip forwards. Raise and lower left leg about 7.5–10 cm/3–4 inches from floor (10b).

It's wrong if . . .
You move body or lean away from extended leg as you roll hip forwards. If you are doing this exercise properly, you'll only be able to raise leg a few cm and you'll feel the pull on the muscles from the back of knee to top of leg.

5 Repeat the exercise five times, then change to other leg and repeat a further five times.

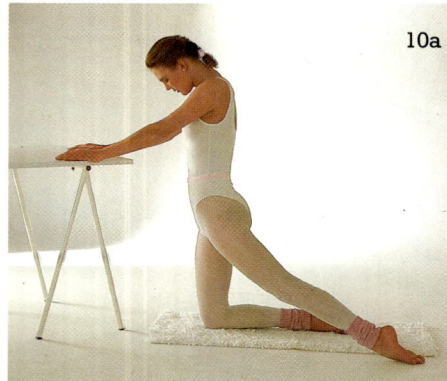

10a

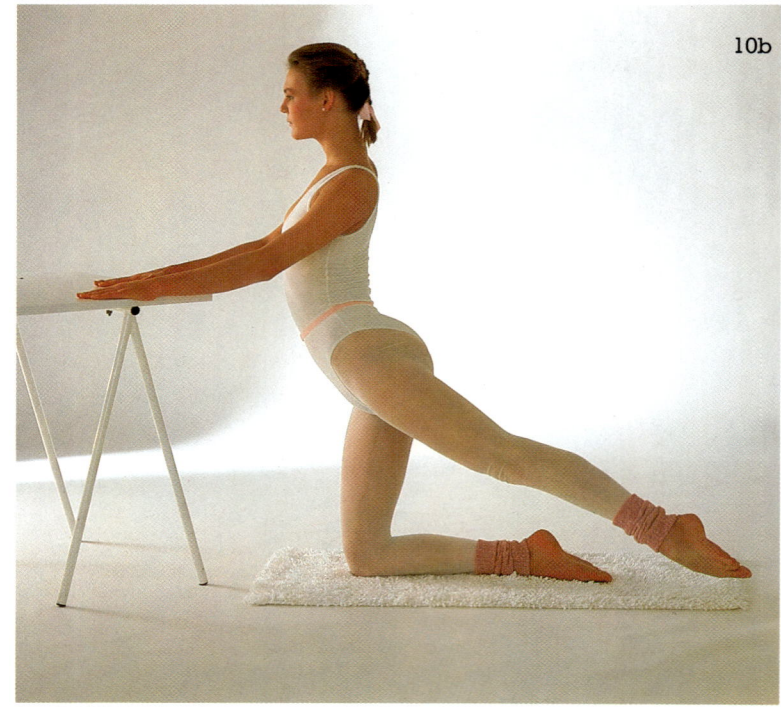

10b

Exercise 11

What it does
Firms the thighs

How you do it
1 Stand sideways to any firm object – table or chair – which can give hand support at waist level. Using right hand to steady yourself, hold left arm at shoulder level and squat on balls of feet, knees apart. Make sure knees are over feet and do not roll inwards (11).

It's wrong if . . .
Bottom sticks out, heels are apart and knees pointing to front. Knees should be as wide apart as possible, heels firmly together.

2 Keeping back absolutely straight, do small bounces up and down. Do five bounces, straighten legs completely, then do another five bounces. Gradually build up to 40 bounces.

It's wrong if . . .
You lean forwards as you bounce, sticking out bottom.

3 In squatting position – knees wide, heels firmly together – raise body until bottom is about 30 cm/12 inches off the floor. Keeping back straight, hold position and open knees wider. Keep pushing with small movements to a count of 10.

It's wrong if . . .
You don't keep body raised as you do the exercise. Don't let heels fall backwards, keep them together.

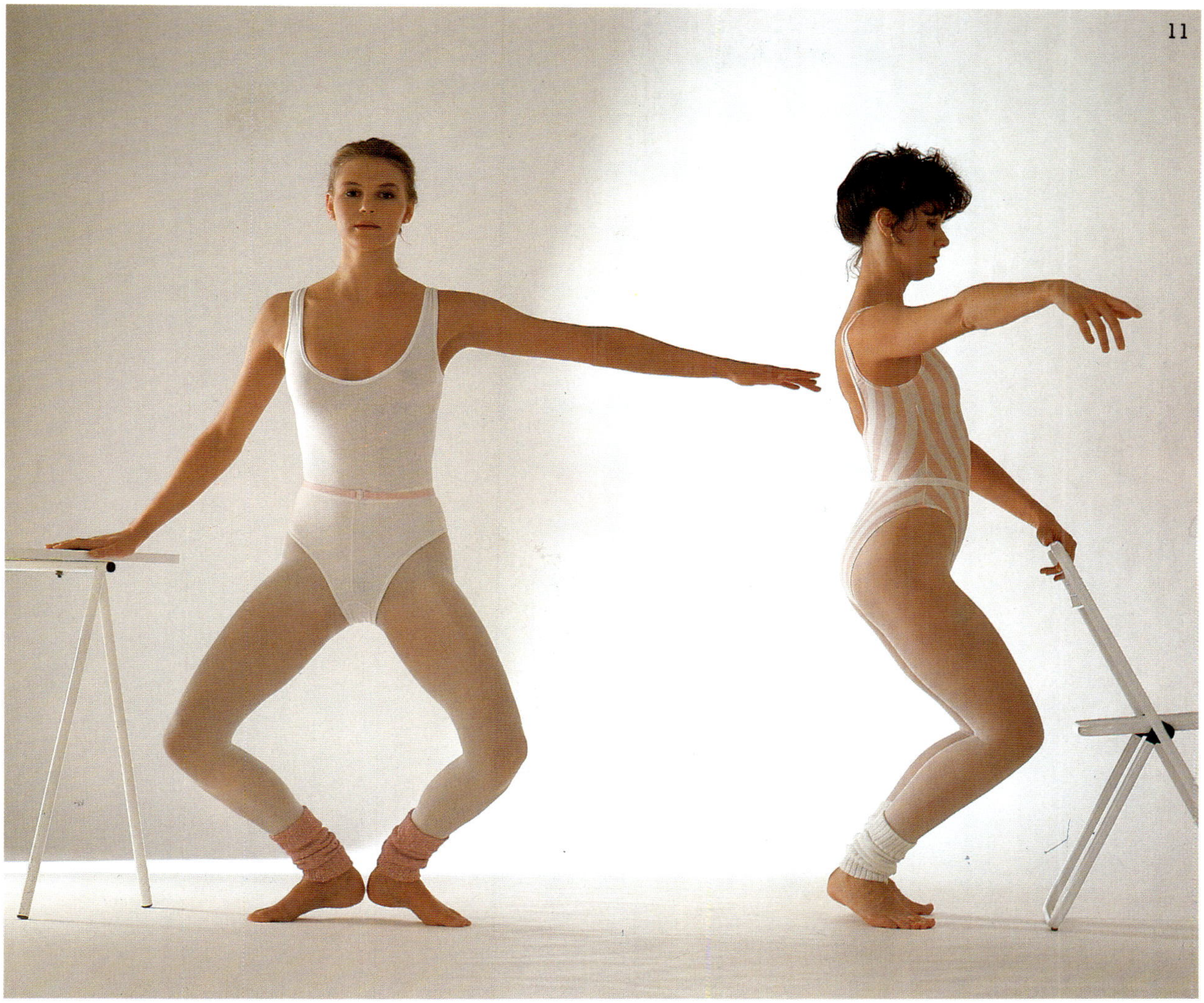

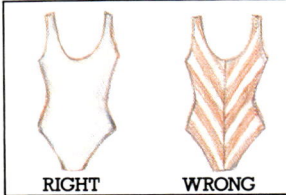
RIGHT   WRONG

Relax

1 Lie flat on your back on the floor. Make sure you are lying in a straight line with head straight and chin tucked in.
2 Raise shoulders away from floor and up to ears, then relax them as you lower them back to floor.
3 Raise bottom, press lower back into floor, clench buttocks, then relax as you lower them again.
4 Tense leg and feet muscles, then relax them allowing feet to flop outwards.
5 Stretch arms about 30 cm/12 inches from your body, stretching fingers outwards, then relax arms and place palms upwards with fingers slightly curled in a relaxed position.
6 Tighten muscles in face, then relax. Close eyes and breathe in and out very deeply for about five minutes.
7 Roll over on your side and very slowly get to your feet.

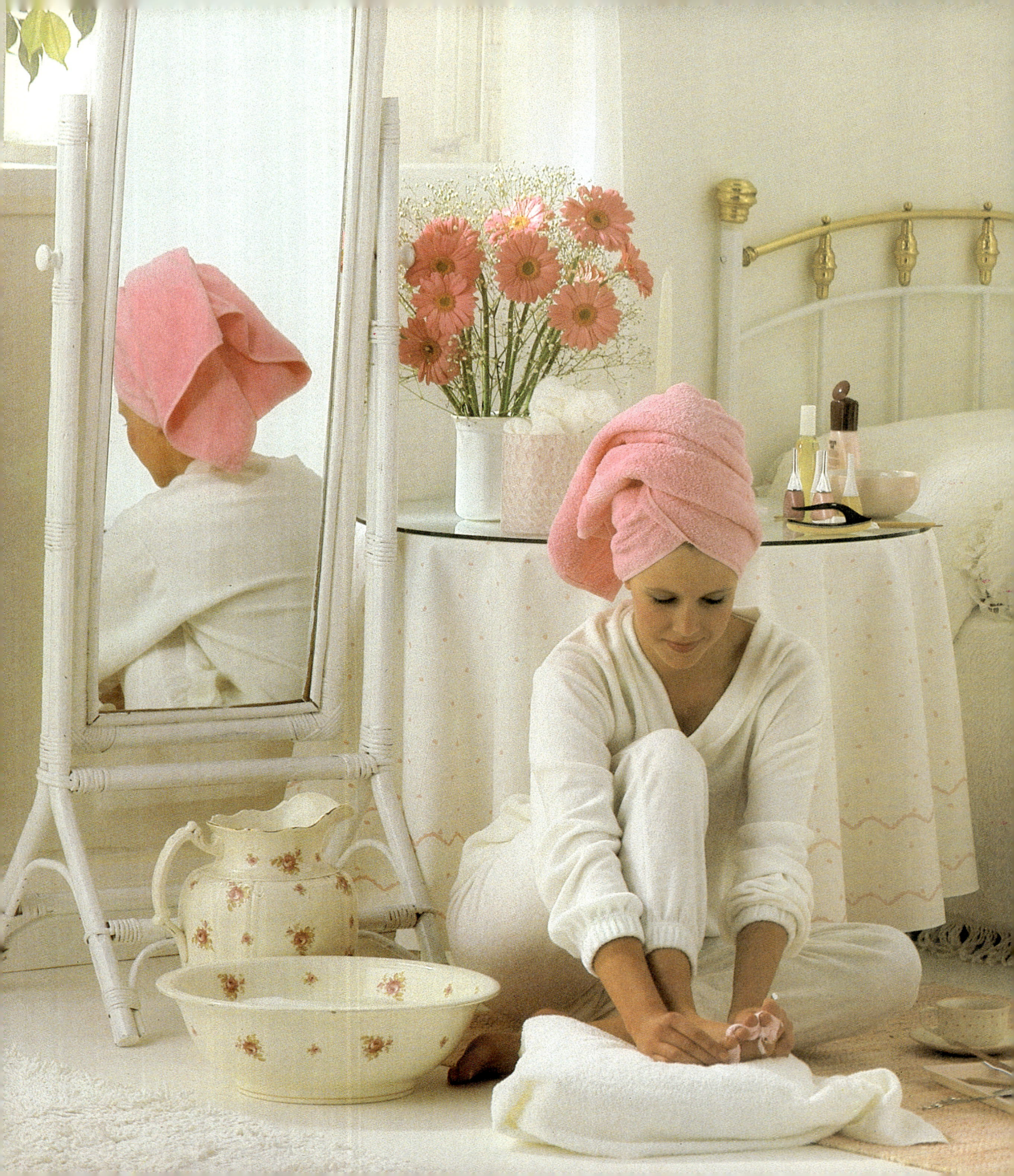

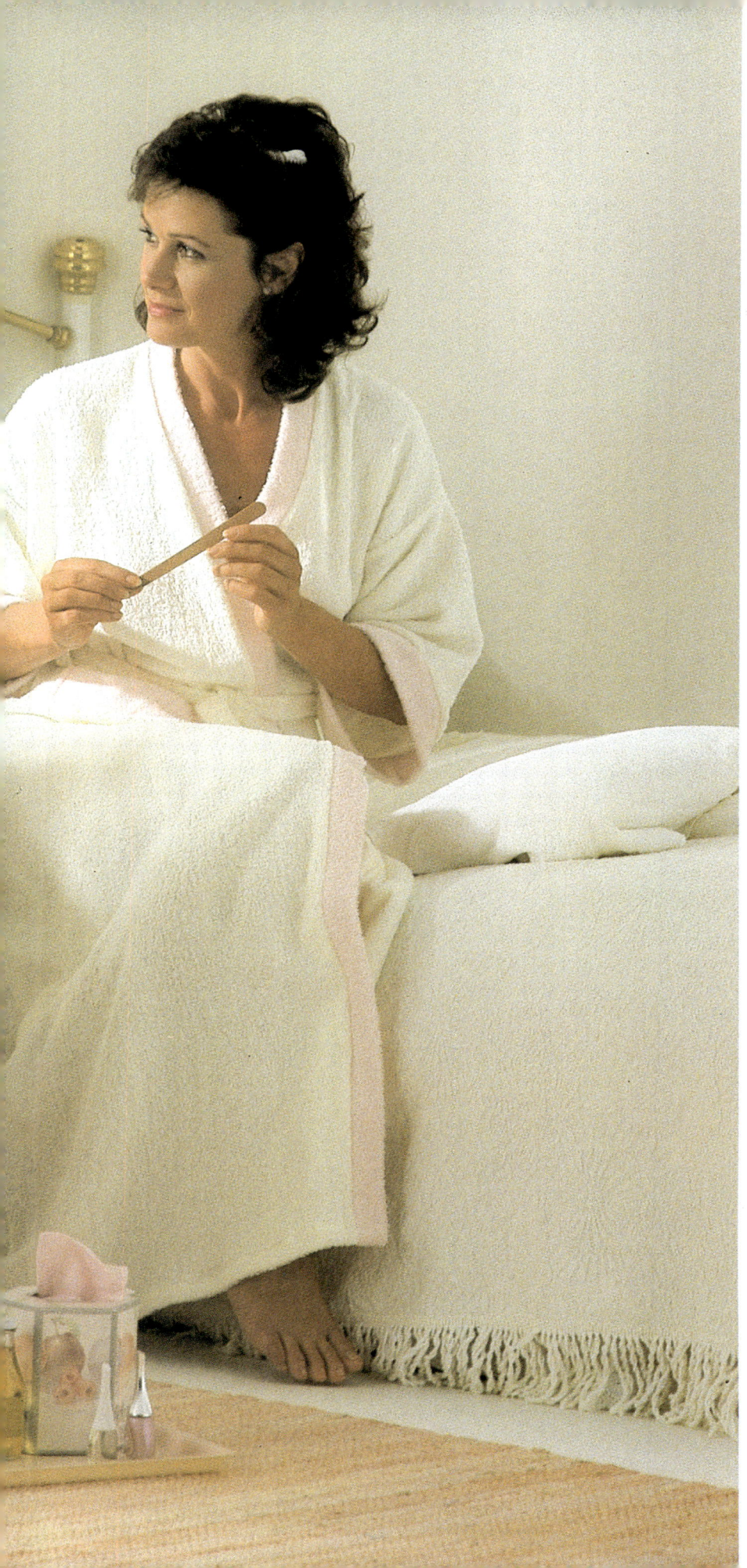

BEAUTY

The various Home Health Farm beauty treatments enable you to improve your appearance without spending too much money. But remember, good looks are not just a matter of using the right makeup or selecting a flattering hairstyle. They also depend upon the attitude you have towards yourself.

Learning to love your body, wearing becoming clothes and radiating an air of confidence are sure ways of making yourself more attractive. Keeping yourself well groomed is another.

It is possible to achieve a new look by following our Complete Makeover (see page 68), and even if you are relatively content with your looks we suggest you set aside plenty of time to tackle the Bare Essentials . . .

Hands and nails are always on show and a good manicure and regular care can make you proud to show them off. If you want good-looking hands you should faithfully use rubber gloves when you do housework and keep your nails nicely shaped and in good condition. Buff nails to give them a pretty gleam and run a white nail pencil gently under the tips to whiten them. If your hands are often in water, use hand cream liberally, and rub cream into your hands before you go to bed each night.

Feet are out of view most of the time and are a part of the body many people neglect but discomfort in the feet shows in your face, so make sure you pamper them regularly. The pedicure in Bare Essentials keeps your feet nicely in trim.

Even if you don't wear makeup every day you should follow the cleanse, tone and nourish programme as given in the facial treatment on page 65. If your skin is very dry use a good night cream and a daytime moisturizer, too. A cleansing cream or creamy lotion is usually far kinder to a dry complexion for removing the day's grime than soap and water. If you have an oily skin choose a light-textured cream or lotion and apply the very thinnest layer. Toning with a good astringent after cleansing is vital in your case. A moisturizer may help to make a better base for foundation by evening out greasy and less greasy areas.

Bare Essentials

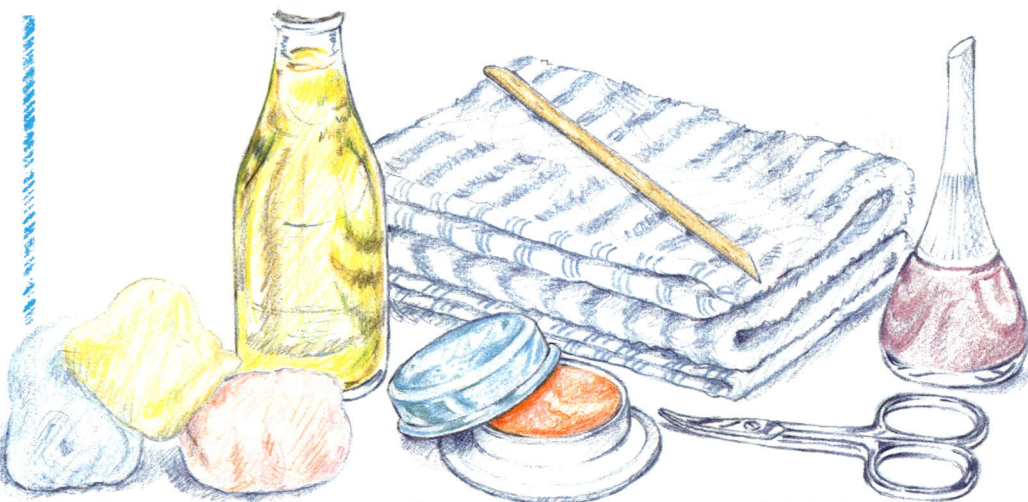

Manicure

It will take
30 minutes

You will need
a towel
cotton wool
nail polish remover
an emery board
cuticle cream
a small bowl of soapy
  water
almond or olive oil
  (optional)
cuticle remover
an orange stick
nail scissors or cuticle
  nippers
hand lotion
nail glue (optional)
nail buffer (optional)
nail strengthener
  (optional)
basecoat
nail polish
topcoat (optional)

Remove all rings and bracelets before you start. Work at a table, or on a cushion covered with a towel on your lap.

1 Remove nail polish with a pad of cotton wool soaked in nail polish remover. Work from the base to the tip of the nail to avoid staining the fingers. Make sure all polish is removed from around the cuticles. If polish is a stubborn, deep shade, or has been thickly applied, let the remover pad soak into the nail for a couple of seconds before you start rubbing.

2 Before filing, take an objective look at your nails, then follow the professionals' advice and level them all off to the same length. Use the fine side of the emery board to file your nails, with your hand clenched towards you. (Unless your nails are particularly long and strong, the darker side of the emery board will be too rough. Incorrect usage can split nails.)

Almond-shaped nails: file in one direction only, using short, rapid strokes from the sides to the centre of the nail. (See-saw movements increase splitting and weaken nails.) Don't file the sides down, they should be left to give support to the nail. Finish by rounding off at the tip. *Square-shaped nails:* file across the top of the nail in one direction only, then soften the corners. (The advantage of keeping nails square is that it helps strengthen them; filing the sides weakens the nails.)

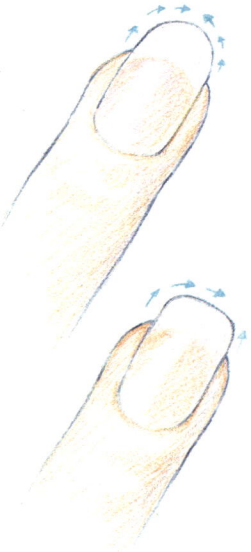

3 When the nails on both hands have been filed, massage cuticle cream into the base of each nail with firm, circular movements. (This will help soften and nourish the cuticles and makes them more flexible too.) Then soak your hands in warm, soapy water for 5 minutes. (If your nails and cuticles are dry or flaky, you may like to add a teaspoon of almond or olive oil to the water.) Dry your hands, gently smoothing the cuticles back with the towel.

4 Cover the cuticles with cuticle remover. Then dip the 'hoof' end of an orange stick in water, wrap it in a little cotton wool and use it to free the cuticle gently from the nail bed, pushing it back with circular movements. Use the pointed end of the orange stick to clean under the nails.

5 Tidy up your nails by bevelling away the frayed edges with light, upward strokes, using the fine side of the emery board. (This will also help prevent nail layers splitting apart.) Carefully trim away any loose, dead skin or hangnails with scissors or cuticle nippers. *Never* cut your cuticles.

6 Apply hand lotion to your hands, smoothing it into the skin with wide, circular movements from the fingertips to the wrist and between your fingers. Then rub over your nails with a little nail polish remover to remove all soap, oil, cream, etc. (If you apply polish to greasy nails it will chip very quickly.)

7 Various corrections can be made at this stage to improve the appearance of your nails. Nail strengthener can be applied to reinforce weak nails. Nail glue can be used to repair splits and breakages, but you must be careful not to drip any on the skin or cuticles and to wait at least one minute for the glue to dry.

It is said that a nail buffer will increase blood circulation to the nail bed and stimulate growth, as well as helping to remove any ridges and discoloration. Always buff in one direction only, from cuticles to tips. This will give the nails such a healthy sheen that you may prefer to end the manicure here.

8 Apply basecoat to your nails, taking care not to cover the cuticles. (This acts as an 'undercoat', prolonging the life of the polish and smoothing over dents and ridges.) Use light, rapid strokes to achieve even coverage.

Application: always apply basecoat, enamel and topcoat in three strips – the first down the centre of the nail from cuticle to tip, then one on either side, flexing the brush to spread the colour to the outer edges of your nails. Allow each coat to dry completely before adding the next.

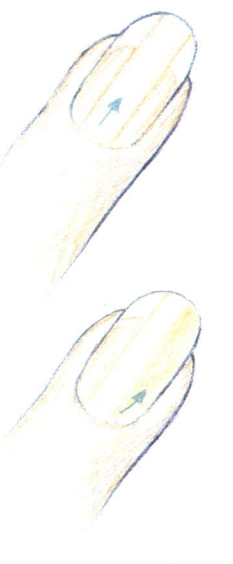

9 Apply two coats of nail polish wiping the brush on the inside of the bottle to remove excess polish. (Test by holding up the brush: it should not drip.) The choice of nail polish colour is important: if you have short nails, avoid dark or bright colours which will accentuate the fact. A polish-free gap either side of your nails will make them look longer and slimmer. Any polish which touches the cuticles should be removed immediately as once it dries it is impossible to remove without leaving tell-tale smudges. Leave nails to dry for at least 3 minutes before applying the second coat of polish.

10 A colourless topcoat may be applied once the polish is completely dry, this adds lustre to your nails. Allow your nails to dry for 10–15 minutes before touching anything.

Applying false nail tips

You may prefer to use full false nails instead of nail tips, but nail tips tend to look more genuine. They are also better for your nails as they allow the base of the nail to breathe.

If you are careful, your false nail tips should last 1–3 weeks.

It will take
1 hour

You will need
a towel
cotton wool
nail polish remover
an emery board
cuticle cream
a small bowl of soapy
  water
almond or olive oil
  (optional)
cuticle remover
an orange stick
nail scissors or cuticle
  nippers
hand lotion
a pack of false nail tips
  complete with nail glue
  (available from
  chemist)
a nail buffer (often
  enclosed in pack)
a ridge-smoothing
  basecoat (optional)
nail polish (optional)
topcoat (optional)

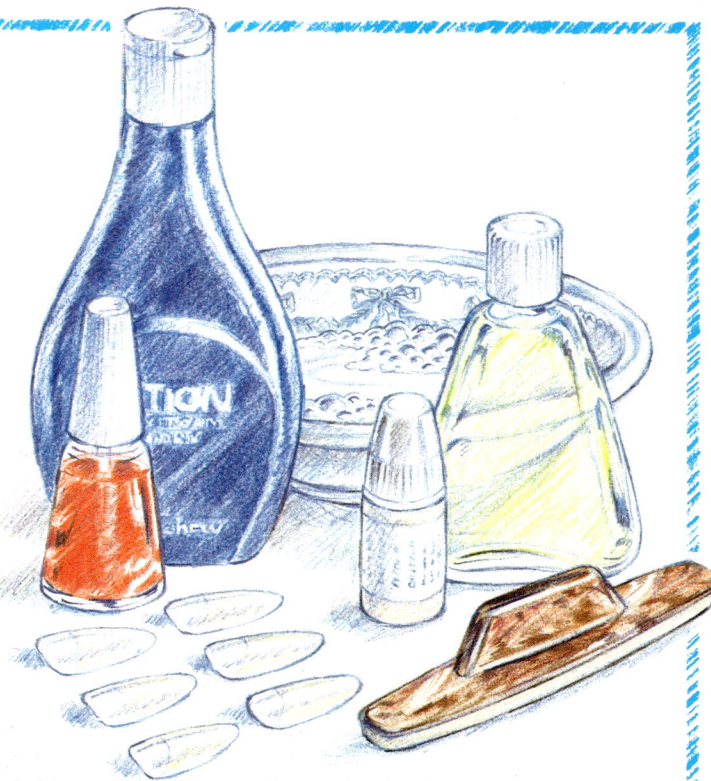

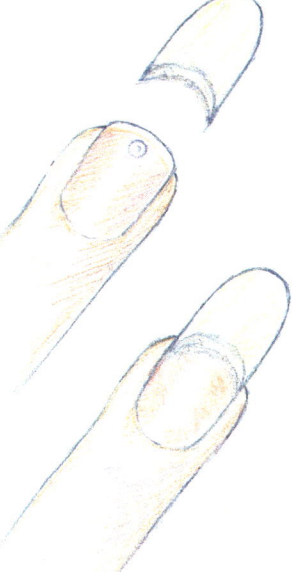

1 Manicure your nails up to the basecoat stage (see left).

2 Using the dark side of the emery board, slightly roughen the tip of each nail. (This makes it easier for the false nail to adhere and ensures it stays in place longer.)

3 You will probably find varying size nail tips in your pack, so now match the size of the tips to your own nails.

4 Starting with the thumb of your right hand (left if you are left-handed), apply one drop of glue to the centre of your nail.

5 Apply the nail tip, covering the top third of your nail, and hold it firmly in position for 15–20 seconds.

6 Using the dark side of the emery board, file the nail tip into the desired shape. (For once, see-sawing is allowed!) Buff over the join until it is smooth.

7 Apply nail tips to remaining nails in the same way.

8 In case you haven't buffed your nails sufficiently, it is a good idea to apply a basecoat to hide any ridges. Apply nail polish and topcoat if desired (see Manicure left).

Pedicure

It will take
40 minutes

You will need
nail polish remover
cotton wool
a large bowl of warm,
   soapy water
disinfectant (optional)
almond or olive oil
   (optional)
a towel
pumice stone
small scissors or nail
   clippers
an emery board
cuticle remover
an orange stick
hand lotion
tissues
nail buffer (optional)
basecoat
nail polish
topcoat (optional)

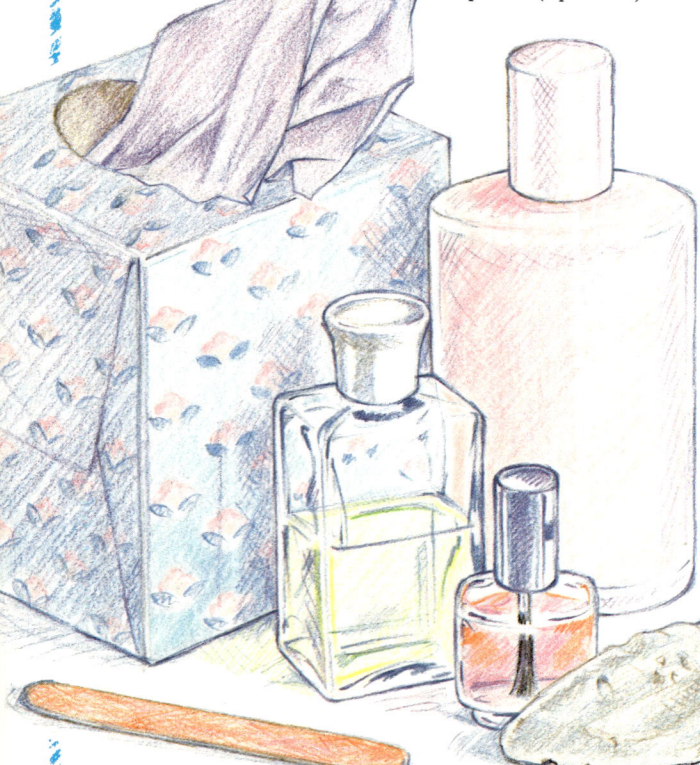

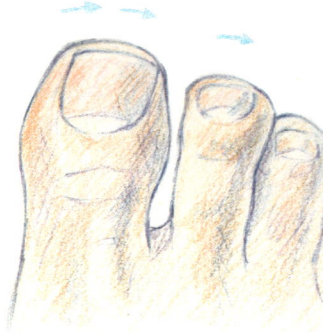

3 Remove your feet from the water, dry them thoroughly on a towel and rub away any hard skin on the soles and heels with a pumice stone. (This is the best time to deal with hard skin as the feet have been softened.)

4 Using small scissors or nail clippers, cut your toenails straight across, with a gentle curve at the sides to prevent ingrowing toenails. Then file the nails in one direction only with short, firm strokes, using the dark side of the emery board. Round off any sharp corners and rough edges.

5 Massage cuticle remover into the base of each toenail, using circular movements. Then gently push back the cuticles with the 'hoof' end of an orange stick wrapped in a little damp cotton wool. Clean carefully under the nails with the pointed end of the orange stick. This will also release any frayed edges which should be bevelled away with light, upward strokes, using the dark side of the emery board.

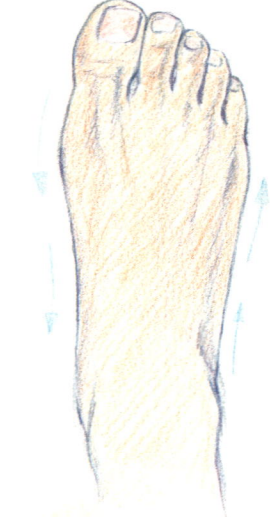

6 Trim away any loose skin with scissors or clippers. *Never* cut your cuticles.

7 Massage your feet with hand lotion, smoothing it in from the toes to the ankles on the top of the foot. On the underneath, work from heel to toe. Rub over your toenails with a little nail polish remover to remove any grease.

8 Roll up a tissue lengthways and weave it between your toes. (This separates your toes and prepares them for painting.) Apply basecoat thinly and evenly to toenails from the cuticles to the tips of the nails, taking care not to cover the cuticles. Then apply two coats of polish and one of topcoat (for additional sheen), leaving 3 minutes between each application for the polish to dry. Bold, bright colours look particularly good on toenails.

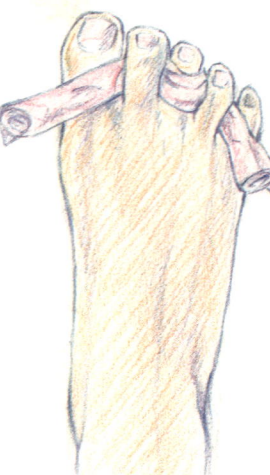

Alternatively, buff your nails – in one direction only – to help remove ridges and discoloration and to make them shine.

9 When the polish is dry you can remove the tissues. But try to leave about one hour before putting your tights and shoes back on – the nails on the big toes have a tendency to smudge.

You will probably find it easiest to work sitting on the floor, with your foot on a cushion covered with a towel.

1 Remove any nail polish from toenails with a pad of cotton wool soaked in nail polish remover. Rubbing from the base to the tip of your nails will prevent staining around the toes. Make sure you remove all polish from around the cuticles.

2 Soak your feet in a bowl of warm, soapy water (or dangle them over the edge of the bath) for 5–10 minutes. You may like to add a little mild disinfectant, and maybe a few drops of almond or olive oil to the water to moisturize your feet.

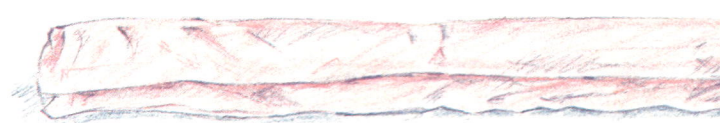

Bleaching body and facial hair

Fine facial down is a very common cause for concern; but unless it is truly disfiguring, bleach rather than removal is preferable. There are good cream bleaches sold specially for use on the face.

● Make sure the area to be bleached is clean and dry.
● Never apply bleach after a hot bath.
The bleached effect should last 4–6 weeks.

It will take
30 minutes

You will need
a bleach specifically for facial and body hair (available from chemist)
a spatula (usually enclosed with bleach)
a bowl (for the bleach)
a bowl of lukewarm water
a towel

1 Follow the packet directions to make up the required amount of bleach. (This will usually involve blending a cream and a powder, or two creams.)

2 Using the spatula, apply a fairly thick layer of bleach to the skin. Make sure that all the hair is completely covered.

3 Leave the bleach on your skin for the required amount of time: usually 5–10 minutes for upper lip or face, and 10–15 minutes for arms, legs or tummy. If there is a stinging sensation, remove the bleach, wash the area with cool water and reapply. If the discomfort persists, discontinue use.

4 Remove a little of the bleach with the spatula, and reapply if the hair is not light enough.

5 When the hair is completely bleached, remove the bleach with the spatula, rinse with lukewarm water and dry with the towel. (Body bleach is quite expensive, so to economize mix up enough bleach for, say, one arm, bleach then remove and apply to the other arm.)

6 Apply a soothing lotion such as an aftersun or light moisturizer.

Deep-cleansing Facial

It will take
1 hour

You will need
a headband or scarf
a mirror
cotton wool

cleansing cream (for normal and dry skin) *or* cleansing milk (for oily and combination skin)
skin tonic or freshener (for normal and dry skin) *or* astringent (for oily and combination skin)
rich moisturizer (for normal and dry skin) *or* lightweight moisturizer (for oily and combination skin)
a large basin of boiling water
herbs or perfume (optional)
a towel
tissues
a face pack
a soft blusher brush
eye lotion or two slices of chilled cucumber
a sponge or soft flannel

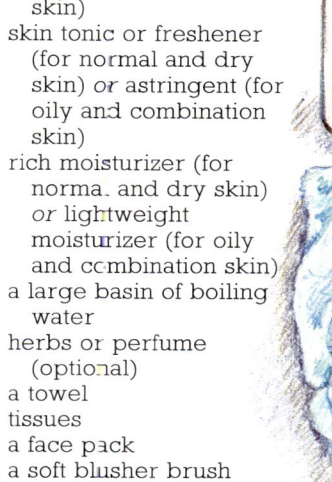
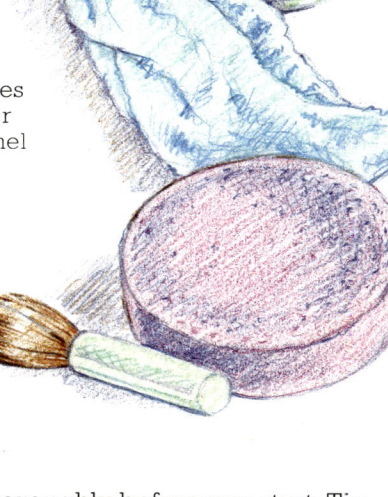

Wash your hands thoroughly before you start. Tie your hair off your face with a headband or scarf. Now take an objective look at your face in the mirror, to assess your skin type.

Skin types

Normal 'balanced' skin is smooth, finely textured and rarely erupts into spots. If you have it, congratulations – it's what the rest of us spend our lives trying to attain!
Dry skin tends to flake and has a matt texture with no apparent pores.
Oily skin shines, tends to break out in spots and is the type most likely to suffer from acne.
Combination skin is a combination of oily and dry skin, usually with a T-shaped panel of oiliness across the forehead and down the centre of the face, and dry patches on the cheeks.

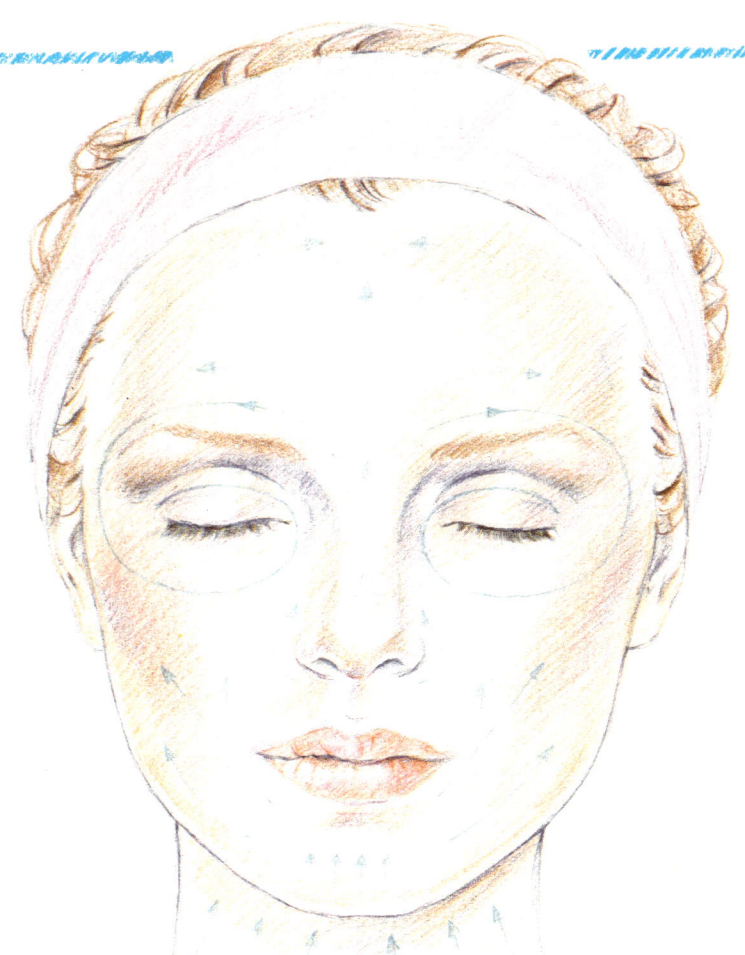

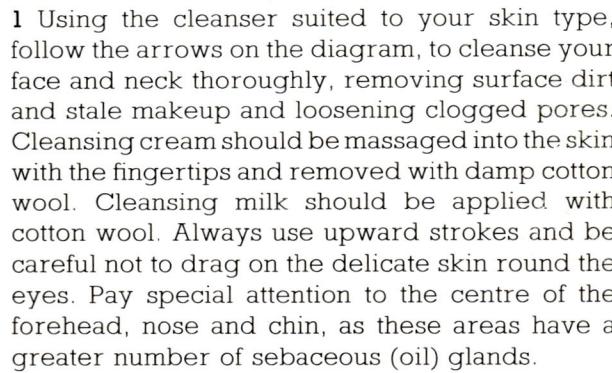

3 Dot about a teaspoonful of moisturizer all over your face and neck, using your fingertips. Now spend 10 minutes massaging it into your skin, following the arrows on the diagram. (Massage helps increase blood circulation and is also good for muscle toning.) For a professional massage your hands should work in unison, following each other across the face, massaging 10 to 15 strokes in one place at a time and exerting even pressure in a rhythmical fashion. Remember to work very gently around the eyes: it is best to use the third finger in this area as it has the lightest pressure.

If your skin is dry or normal, gently dab off excess moisturizer with a tissue, leaving just a residue on your face. If you have oily skin, remove any remaining moisturizer with damp cotton wool.

4 Sit at a table with your face above a bowl of boiling water. Drape a towel over your head to form a 'tent' over the bowl. Steam your face.
Dry skin
Steam for 4–5 minutes.
Normal skin
Steam for 6–8 minutes.
Oily or combination skin
Steam for 8–10 minutes.

You may like to sprinkle some herbs (mint is especially good) or a few drops of your favourite perfume into the water, to give a pleasant fragrance.

5 Tissue your face dry. If you have any blackheads, this is the time to deal with them. Cushion your fingers with damp cotton wool and carefully apply pressure around the blackheads, to squeeze them out gently.

6 Smooth a face pack suited to your skin type evenly over your face and neck, avoiding the eyes, lips and nostrils. (This will tone the skin.) It is a good idea to apply the mask with a clean blusher brush (or a soft paint or pastry brush) rather than your fingertips. Leave the face mask in position for the time stated on the pack.

After application, make the most of this time by lying down and refreshing your eyes: place 2 large pads of cotton wool soaked in eye lotion or cold water, or 2 slices of chilled cucumber over your closed eyes.

You can make your own face pack or mask to suit your skin type, using natural ingredients, see above right.

1 Using the cleanser suited to your skin type, follow the arrows on the diagram, to cleanse your face and neck thoroughly, removing surface dirt and stale makeup and loosening clogged pores. Cleansing cream should be massaged into the skin with the fingertips and removed with damp cotton wool. Cleansing milk should be applied with cotton wool. Always use upward strokes and be careful not to drag on the delicate skin round the eyes. Pay special attention to the centre of the forehead, nose and chin, as these areas have a greater number of sebaceous (oil) glands.

2 Dampen a pad of cotton wool with skin tonic or astringent and apply to your skin, following the arrows on the diagram to remove the last traces of cleanser, tighten the pores and leave your face feeling fresh. You can make your own toner very cheaply, using rosewater and witch hazel:
Dry skin toner
Mix two parts rosewater and one part witch hazel.
Oily skin toner
Mix one part rosewater and two parts witch hazel.
Normal skin toner
Mix equal parts rosewater and witch hazel.

7 Remove the mask with a sponge or flannel soaked in tepid water. Then immediately splash your face with cold water, or apply skin tonic to close the pores. Dry your face by blotting with a clean towel. *Do not rub the skin.*

8 To protect your skin from the effects of makeup and pollution, finish off your facial by toning and moisturizing your face, following the arrows in the diagram, as before.

Natural skin masks

Normal skin mask
Mash half an avocado pear and mix with 1 egg white and 1 teaspoon lemon juice. Spread evenly over your face and leave for 20 minutes.

Dry skin mask
Add a few drops of fresh orange juice to a tablespoon of clear, warm honey or almond oil. Spread evenly over your face and leave for 15–20 minutes.

Oily and combination skin mask
Mix 2 teaspoons Fullers Earth with 1 tablespoon fresh orange juice and enough witch hazel to make a smooth paste. Spread evenly over your face and leave for 10–15 minutes.

Eyebrow shaping

It will take
20 minutes

You will need
a hairband or scarf
a mirror (magnifying is best)
an eyebrow brush or small toothbrush
an orange stick or pencil
a pair of tweezers (flat or slant-tipped)
cotton wool
tepid water, skin tonic or witch hazel

1 Tie your hair off your face with a hairband or scarf.

2 Using an eyebrow brush or small toothbrush, brush your brows upwards and then across. This will make the hairs fall into their natural line, and they will be easier to pluck.

3 As a general rule, it is best just to tidy your brows and define the natural curve, rather than alter the shape drastically. Thin eyebrows can make you look sharp-featured; very bushy ones tend to overshadow and hide your eyes.

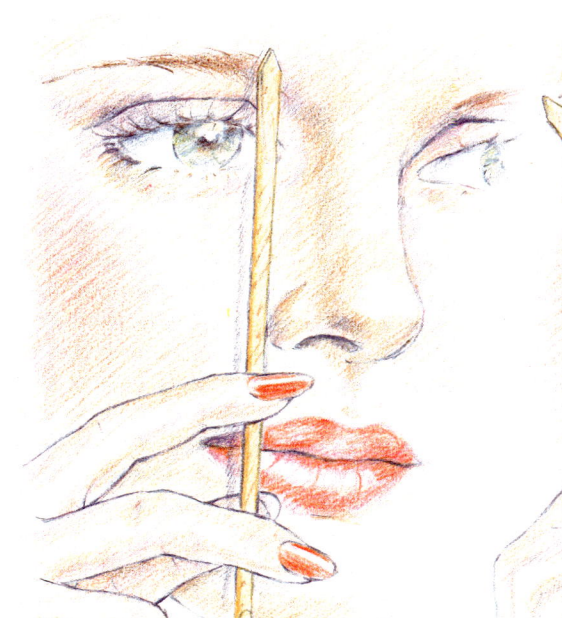

Tweezer out any stray hairs from underneath the natural arch of the eyebrow, but *never* pluck the hairs above the eyebrow or you'll end up with uneven patches.

4 Always pluck one hair at a time, using swift, sharp movements in the direction the hair is growing, and holding the skin taut with your other hand. (This makes plucking easier and ensures the skin does not get caught in the tweezers.) While plucking, smooth away any loose hairs, using cotton wool dampened with tepid water, skin tonic or witch hazel. This also helps soothe the skin.

5 Once you've shaped your eyebrows, you'll probably need to tidy them up every few days as the hairs grow back.

If you ever get tweezer-happy and pluck too much, don't panic. You can draw in a fuller shape while waiting for the hairs to grow back. (A gingery-brown pencil is best. Unless your brows are very dark, black will look artificial.) For a natural effect, draw in the brows with light, upward strokes, then blend gently with your fingertips.

To obtain the ideal shaped eyebrows for your face: hold an orange stick or pencil vertically beside your nostril. The eyebrow should start exactly where the pencil crosses it. Pluck out any hairs that grow beyond this point.
Now hold the orange stick or pencil diagonally beside your nostril and align it with the outer corner of your eye. The eyebrow should stop exactly where the pencil crosses it. Pluck out any hairs that grow beyond this point.

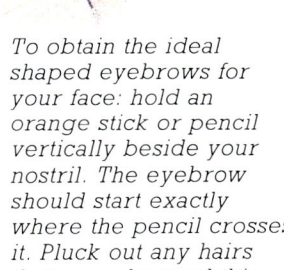

Complete Makeover

Before you start your makeover make an honest appraisal of any face fault. No one is perfect, and even the world's most lovely women have something to hide. The first law of clever camouflage is to underplay problem areas and accentuate good points. Coolly assess all alterable flaws – and make up your mind to correct them. Has your hair lost some of its youthful lustre? Would it benefit from a colour-enhancing rinse? Or have you always hated your mouse-brown hair and would you like to be a natural-looking blonde? It is not too difficult to change your hair colour and in this section we'll tell you about the various ways you can do this.

Before you start your makeover, check the lighting. Fluorescent lighting drains the face and ordinary bulbs are better. But even with these you have to be careful. If the light comes from above and casts shadows over your face your makeup will never look right. It is best to have the light shining evenly from either side of the face. Two table lamps should do the trick. And do remove the shades if you can. If the lighting is too soft and kind when you are making up you will look a dream by that light – but not in the street. The harder and harsher the light you make up by, the better your face will look when you go out.

Unless you have an absolutely flawless skin you'll always look better with a foundation. Today's wonderful variety includes foundations so light that they tone down any imperfections, help hide blemishes, yet give a flawless, 'natural' look. This makes a lovely base for eyeshadows and blusher; all colour makeup lasts better if it is applied over a foundation. To choose a foundation colour try it on the back of your hand. If it blends in naturally, it is usually right for your face, too.

If you want a natural-looking, long-lasting makeup you must use loose powder. You need buy only one sort: the no-colour translucent kind. The most natural-looking makeup effect comes from tinted foundation which gives the right skin tone, 'set' with the translucent powder. This type of powder is designed to let light through, so there is no real colour build-up, as with tinted powders; these should never be used for touch-ups during the day, because if colour goes on colour you will end up with a very 'made-up' look, and that is not what the art of makeup is about.

Accept that you cannot change your face, do your best with a problem, then forget it. The best beautifier at any age is an inward content shining through – and that's something you can't buy in a pot or tube.

Professional makeup

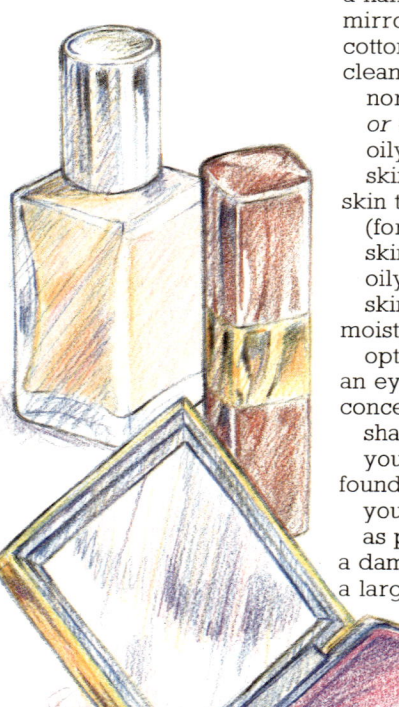

It will take
45–60 minutes

You will need
a hairband or scarf
mirror
cotton wool
cleansing cream (for normal and dry skin) *or* cleansing milk (for oily and combination skin)
skin tonic or freshener (for normal and dry skin) *or* astringent (for oily and combination skin)
moisturizer (tinted optional)
an eye pencil
concealer (two to three shades lighter than your skin tone)
foundation (as close to your natural skin tone as possible)
a damp sponge
a large blusher brush
blusher
shader (a blusher that is a shade darker than your usual blusher)
face powder
a selection of eye makeup brushes and applicators
eyeshadows
eyeliner (optional)
Kohl (optional)
eyebrow brush or small toothbrush
eyebrow pencil (optional)
eyelash curlers (optional)
mascara
combined lash brush and comb or small toothbrush (optional)
cotton bud
highlighter
lip pencil (optional)
lip brush
lipstick
tissues
lip gloss (optional)

Before starting, tie your hair off your face with a hairband or scarf.

Work in front of a mirror in a room where you can see your face in a really good light. (If possible, apply your makeup in the light you are going to be seen by. If it's a daytime makeup take your mirror to a window and use natural light; if it's an evening makeup apply it by electric light.)

1 Cleanse, tone and moisturize

Thoroughly cleanse, tone and moisturize your face and throat (see Facial, page 65). A tinted moisturizer can be useful to help balance out skin tones before applying makeup. (A green tint, for example, will tone down redness.) Let the moisturizer sink into your skin for a few minutes, so that your skin is not shiny or slippery.

2 Assess your face shape

Stand an arm's length away from a mirror. Close one eye and focus on your face in the mirror. Using an eye pencil, draw the outline of your face on the mirror. Open both eyes, and you will be able to see clearly what shape your face is. (This will be useful later.)

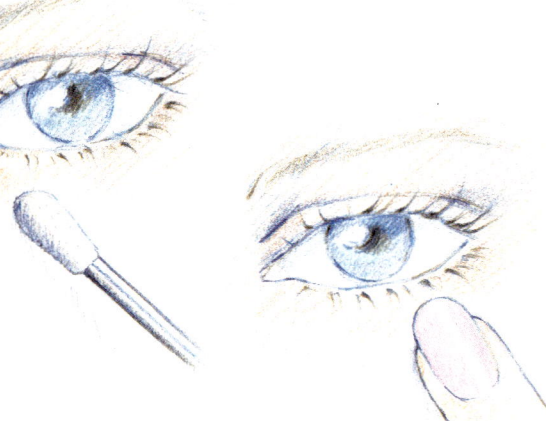

3 Apply concealer

Dot concealer sparingly on the dark circles under your eyes. Blend it into the surrounding skin by patting lightly outwards with your fingertips. Don't rub or drag the skin and don't put concealer over 'bags' – it only accentuates them. Dot concealer over any blemishes, spots, scars or red veins, and blend it outwards as before.

4 Apply foundation

Dot foundation over your face (*not* your neck). Blend it evenly outwards with a damp sponge. Be careful to blend the foundation well around your nose and fade it away under your chin. Don't put much under your eyes, as it can make tiny lines look deeper than they actually are. Check you have no obvious harsh demarcation lines around your jaw.

5 Apply face powder

Dip a large clean blusher brush into a tub of colourless, translucent or tinted powder. (This helps make your makeup last, and should be applied after *any* cream product like foundation or eye colour.) Shake off any excess powder. Lightly dust the powder all over your face, using downward strokes (following the direction in which your downy facial hairs grow).

6 Apply blusher

Blusher colours can be mixed and matched together. Select a shade that tones in with your lipstick and the colour of the clothes you are wearing.

To work out where your blusher should be applied, look straight at yourself in the mirror and place a finger directly below your eyeball on your cheekbone. Apply blusher here, using upward strokes with a large blusher brush, and then blend along the cheekbone towards the hairline. Repeat on the other cheek.

7 Shape and shade your face

Use a blusher a shade darker than the blusher you are using on your cheekbone. Consider the shape of your face and apply in an upwards direction to any areas that you wish to slim down, such as cheeks, nose or jawline, see right. Soften the edges and blend the shader into your blusher to prevent harsh lines.

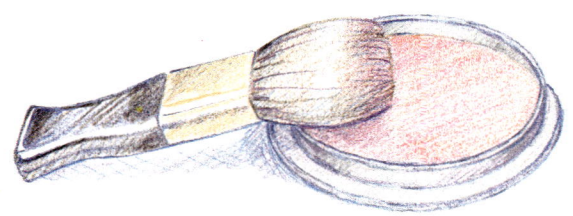

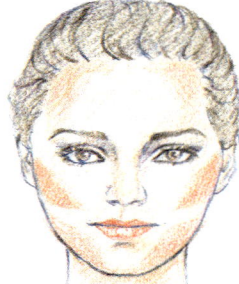

Round Face

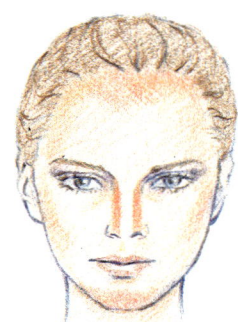

Oval Face

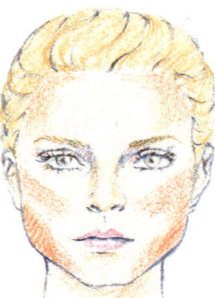

Square Face

8 Make up your eyes

Apply your eyeshadows

If you are new to wearing eyeshadow, start off your collection with shades of grey and brown and add other colours later if you wish.

Cream eyeshadows: apply with a brush and then blend with a brush or your fingertips.

Powder eyeshadows: apply lightly with an applicator or brush and blend carefully at the edges.

Here are a few professional tips to help you correct and emphasize your eyes:

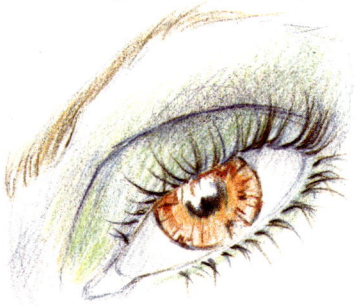

Heavy-lidded eyes
(a) Apply eyeshadow across the entire eyelid, making sure it covers the crease.
(b) Blend the eyeshadow well.
(c) Apply a little colour under the eye for balance.

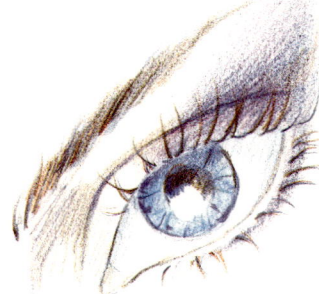

Close-set eyes
(a) Using an eye pencil, draw a triangle of colour from the outer corners of the eyelid halfway across the upper and lower lid and the crease.
(b) Blend the eyeshadow up towards the end of the eyebrow and just under the lower lashes. Smudge for a soft effect.

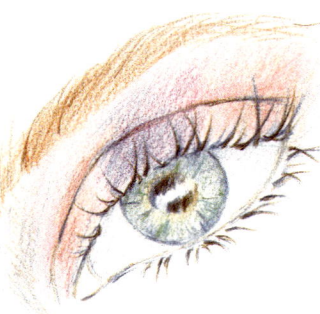

Small eyes
(a) Apply a bright but soft colour eyeshadow over the entire lid to enlarge the eye.
(b) Accentuate the centre of your eyelid with a more definite and slightly contrasting shade.
(c) Blend well.

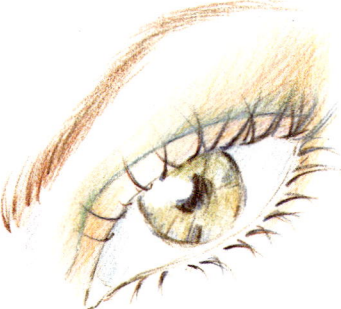

Small-lidded eyes
(a) Apply a light eyeshadow to the eyelid.
(b) Draw a dark line in the crease.
(c) Blend upwards and outwards.

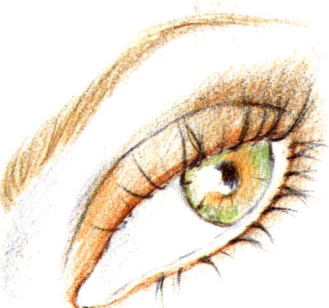

Protruding eyes
(a) Using a medium to deep coloured eye pencil, draw a line round your eye close to the lashes.
(b) Smudge lightly to avoid too hard a line.

Apply eyeliner

Draw a line close to the lashes from the inner to outer corner of the eye, if desired. Brown or grey eyeliner will give a softer line than black.

You can also use Kohl in the inner rim of your eye, being careful to pull the eye down *gently* so that the pencil does not touch the eyeball.

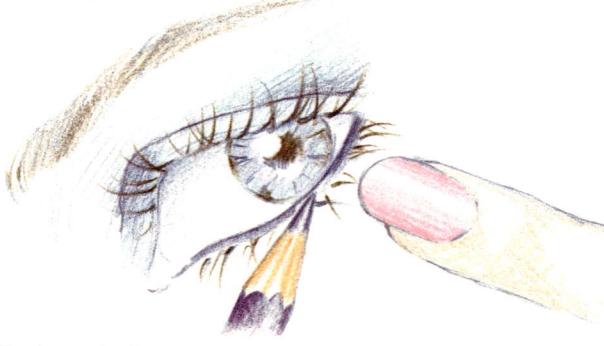

Curl eyelashes

If you want to use eyelash curlers, do so now. (They are a scissor-like contraption to make your lashes look longer and thicker.) Just one gentle squeeze should be enough. Be *very* careful not to take the curlers off the lashes before your eyes are fully opened or you will pull the lashes out. (Be careful not to blink either, as this will have a similar effect.)

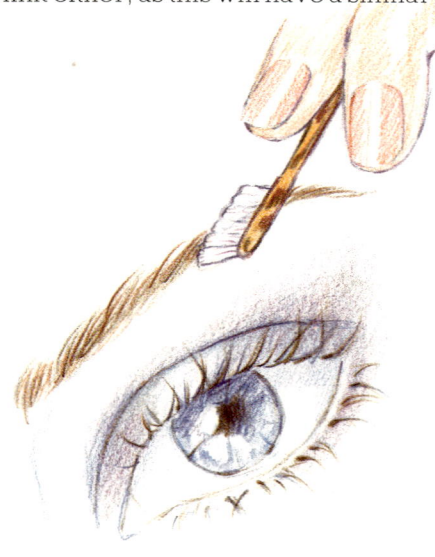

Tidy your eyebrows

Using an eyebrow brush or small toothbrush, brush your eyebrows upwards and then across so that the hairs fall into their natural line.

You can darken or shape your eyebrows with a blunt-ended, grey or brown pencil (black gives too hard a line). Use short, light strokes, and draw on to the hairs, then brush away so that you are not left with any tell-tale lines.

Apply mascara
Use a brown or brownish black mascara, it looks much more natural than black, even if you have dark hair. Lightly coat your bottom lashes by gently running the brush along the lashes. Apply a light coat of mascara to your upper lashes, firstly to the top side, stroking the colour down, and then to the underside, stroking the colour up. Using a combined lash brush and comb or small toothbrush, separate the lashes carefully to avoid clogging.

   Apply a second light coat of mascara to your lashes, as before. Look closely in the mirror and remove any unwanted smudges with a cotton bud.

9 Apply highlighter

Apply on the bone below the eyebrow and on the cheekbone below the outer corner of the eye, to accentuate your features.

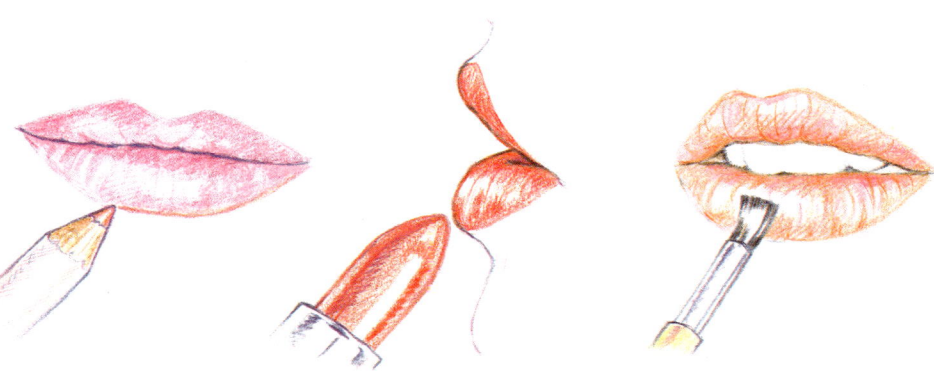

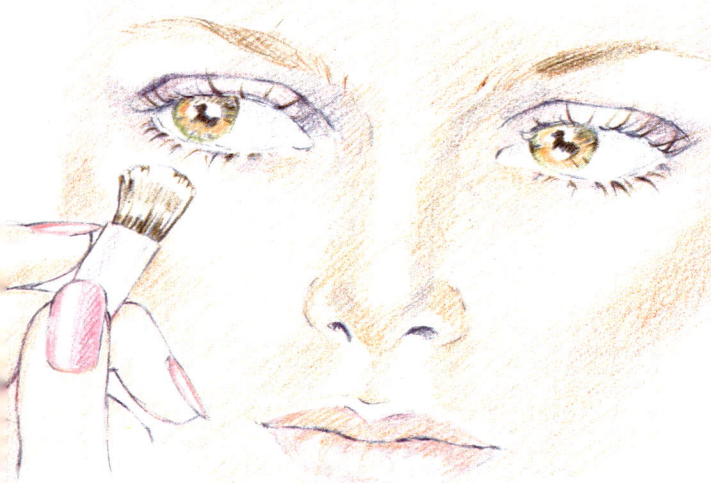

10 Make up your lips

Experiment with shades of lipstick to see which suits you the best. Tones should match what you are wearing, but a soft, natural lipstick will play down the mouth area, while a strong, bright colour will draw attention to it.

   Outline your lips using a sharp lip pencil or a lipbrush and a lipstick a shade darker than the one you're intending to fill in with.

   A lipline gives your lips a good shape and covers up any imperfections. If you have a large bottom lip making the line sit right on the lip will give it a smaller appearance. If you have a thin bottom lip, drawing the line just underneath the natural line will make it look slightly larger.

   Fill in your lips with a lipstick or a lipbrush. (A lipbrush is better for getting into all the nooks and crannies.)
Full lips should be toned down with soft colours.
Uneven or small lips look fuller if you apply matt and pearlized lipsticks to the central areas.

Blot your lips with a tissue. Apply a fresh coat of lipstick, to prolong your lipstick's life. Apply lipgloss if desired.

Look in the mirror and marvel at the new you!

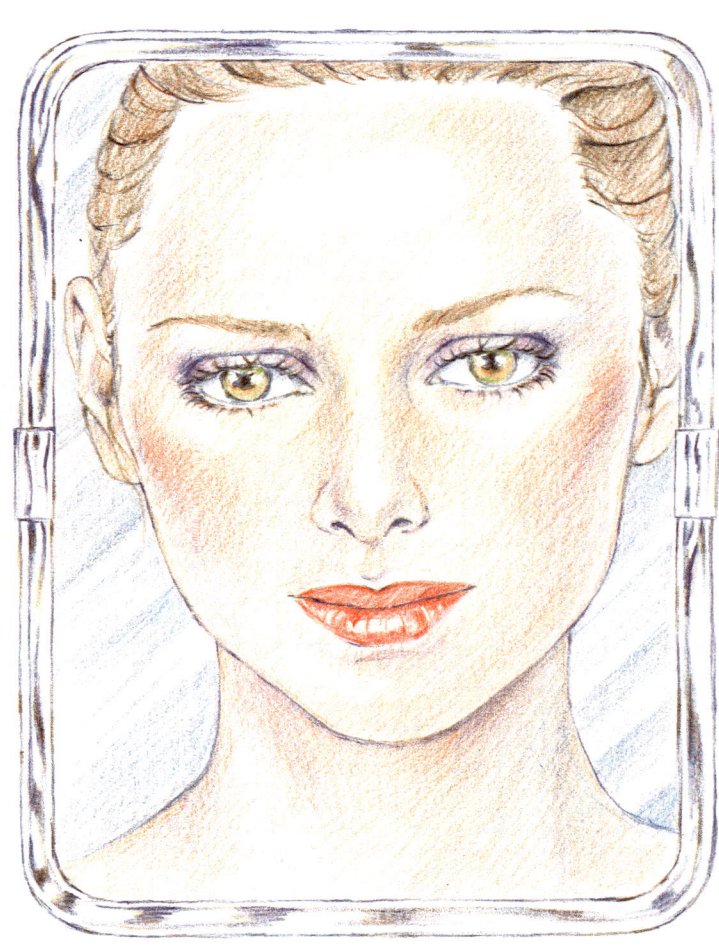

Applying false eyelashes

It will take
30 minutes

You will need
a hairband or scarf
non-oily eye makeup
    remover
cotton wool
a set of individual lashes
    complete with lash
    glue (available from
    chemist)
mirror (magnifying is
    best)
a pair of tweezers

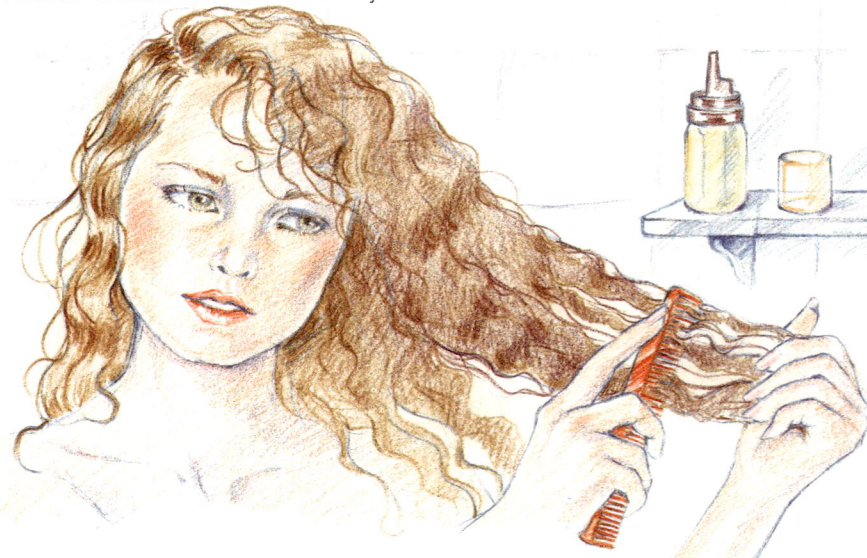

If your eyelashes are very light you can dye them (see page 78). Alternatively you can apply false eyelashes, the individual type are the most effective. You can use false lashes on a backing strip instead of individual lashes, but they look more artificial, and can irritate and feel heavy on the eye.

1 Tie your hair off your face with a hairband or scarf. Thoroughly cleanse your eyes and lashes with a cotton wool pad soaked in non-oily eye makeup remover, to remove all traces of oil.

2 Using tweezers, pick up one false lash and dip the root in the glue.

3 Starting at the centre of the eye, apply one lash at a time, working out to the outer corner first, and then from the centre to the inner corner. Make sure that you attach the false lash to your natural lash, *not* your eyelid. Now apply false lashes to the other eye. Always apply to the top lashes only.

4 Keep your eyes as still as possible, and don't wash or apply makeup for 10–15 minutes, to allow the glue to dry.

5 Blink several times to check that all the lashes are secure. With care, your false lashes may last 2 to 3 weeks, although the odd one or two will inevitably fall out.

Colouring your hair

For a really dramatic colour change, such as dark brown to blonde, it is advisable to visit a hair salon but home treatments can be very effective.

Temporary colours

Temporaries are the mildest form of colorant. They coat only the outer layer (cuticle) of the hair, and usually change the *tone*, rather than the *colour* of the hair.

Temporary colours are available in water rinses, gels, setting lotions and sprays.

Temporaries do not usually require a skin patch test as they are hypo-allergenic.

It will take
5 minutes

You will need
shampoo
a bowl or sink of hot
    water
a towel
a water rinse, gel or
    coloured setting lotion
    (sprays are applied
    straight on to dry hair).

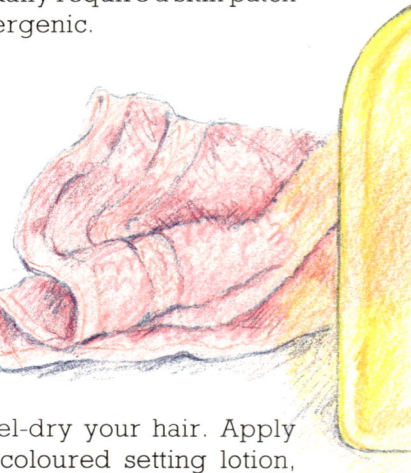

Shampoo, rinse and towel-dry your hair. Apply the water rinse, gel or coloured setting lotion, making sure that all the hair is covered. Comb through the hair if you want an even distribution. (Many people prefer to use temporary colorants just to colour parts of their hair.) Dry and style your hair as usual.

Temporaries are removed in the first wash.

Semi-permanent colours

Semi-permanents give a stronger, richer colour change. They penetrate some way into the hair shaft, so take longer to wash out.

Never use a semi-permanent on bleached or very grey hair as it may give unnatural results. Semi-permanents fade in about 4–6 weeks.

It will take
30 minutes

You will need
a bowl or sink of hot
   water
shampoo (optional)
a pair of plastic gloves
a semi-permanent hair
   colorant
a towel
conditioner (optional)

Wet or shampoo your hair (depending on pack instructions). Wearing plastic gloves for protection, shampoo the colorant into your hair, making sure that all the hair is covered. Leave the colorant on for 5–20 minutes, depending on how strong an effect you want. Rinse off the colorant and condition your hair if desired. Dry your hair in the normal way.

SKIN PATCH TEST
1 Mix up a small amount of colorant.
2 Apply a patch about 2.5 cm/1 inch square to the inside of your elbow. (A hairdresser will normally perform the test behind the ear, but at home the elbow is easier to reach and observe.)
3 Leave the colorant for 24 hours, making sure it is not rubbed or washed off.
4 Wipe off the colorant. If there is any reaction, such as redness, irritation or soreness, do not use the colorant.

STRAND TEST
1 Cut off 30–40 strands of hair close to the scalp.
2 Apply the colorant to these strands. (Economize by using the left-over mixture from the skin patch test.)
3 Leave for the length of time specified in the pack instructions.
4 Wash off the colorant and study the results in strong daylight. Remember, everyone's hair is different, so it is unlikely to be identical to the colour on the pack.

Permanent tints

Permanents penetrate right through into the hair shaft and are locked in, so they don't wash out although the colour may fade a little with shampooing.

Permanents are ideal for covering grey hair.

Always carry out a skin patch test 24 hours in advance to check that the dye will not cause a reaction. It is a good idea to do a strand test at the same time.

It will take
1 hour

You will need
a permanent colorant
a pair of plastic gloves
a bowl or sink of hot
   water
a wide-toothed, non
   metal comb
conditioner
a towel

Mix up the colorant. (This will usually involve combining a bleaching agent – to open up the cuticle of the hair – and a dye.) Wearing plastic gloves for protection, apply the mixture to your dry hair. Make sure that the roots and hairline are covered with colorant. (When applying colorant to your hairline, make sure that the dye does not mark the skin on your face or neck. If it does, wash off immediately.) Comb the dye through your hair, ensuring by gentle massage that every hair is covered. Wait for the length of time specified in the pack instructions. Wet your hair and lather up the colorant, or apply shampoo according to pack instructions. Rinse your hair until the water runs clear. Apply conditioner to fix the new colour and to leave your hair shiny. Dry and style your hair as usual. If you are left with any colorant on your hands, gently rub over them with a pumice stone.

When new hair grows through it will have to be coloured too. But normally this just involves reapplying the colorant all over your hair, rather than fiddly root retouching.

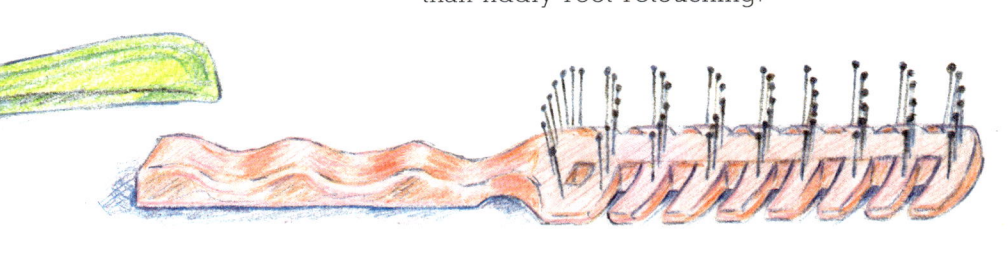

Lightening your hair

Lighteners work by taking away some of the coloured pigment from each hair shaft. The more pigment removed, the lighter the hair will be.
- Medium brown to fair hair will become blonde.
- Dark hair will lighten to medium brown.
- Redheads will not change to blonde easily.
Carry out a skin patch test 24 hours in advance (see page 73).

It will take
40 minutes

You will need
a lightener
a pair of plastic gloves
cotton wool
a bowl or sink of hot
  water
a wide-toothed, non-
  metal comb
conditioner
a towel

1 Wearing plastic gloves for protection, apply the lightener to your dry hair. (If you get any lightener in your eyes rinse with warm water immediately.) Make sure that the roots and hairline are covered with lightener.

2 Comb the lightener through your hair, ensuring by gentle massage that every hair is covered.

3 Following pack instructions, wait for the lightener to take effect, checking every 5 minutes by completely cleaning a strand of hair with cotton wool.

4 Rinse your hair until the water runs clear.

5 Apply conditioner to fix the new colour and leave your hair shiny.

6 Dry and style your hair as usual.

When darker roots appear, reapply lightener to the roots only. If you reapply lightener to already lightened hair you will overbleach it, making the hair excessively dry and prone to breakage and split ends.

Restoring colour to bleached hair

This is a gradual process in which you apply a permanent colorant to your hair every 2–3 weeks, gradually building up the colour until you find the shade that matches your natural colour. Always check the pack to ensure that the colorant is suitable for use on bleached hair.

Carry out a skin patch and strand test 24 hours in advance (see page 73).

Apply the colorants (see page 72) in the following order:

1 Dark blonde. (This first colorant may not noticeably alter the colour of your hair, but it will provide a base for the rest of the colorants to build on)

2 Very light brown

3 Light brown

4 Medium brown

You will have to reapply the final colorant of your choice every 6–8 weeks until all the bleached hair has been cut out.

Highlighting your hair

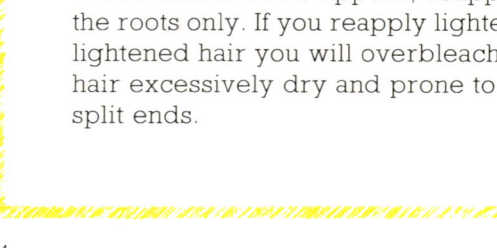

It will take
1 hour

You will need
a friend to do the
  highlighting
a plastic cap pierced
  with holes (optional)
a crochet hook (optional)
aluminium foil
lightener
a pair of plastic gloves
cotton wool
a bowl or sink of hot
  water
semi-permanent colorant
  (optional)
conditioner
a towel

1 Put the plastic cap over your dry hair. (You can make your own highlighting cap by piercing holes in a very thin bathing cap.)

2 Using the crochet hook, draw small sections of hair through the holes in the plastic cap.

3 Wearing gloves, apply lightener to the strands of hair that have been drawn through.

4 Wrap the strands in aluminium foil. (Highlighting can also be done without the cap: just lighten selected strands and wrap them in foil.) The foil seals in the heat and speeds up the tinting process.

5 Wait for the lightener to take effect, checking every 5 minutes by cleaning a strand of hair with cotton wool. (The lightener usually needs to be left on for between 20 and 45 minutes.)

6 When the desired colour is achieved, remove the foil and thoroughly rinse off the lightener.

7 Shampoo in a semi-permanent colorant (see page 73) or simply shampoo, rinse and condition your hair. (Remove the cap when you have shampoo on your head, it will then slide off easily.)

8 Dry and style your hair as usual.

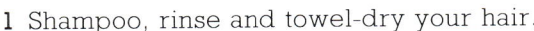

Dyeing your hair naturally

There are several natural dyes available.

HENNA TREATMENT
Henna is an excellent conditioner that enriches and reddens dark hair. It should never be used on grey or blonde hair, nor hair that has been chemically tinted. Henna fades in about 6–8 weeks.

It will take
40 minutes to 1 hour

You will need
shampoo
a towel
heavy moisturizer
a cup for measuring
henna powder
very hot water
a bowl to mix in
a spoon
a pair of plastic gloves
tea or coffee (optional)
aluminium foil
a hair drier (optional)
a bowl or sink of hot
water

1 Shampoo, rinse and towel-dry your hair.

2 Apply a thick layer of moisturizer around your hairline to act as a barrier against the henna.

3 Mix 1 cup of henna and 1 cup of hot water into a smooth paste. You can also add a few tablespoons of tea leaves (to bring out the red) or coffee grains (to dull down the red). Add a little more water if the paste is too thick.

4 Wearing plastic gloves for protection, apply the henna mixture to your hair, gently massaging to ensure that every hair is covered.

5 Cover all your hair with a sheet of aluminium foil to seal in the heat.

6 Leave for the length of time specified in pack instructions. (Using a hair drier will speed up the process.)

7 Shampoo the henna off and rinse your hair until the water runs clear.

8 Dry and style your hair as usual.

SAGE TREATMENT
This will dull grey hair, producing a brown tone. Use once a week.

It will take
40 minutes

You will need
4 tablespoons sage
   leaves
1 cup boiling water
a sieve
a comb
a bowl or sink of hot
   water
a towel

1 Put the sage leaves in the water and leave to infuse for about 15 minutes, or until cool enough to apply to the head. Strain through the sieve.

2 Apply the sage liquid to your hair and roots, combing through to ensure that all the hair is covered.

3 Leave for 15 minutes to 1 hour, depending on how strong an effect you want.

4 Rinse off thoroughly until the water runs clear.

5 Dry and style your hair as usual.

CAMOMILE TREATMENT

This lightens hair. It is especially good on blonde hair and brings out the highlights in brown hair. Use once a week.

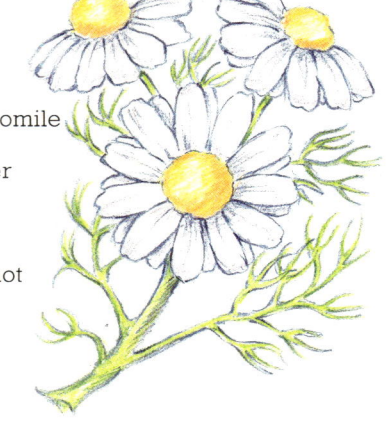

It will take
40 minutes

You will need
2 tablespoons camomile
  flowers
1 pint boiling water
a sieve
a jug
a comb
a bowl or sink of hot
  water
a towel

1 Put the camomile flowers in the water and leave to infuse for about 15 minutes, or until cool enough to apply to the head. Strain through the sieve into a jug.

2 Apply the camomile liquid to your hair and roots, combing through to ensure that all the hair is covered.

3 Leave for 15 minutes to 1 hour, depending on how strong an effect you want.

4 Rinse off thoroughly until the water runs clear. Dry and style your hair as usual.

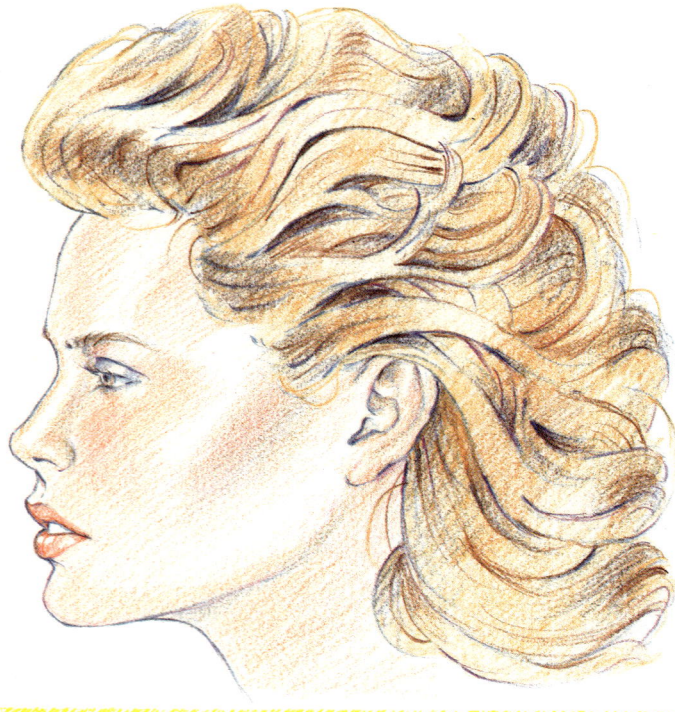

Conditioning your hair

A new hairstyle can crop off the years quicker than any other beauty treatment in the world but whatever style you choose, your hair will only look good if it is in tip-top condition. The home conditioning treatments that follow help you to keep your hair looking healthy without spending a fortune on commercial products. First assess your hair type:

Oily hair almost always accompanies oily skin. It is often very fine and becomes lank and greasy soon after shampooing.
Dry hair tends to be full of electricity and is dull, brittle and can be hard to control.
Normal hair is shiny, well-balanced and does not require washing as frequently as greasy hair.

Lemon and vinegar treatment for greasy hair

It will take
10 minutes

You will need
shampoo
a towel
½ cup fresh lemon juice
½ cup vinegar
a jug
a wide-toothed comb
a bowl or sink of warm
  water

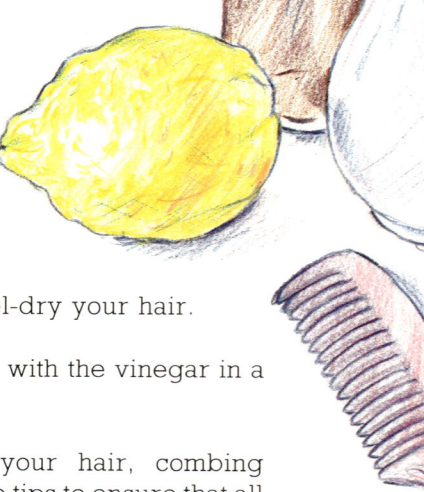

1 Shampoo, rinse and towel-dry your hair.

2 Combine the lemon juice with the vinegar in a jug, blending thoroughly.

3 Apply the mixture to your hair, combing through from the roots to the tips to ensure that all the hair is covered.

4 Leave on for as long as possible, at least 1 minute. (If your scalp starts to feel itchy rinse off immediately.)

5 Rinse off with warm water. (Never use very hot water on oily hair as it stimulates the sebaceous glands, thus producing more oil.)

6 Dry and style your hair as usual.

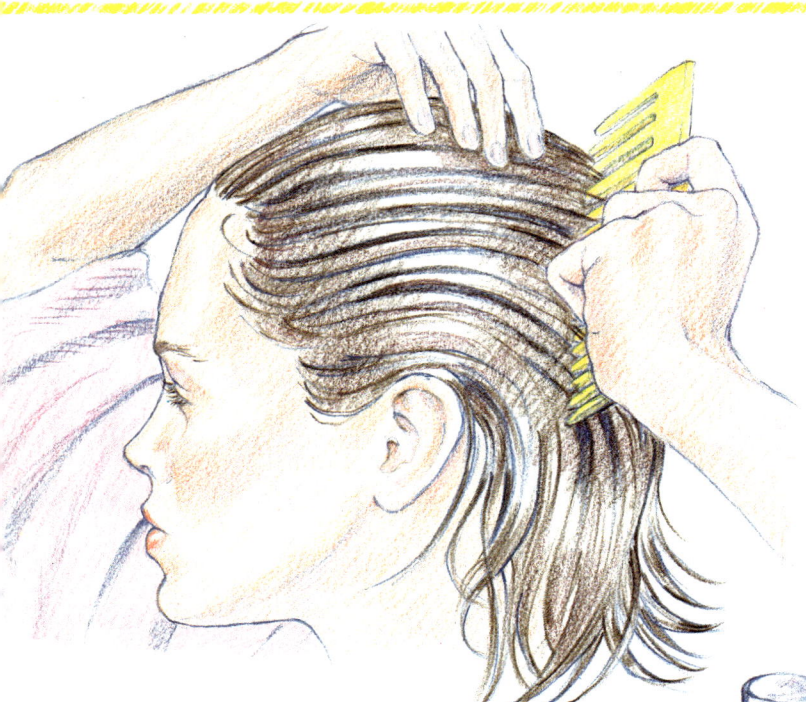

Warm oil treatment for dry hair

It will take
20 minutes

You will need
1–2 50ml bottles of
   vegetable, almond or
   coconut oil
a wide-toothed comb
cling film or aluminium
   foil
a warm towel
shampoo
a bowl or sink of hot
   water

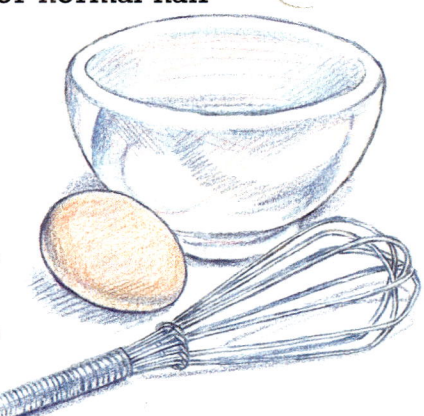

1 Heat the oil to blood temperature in a small saucepan.

2 Massage the oil into your hair and scalp until your whole head is saturated.

3 Comb through to ensure that all the hair is covered.

4 Wrap all your hair in cling film or foil, and cover with the warm towel.

5 Leave the oil on for as long as possible, (at least 20–30 minutes or overnight if you can).

6 Thoroughly wash off the oil. (Two shampoos should be sufficient.)

7 Dry and style your hair as usual.

Egg treatment for normal hair

It will take
30 minutes

You will need
1 egg
1 tablespoon castor
   oil
1 teaspoon vinegar
1 teaspoon glycerine
a mixing bowl
a hand beater
a wide-toothed comb
cling film
a warm towel
shampoo

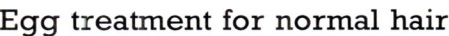
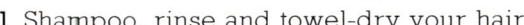

1 Shampoo, rinse and towel-dry your hair.

2 Mix all the ingredients for the conditioner in the mixing bowl with the hand beater.

3 Massage the mixture into your scalp.

4 Comb through with the comb, to ensure that all the hair is covered.

5 Cover your hair with cling film then a warm towel.

6 Leave for 10–30 minutes.

7 Rinse off thoroughly and shampoo.

8 Dry and style your hair as usual.

Eyelash tinting

It will take
30 minutes

You will need
a hairband or scarf
non-oily eye makeup
 remover
cotton wool
a mirror (magnifying is
 best)
an orange stick
petroleum jelly or heavy
 moisturizer
an eyelash dye kit
 (available in most
 chemists)
a bowl of lukewarm
 water
tissues

If you have a history of sensitivity or allergy to eye makeup, or suffer from conjunctivitis, eczema or psoriasis in the eye area, consult a doctor before carrying out this treatment. Contact lenses *must* be removed.

1 Tie your hair off your face with a hairband or a scarf.

2 Cleanse your eyes and lashes thoroughly with a non-oily eye makeup remover.

3 To avoid staining the skin while tinting, use an orange stick to apply a fairly thick layer of petroleum jelly or heavy moisturizer to the skin surrounding the lashes. Make sure the petroleum jelly or moisturizer goes right up to the roots of the lower lashes and along the top lid.

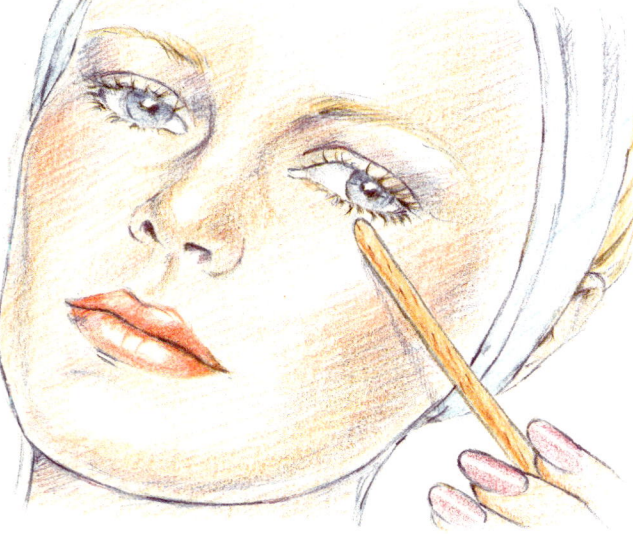

4 Follow the packet directions to make up the tint. (This will probably involve mixing the dye with a weak solution of hydrogen peroxide.)

5 Very carefully apply a thin coat of tint to the lashes and roots, using a clean, oil-free orange stick. You will probably find it easier to coat your bottom lashes first. If any tint touches the skin remove it immediately with damp cotton wool.

6 Leave the tint for 10–15 minutes (depending on your natural colour and the finished shade required). Then carefully wipe it away with pads of damp cotton wool.

7 Gently dry your lashes with tissues. If your eyes feel a little irritated apply a few eye drops – and don't worry!

The tint will last for 4–6 weeks.

Eyebrow tinting

It will take
20 minutes

You will need
a hairband or scarf
non-oily eye makeup
 remover or witch hazel
cotton wool
a mirror (magnifying is
 best)
petroleum jelly or a
 heavy moisturizer
an eyelash dye kit
 (available in most
 chemists)
an orange stick
a bowl of lukewarm
 water
tissues

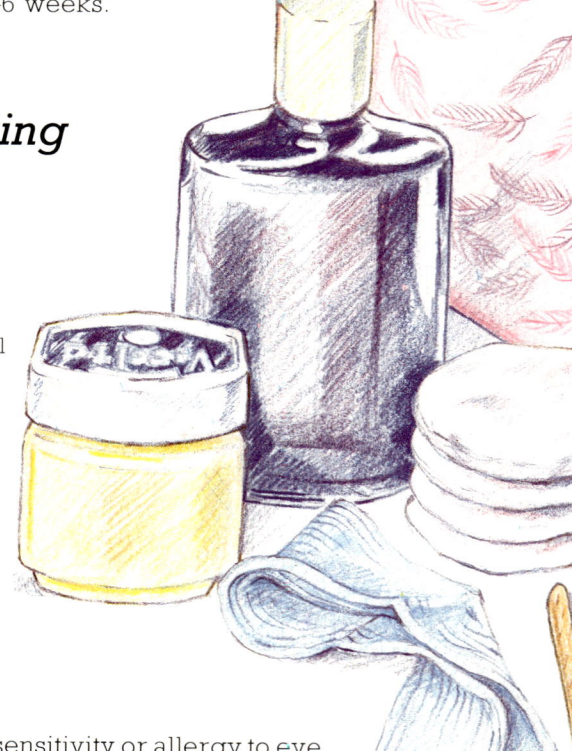

If you have a history of sensitivity or allergy to eye makeup, or suffer from conjunctivitis, eczema or psoriasis in the eye area, check with a doctor before carrying out this treatment.

1 Tie your hair off your face with a hairband or a scarf.

2 Thoroughly cleanse your eyebrows with a non-oily eye makeup remover or witch hazel to remove natural oils.

3 To avoid staining the skin while tinting, apply a thick layer of petroleum jelly or heavy moisturizer to the skin all round your eyebrows. Be very careful not to get any grease on the eyebrow hairs.

4 Follow the packet directions to make up the tint

5 Apply the tint to your eyebrows with an orange stick, making sure you cover the hairs and roots completely.

6 Leave the tint for 3 minutes only. Brow hairs take very quickly, and if you tint them too dark they will look artificial. (Red hair is the most resistant to tinting and *may* require double the exposure time to achieve satisfactory results.) Remove the tint with pads of damp cotton wool, using firm strokes.

7 Gently blot your brows dry with tissues.

8 Reapply the dye if you require a darker shade. But don't leave it on for longer than an additional 3 minutes before removing and checking the colour again.

The dye will last for 4–6 weeks.

Eyebrow bleaching

It will take
20 minutes

You will need
a hairband or scarf
non-oily eye makeup
  remover or witch hazel
cotton wool
a mirror (magnifying is
  best)
cream bleach specifically
  for facial and body hair
  (available in most
  chemists)
a wooden spatula
a bowl of lukewarm
  water
a towel

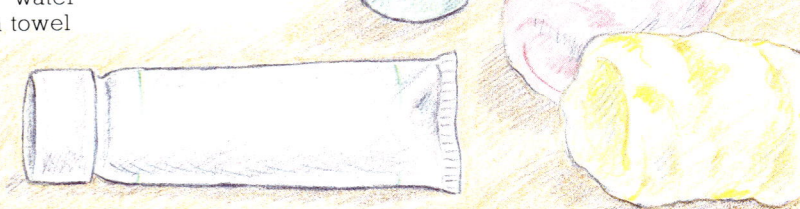

If you have a history of sensitivity or allergy to eye makeup, or suffer from conjunctivitis, eczema or psoriasis in the eye area, check with a doctor before carrying out this treatment.

1 Tie your hair off your face with a hairband or scarf.

2 Thoroughly cleanse your eyebrows with a non-oily eye makeup remover or witch hazel.

3 Follow the packet directions to make up the required amount of bleach. (It is not necessary to protect the surrounding skin with a heavy barrier cream as with tinting.)

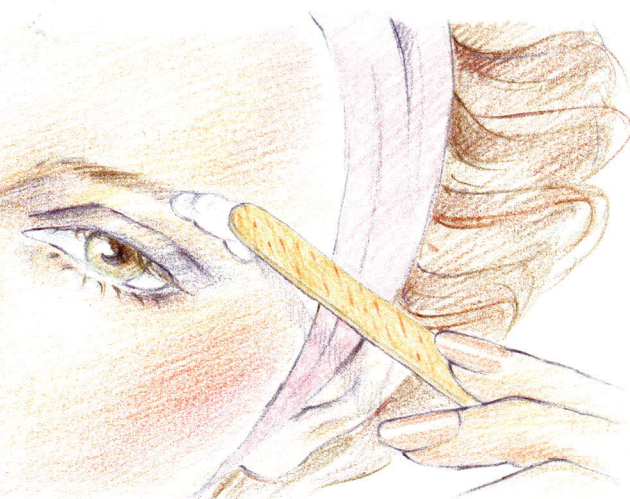

4 Using a wooden spatula, apply a fairly thick layer of bleach to your eyebrows, making sure you completely cover all the hairs and roots. If there's a stinging sensation, remove the bleach, wash the area with cool water and reapply. If this discomfort persists, discontinue use.

5 After 3 minutes remove the bleach with the spatula and check the colour. Don't worry if your brows look ginger – this is the halfway house between black and blonde.

6 Reapply the bleach if necessary, and check again in 3 minutes.

7 When the colour is satisfactory, remove as much bleach as possible with the spatula, and rinse off the residue with lukewarm water.

8 Dry gently with a towel.

The bleach should last 2–4 weeks.

You'll need help with the treatments in this section, so why not plan to have a home health farm day with a friend? There is also another advantage, it means there is far less chance that you will cheat on your diet or your exercises if you have someone who is following a similar programme with you! Plan your day's programme allowing time for you to help each other with your treatments.

A slim and youthful shape moves easily, without apparent effort; there's nothing stiff or rigid or ponderous about it. The combination of exercise and massage helps make your body supple.

Take lots of time over the luxurious massage. It should make you feel relaxed, so don't plan to do it just before you launch into a rigorous exercise session. It's best to exercise first, have a long bath and then relax with the massage.

Feet are all too often allowed to get completely set in their ways with many muscles going to waste, and will greatly benefit if you work at getting them dextrous. In the bath use your toes to turn the taps on and off, fish up the flannel and haul out the plug. As you dry your feet, try toe traction. Pull each toe firmly to left and right, then stretch it straight ahead. Feel that you own ten separate toes: stand up and waggle your big toe away from the rest, then try to separate the others one by one. All this improves the circulation, peps up neglected muscles and helps you beat bunions. To help give your feet suppleness and spring, go for 'funny walks' through the house. Set off barefoot, walking on tiptoe: this boosts your underfoot arches. Walk on the sides of your feet with your toes curled in, then walk on your heels.

Hands and feet can get very dry if you haven't bothered with them for a long time. The paraffin wax treatment (see right) helps to keep them soft and in better condition. A whole body wax treatment tends to be rather messy, so we don't suggest you attempt this. You will be using hot wax, so be very careful that it is comfortably cool before you immerse hands or feet. If you have a cooking thermometer wait until the wax is at 68°C/155°F before you touch it. Either cover your carpet with polythene or sit in a place where you can easily mop up any drips.

This has to be the luckiest era for legs. If you've got good ones, then today's fashions let you show

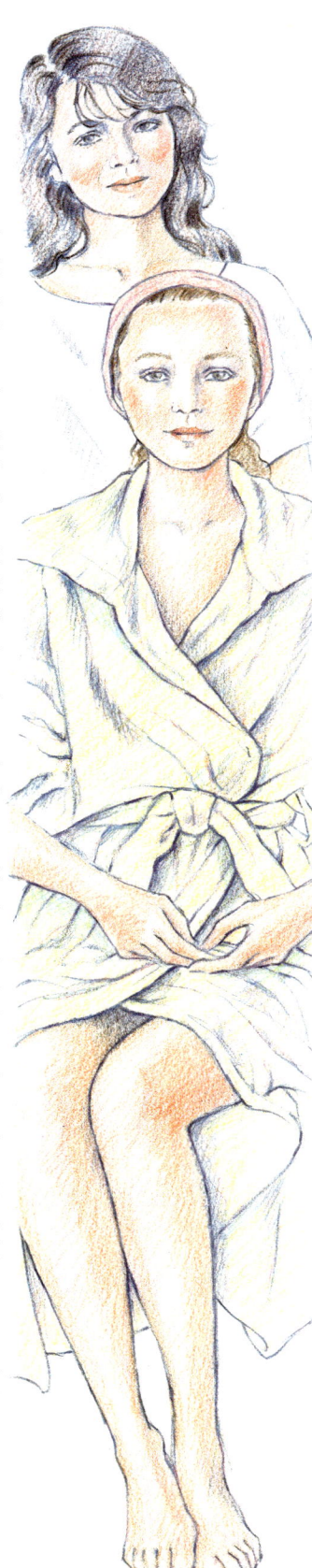

them off. It is absolutely essential, though, that elegant legs are not marred by unsightly hair. Unwanted leg hair can be removed by shaving, but this tends to grow back very quickly because you are not removing the hair below the surface of the skin. You could use a depilatory cream which does dissolve the hair below the surface, but a leg wax gives the deepest hair removal. Don't attempt this, though, if your pain threshold is low, as it does hurt for a few minutes when the hairs are plucked out. You also need a friend who isn't squeamish about helping you with this. The advantage of waxing is that the hair is removed further down towards the follicle than when using depilatory creams so it takes longer for the hair to grow back. It doesn't stop the hair growing, however: only electrolysis can do this. Be very careful when you apply the warm wax. It should be at 68°C/155°F if you test it with a cooking thermometer. You will get the best results if the hairs you are waxing are not very short, so that the wax has something to hold on to.

Even if you loathe the size of your legs, you still need to keep them in hairless condition. But aim at distraction rather than drawing attention to them. Heavy legs call for every lengthening trick you can play. Pale colours enlarge so wear dark rather than neutral tights (but do not wear black), and ankle-interrupting straps on shoes are out. So are flat shoes except with trousers. Plain court shoes in a dark shade are the most flattering. Don't forget the first rule of fashion is to keep comfortable. You can't look really good unless you feel relaxed, so suffering from sadistic shoes isn't sense. A happy face enhances a woman far more than the costliest outfit.

If you enjoy your home health farm treatments, be sure you make time to repeat them regularly. However much you are at others' beck and call, set aside an hour or two every week just for you and use it to repeat your favourite treatments. Make it plain that you've earned this private time and insist it is respected. Knowing that your body is as immaculate as you can make it is a big confidence-booster.

Remember this final tip. There's an instantly available face-lift with an effect that no cosmetic surgeon can achieve. It's a wide, warm smile. . .

Paraffin wax treatment for hands and feet

This treatment cleanses and softens the skin. Professionals often cover the whole body with paraffin wax, but this is a very messy treatment, and you should not attempt it unless you have a friend to help with the application, a clean paintbrush to apply the wax and a well-protected bed to lie on. Never cover your neck and face with wax.

It will take
30 minutes

You will need
1–2 kg/2¼–4½ lb paraffin
　wax (can be ordered
　from chemist)
a large saucepan
greaseproof paper
a bowl of lukewarm
　water (optional)
a towel (optional)

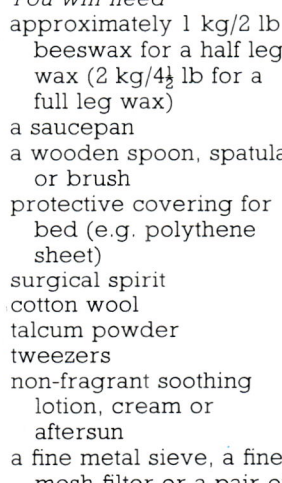

1 Make sure the area to be treated is clean, and remove all jewellery.

2 Heat the wax in a saucepan until it melts. Let the wax cool until it is comfortable to the touch.

3 Immerse your hands and/or feet in the wax.

4 Remove hands and/or feet from the pan and allow the wax to dry for a few minutes.

5 Repeat this procedure three or four times until you have a thick build-up of wax covering the skin.

6 Wrap your hands and/or feet in greaseproof paper to seal in the heat.

7 Leave the wax to harden for 10–15 minutes.

8 Peel the wax off gently in one piece.

9 Rinse the area with warm water and pat dry with the towel. (If your skin is dry, you may prefer to leave on the oily residue.)

Wax treatment for unwanted hair

Waxing is an effective way of removing unwanted hair and is suitable for most parts of the body, but *not* the face.

Like plucking, waxing pulls the hair out from beneath the skin's surface (although it doesn't destroy the roots), so regrowth takes longer than with shaving and many people find their hairs grow back sparser and softer in texture.

You will need
approximately 1 kg/2 lb
　beeswax for a half leg
　wax (2 kg/4½ lb for a
　full leg wax)
a saucepan
a wooden spoon, spatula
　or brush
protective covering for
　bed (e.g. polythene
　sheet)
surgical spirit
cotton wool
talcum powder
tweezers
non-fragrant soothing
　lotion, cream or
　aftersun
a fine metal sieve, a fine
　mesh filter or a pair of
　nylon tights

It is best to work on a bed or raised surface, ideally with a friend to help you get at all the awkward areas.

1 Heat the wax gently in a saucepan for about 30 minutes until it has a syrup-like consistency. Remove the pan from the heat and test the temperature by spooning a little wax on to the inside of your wrist. If it is very hot, wait a few minutes for it to cool down to a comfortable temperature (68°C/155°F).

2 Dampen a pad of cotton wool with surgical spirit and clean over the area to be waxed, to remove natural oils, moisturizers, etc. (If the area is greasy the wax will not adhere properly.) Always stroke upwards, lifting the hairs away from the skin's surface.

3 Dust over with talcum powder, stroking upwards to make the hairs stand erect.

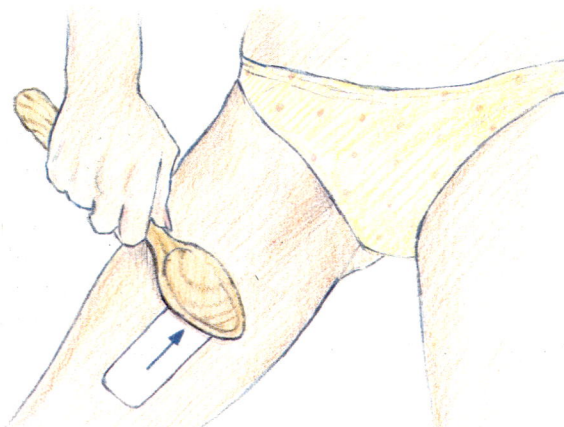

4 Using a wooden spoon apply the wax evenly in 2 mm/$\frac{1}{4}$ inch thick strips with thick edges for easy removal. Position the strips in the sequence shown on the relevant diagram (see opposite). For best results apply the wax in the *opposite* direction to the natural hair growth.

5 Allow the wax to cool and set, but do not leave it too long or the wax will become brittle and shatter when you remove it. (The wax takes about 30 seconds to set. A good test is to tap the wax every 10 seconds – it is ready when it no longer sticks to your finger. If you leave the wax on for too long simply apply another layer of hot wax and peel them off together.)

6 Quickly rip off the wax with decisive movements in an upward direction. The wax will take the hairs with it.

7 After waxing the entire area, rub away any fragments of wax with your fingertips. Then tweezer away any stray hairs, or you may be able to pull them out with your fingers.

8 Massage soothing lotion gently into the skin. (If you have sensitive skin a scented lotion may make you itch.) Any redness or blotches will fade.

Professional tip: the faster you pull off the wax the less painful it will be. Waxing can be painful, particularly if you retain water – just before a period, for example – but rubbing the area immediately after each removal will soothe smarting.
   If the wax in the pan cools during the application, reheat to melt again, and retest before applying. You may find you need to go over the same patch more than once, but once most of the hair is removed, you'll find it less painful.

Half leg wax (from ankle to knee)

It will take
30 minutes (plus 30 minutes to heat the wax)

Apply the strips of wax in the order shown below

Regrowth
Approximately 4–6 weeks

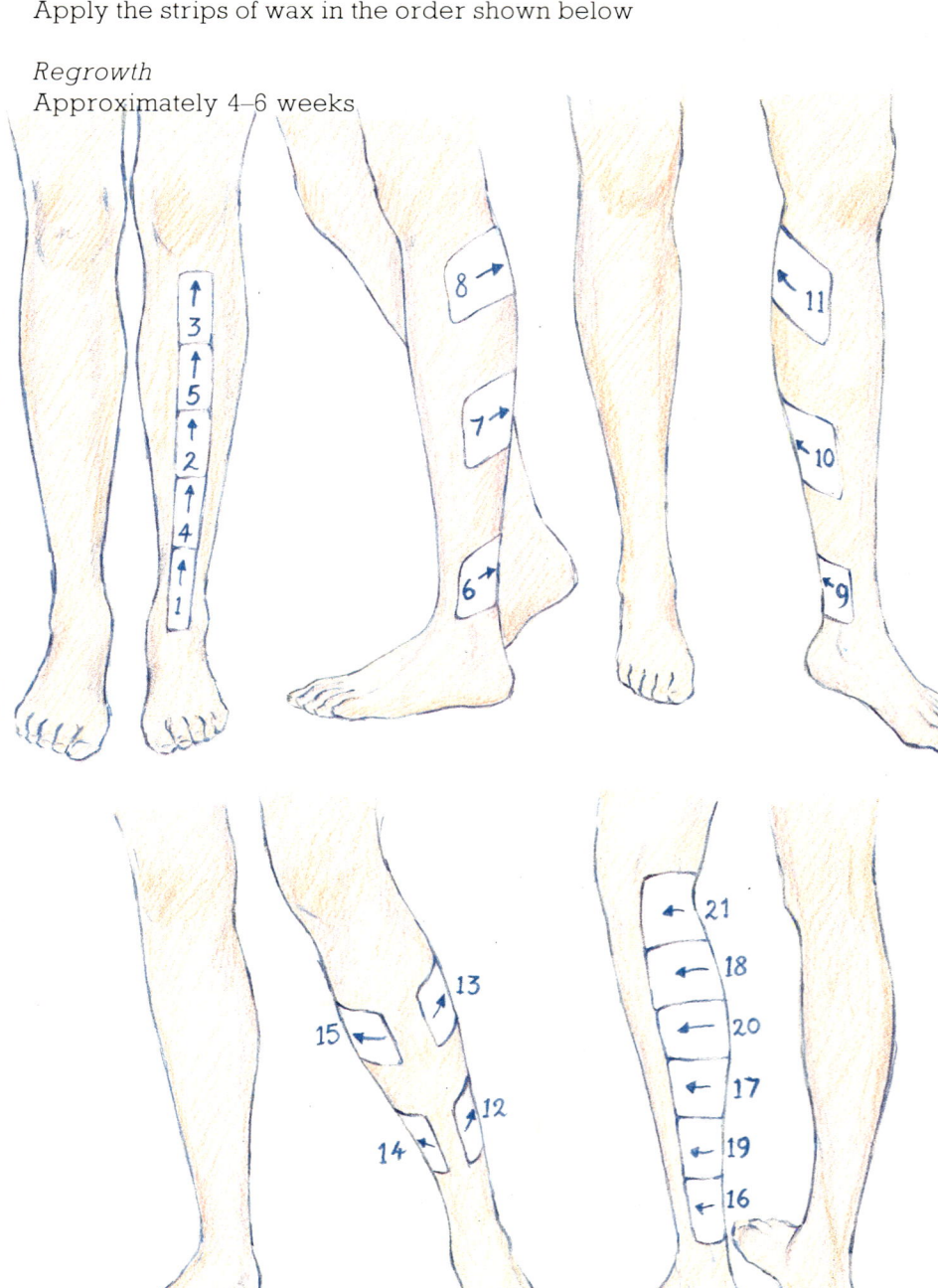

Full leg wax

It will take
1 hour (plus 45 minutes to heat the wax)

Follow the sequence for the half leg wax (left) then follow the order shown below

Regrowth
Approximately 4–6 weeks

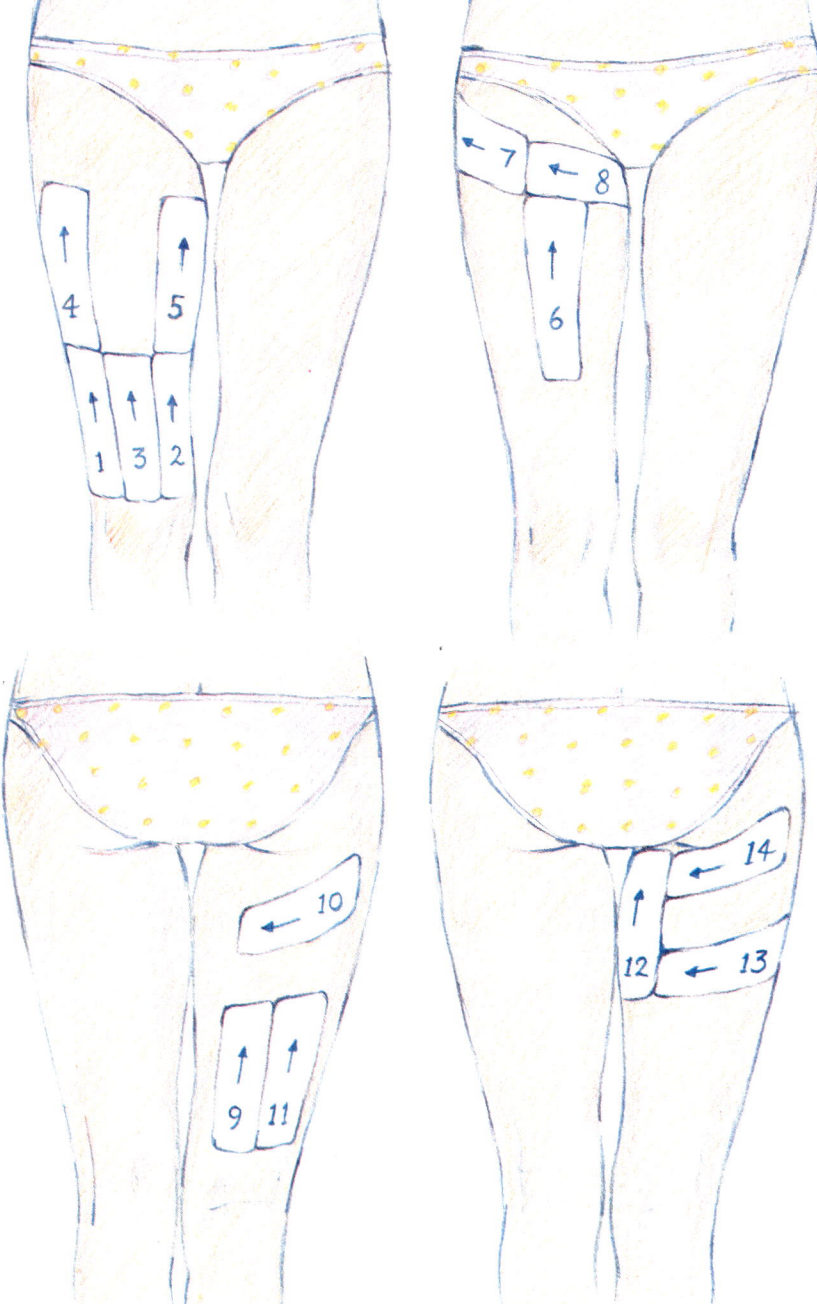

Bikini line wax

It will take
20 minutes (plus 30 minutes to heat the wax)

If the hair is long and thick, trim it with scissors before waxing. It helps to hold the skin taut when applying the wax. Small patches of wax will cause less discomfort, but this area is particularly sensitive, and if you have strong hair growth minute blood spots may appear.

Regrowth
Approximately 3–4 weeks

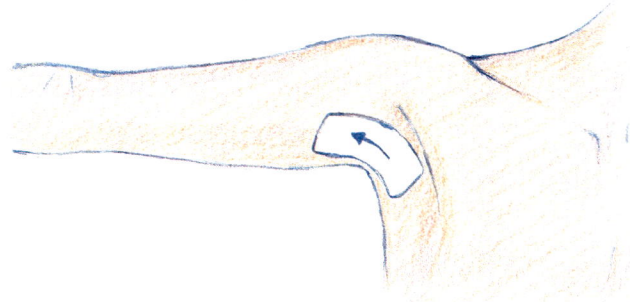

Underarm wax

It will take
20 minutes (plus 30 minutes to heat the wax)

To prevent irritation, do not apply deodorant for 6–12 hours after waxing. (You can use unscented talcum powder instead.)

Regrowth
Approximately 3–4 weeks

After use

Wax may be reused, but it must be cleaned and filtered to remove dead skin and hairs. Heat the wax in a saucepan until it is very liquid, then pour through a fine metal sieve with small holes or a fine mesh filter (try using nylon tights). *Be careful* not to spill the wax on your skin, as at this temperature it will scald you. Leave the wax to cool and harden before storing it away for future use.

Cool wax

Cool wax kits consisting of pre-waxed strips are available from your chemist. They are not as effective as hot wax but are easy to use, simply follow the packet directions.

Massage

It will take
1 hour

You will need
a friend to do the
    massaging or to
    massage
coconut, olive or almond
    oil
a few drops of perfume
    (optional)
a high, firm table or bed
    (if neither is available
    you can work on the
    floor)
cotton wool
skin tonic, freshener or
    astringent
tissues or a towel
perfumed talc

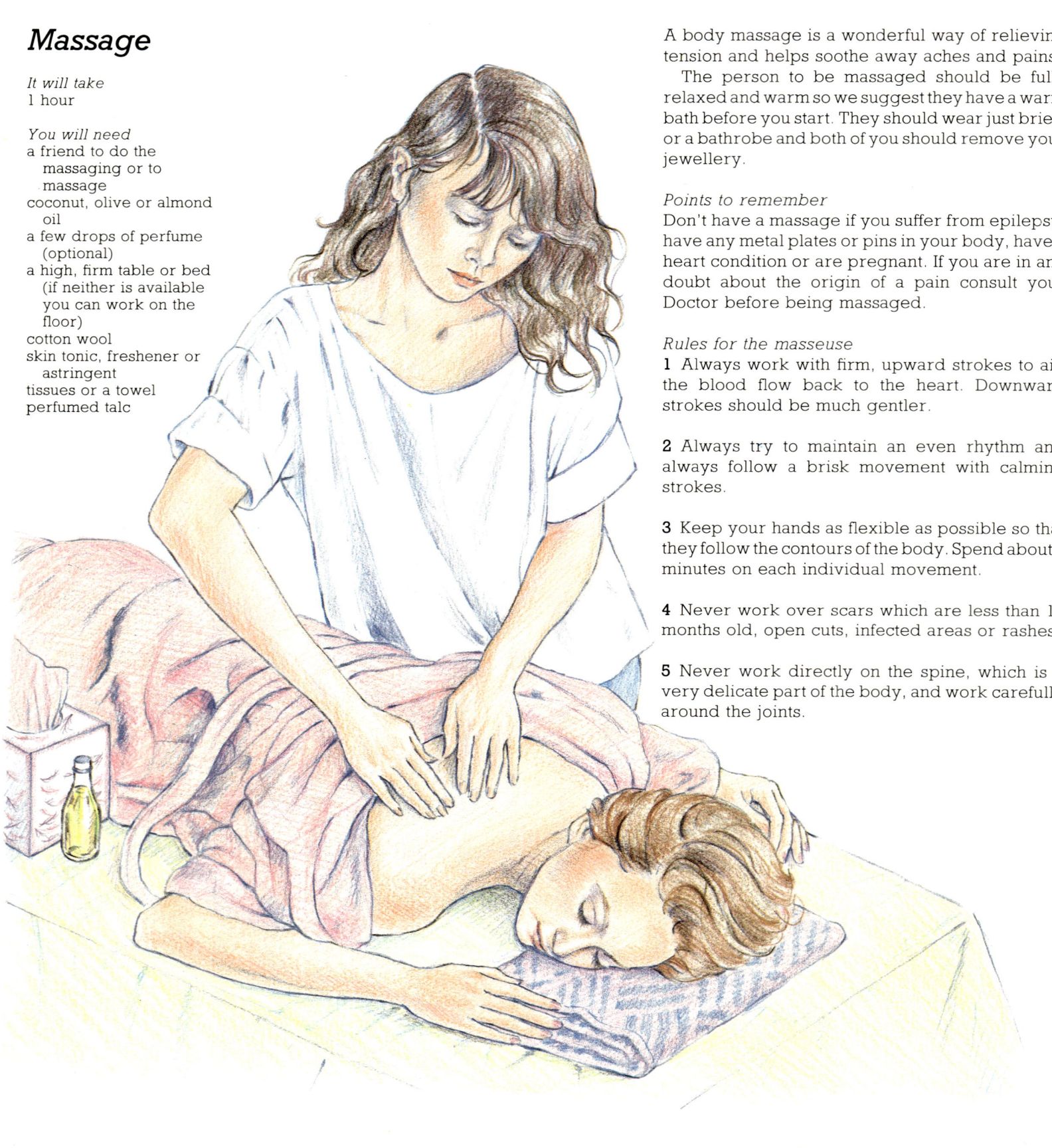

A body massage is a wonderful way of relieving tension and helps soothe away aches and pains.

The person to be massaged should be fully relaxed and warm so we suggest they have a warm bath before you start. They should wear just briefs or a bathrobe and both of you should remove your jewellery.

Points to remember
Don't have a massage if you suffer from epilepsy, have any metal plates or pins in your body, have a heart condition or are pregnant. If you are in any doubt about the origin of a pain consult your Doctor before being massaged.

Rules for the masseuse
1 Always work with firm, upward strokes to aid the blood flow back to the heart. Downward strokes should be much gentler.

2 Always try to maintain an even rhythm and always follow a brisk movement with calming strokes.

3 Keep your hands as flexible as possible so that they follow the contours of the body. Spend about 5 minutes on each individual movement.

4 Never work over scars which are less than 12 months old, open cuts, infected areas or rashes.

5 Never work directly on the spine, which is a very delicate part of the body, and work carefully around the joints.

3 To avoid staining the skin while tinting, apply a thick layer of petroleum jelly or heavy moisturizer to the skin all round your eyebrows. Be very careful not to get any grease on the eyebrow hairs.

4 Follow the packet directions to make up the tint

5 Apply the tint to your eyebrows with an orange stick, making sure you cover the hairs and roots completely.

6 Leave the tint for 3 minutes only. Brow hairs take very quickly, and if you tint them too dark they will look artificial. (Red hair is the most resistant to tinting and *may* require double the exposure time to achieve satisfactory results.) Remove the tint with pads of damp cotton wool, using firm strokes.

7 Gently blot your brows dry with tissues.

8 Reapply the dye if you require a darker shade. But don't leave it on for longer than an additional 3 minutes before removing and checking the colour again.

The dye will last for 4–6 weeks.

Eyebrow bleaching

will take
20 minutes

You will need
a hairband or scarf
non-oily eye makeup
 remover or witch hazel
cotton wool
a mirror (magnifying is
 best)
cream bleach specifically
 for facial and body hair
 (available in most
 chemists)
a wooden spatula
a bowl of lukewarm
 water
a towel

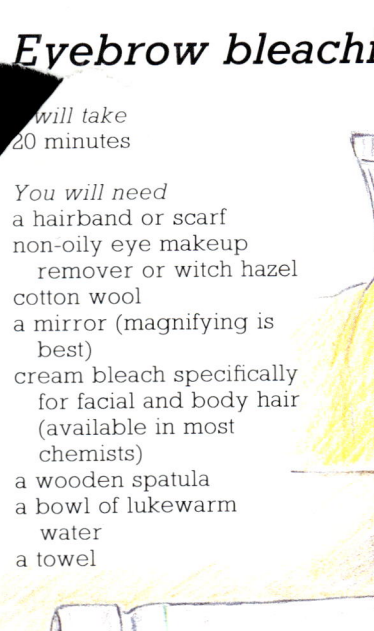

If you have a history of sensitivity or allergy to eye makeup, or suffer from conjunctivitis, eczema or psoriasis in the eye area, check with a doctor before carrying out this treatment.

1 Tie your hair off your face with a hairband or scarf.

2 Thoroughly cleanse your eyebrows with a non-oily eye makeup remover or witch hazel.

3 Follow the packet directions to make up the required amount of bleach. (It is not necessary to protect the surrounding skin with a heavy barrier cream as with tinting.)

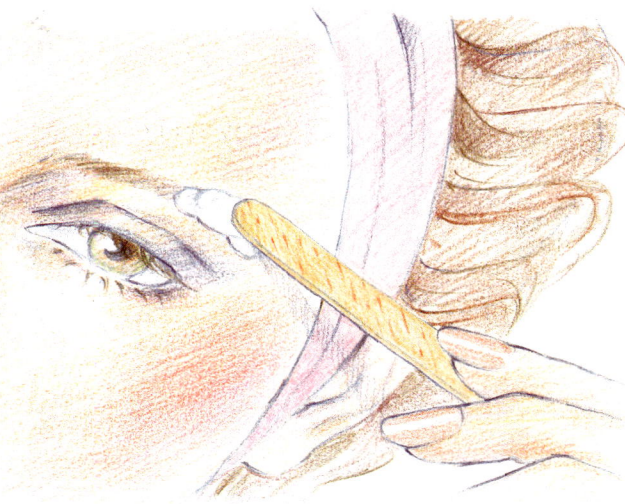

4 Using a wooden spatula, apply a fairly thick layer of bleach to your eyebrows, making sure you completely cover all the hairs and roots. If there's a stinging sensation, remove the bleach, wash the area with cool water and reapply. If this discomfort persists, discontinue use.

5 After 3 minutes remove the bleach with the spatula and check the colour. Don't worry if your brows look ginger – this is the halfway house between black and blonde.

6 Reapply the bleach if necessary, and check again in 3 minutes.

7 When the colour is satisfactory, remove as much bleach as possible with the spatula, and rinse off the residue with lukewarm water.

8 Dry gently with a towel.

The bleach should last 2–4 weeks.

Professional Treatments

You'll need help with the treatments in this section, so why not plan to have a home health farm day with a friend? There is also another advantage, it means there is far less chance that you will cheat on your diet or your exercises if you have someone who is following a similar programme with you! Plan your day's programme allowing time for you to help each other with your treatments.

A slim and youthful shape moves easily, without apparent effort; there's nothing stiff or rigid or ponderous about it. The combination of exercise and massage helps make your body supple.

Take lots of time over the luxurious massage. It should make you feel relaxed, so don't plan to do it just before you launch into a rigorous exercise session. It's best to exercise first, have a long bath and then relax with the massage.

Feet are all too often allowed to get completely set in their ways with many muscles going to waste, and will greatly benefit if you work at getting them dextrous. In the bath use your toes to turn the taps on and off, fish up the flannel and haul out the plug. As you dry your feet, try toe traction. Pull each toe firmly to left and right, then stretch it straight ahead. Feel that you own ten separate toes: stand up and waggle your big toe away from the rest, then try to separate the others one by one. All this improves the circulation, peps up neglected muscles and helps you beat bunions. To help give your feet suppleness and spring, go for 'funny walks' through the house. Set off barefoot, walking on tiptoe: this boosts your underfoot arches. Walk on the sides of your feet with your toes curled in, then walk on your heels.

Hands and feet can get very dry if you haven't bothered with them for a long time. The paraffin wax treatment (see right) helps to keep them soft and in better condition. A whole body wax treatment tends to be rather messy, so we don't suggest you attempt this. You will be using hot wax, so be very careful that it is comfortably cool before you immerse hands or feet. If you have a cooking thermometer wait until the wax is at 68°C/155°F before you touch it. Either cover your carpet with polythene or sit in a place where you can easily mop up any drips.

This has to be the luckiest era for legs. If you've got good ones, then today's fashions let you show

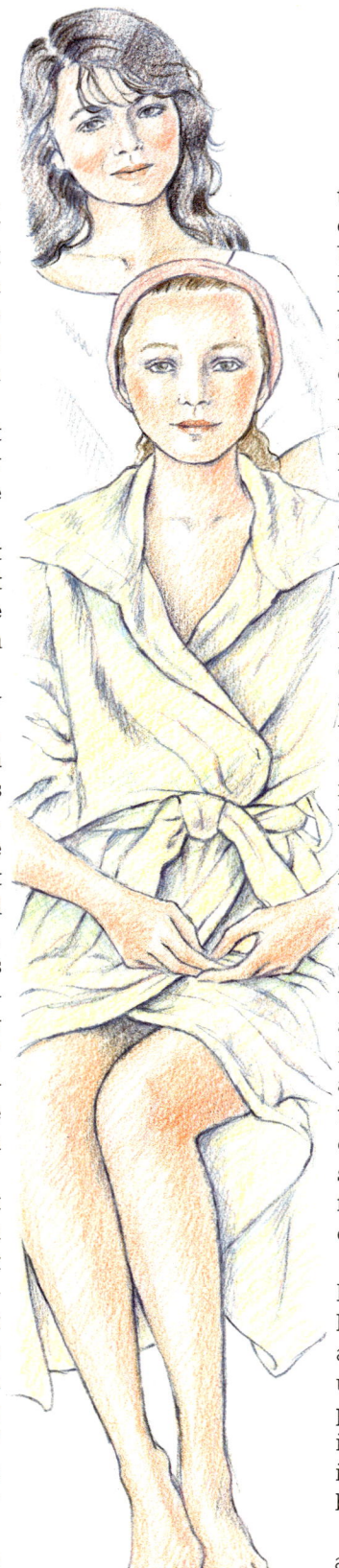

them off. It is absolutely essential, though, that elegant legs are not marred by unsightly hair. Unwanted leg hair can be removed by shaving, but this tends to grow back very quickly because you are not removing the hair below the surface of the skin. You could use a depilatory cream which does dissolve the hair below the surface, but a leg wax gives the deepest hair removal. Don't attempt this, though, if your pain threshold is low, as it does hurt for a few minutes when the hairs are plucked out. You also need a friend who isn't squeamish about helping you with this. The advantage of waxing is that the hair is removed further down towards the follicle than when using depilatory creams so it takes longer for the hair to grow back. It doesn't stop the hair growing, however: only electrolysis can do this. Be very careful when you apply the warm wax. It should be at 68°C/155°F if you test it with a cooking thermometer. You will get the best results if the hairs you are waxing are not very short, so that the wax has something to hold on to.

Even if you loathe the size of your legs, you still need to keep them in hairless condition. But aim at distraction rather than drawing attention to them. Heavy legs call for every lengthening trick you can play. Pale colours enlarge so wear dark rather than neutral tights (but do not wear black), and ankle-interrupting straps on shoes are out. So are flat shoes except with trousers. Plain court shoes in a dark shade are the most flattering. Don't forget the first rule of fashion is to keep comfortable. You can't look really good unless you feel relaxed, so suffering from sadistic shoes isn't sense. A happy face enhances a woman far more than the costliest outfit.

If you enjoy your home health farm treatments, be sure you make time to repeat them regularly. However much you are at others' beck and call, set aside an hour or two every week just for you and use it to repeat your favourite treatments. Make it plain that you've earned this private time and insist it is respected. Knowing that your body is as immaculate as you can make it is a big confidence-booster.

Remember this final tip. There's an instantly available face-lift with an effect that no cosmetic surgeon can achieve. It's a wide, warm smile. . .

Arm massage

1 Lie the person to be massaged on their back.

2 Pour a small amount of oil into your hands, rub them together, then spread it over the arm to be massaged.

3 Hold the right hand and shake the arm vigorously.

4 Using your whole hand, stroke lightly and evenly over the right arm in a rhythmical, continuous movement (1 and 2). This spreads the oil evenly and aids relaxation.

5 Using your thumbs, rub firm circles around the wrist (3). This increases circulation and helps prevent stiffness.

6 Firmly knead the palm of the hand (4).

7 Turn the hand over and using brisk, circular movements with the thumbs, apply friction between the tendons of the fingers and thumb in an upwards direction towards the wrist (5).

8 Using circular movements, knead the joints at the base of the thumb and each finger (6 and 7).

9 Using circular movements with the thumb, slowly and rhythmically knead the arm, lifting and pinching the flesh at the same time (8). (It is easier than it sounds!) Remember that the pressure should always be upwards. This helps tone the muscles.

10 Using your thumbs, and moving the skin over the bones, rub firm circles around the elbow (9).

11 Lift the arm into an upright position and rotate the wrist three or four times to the left, then to the right (10). Stop and relax in between to prevent discomfort. The wrist should be rotated as far as possible.

12 Finish off the arm massage by stroking evenly with your whole hand over the elbow, arm, wrist and hand, finishing at the fingertips (11).

13 Repeat on the left arm.

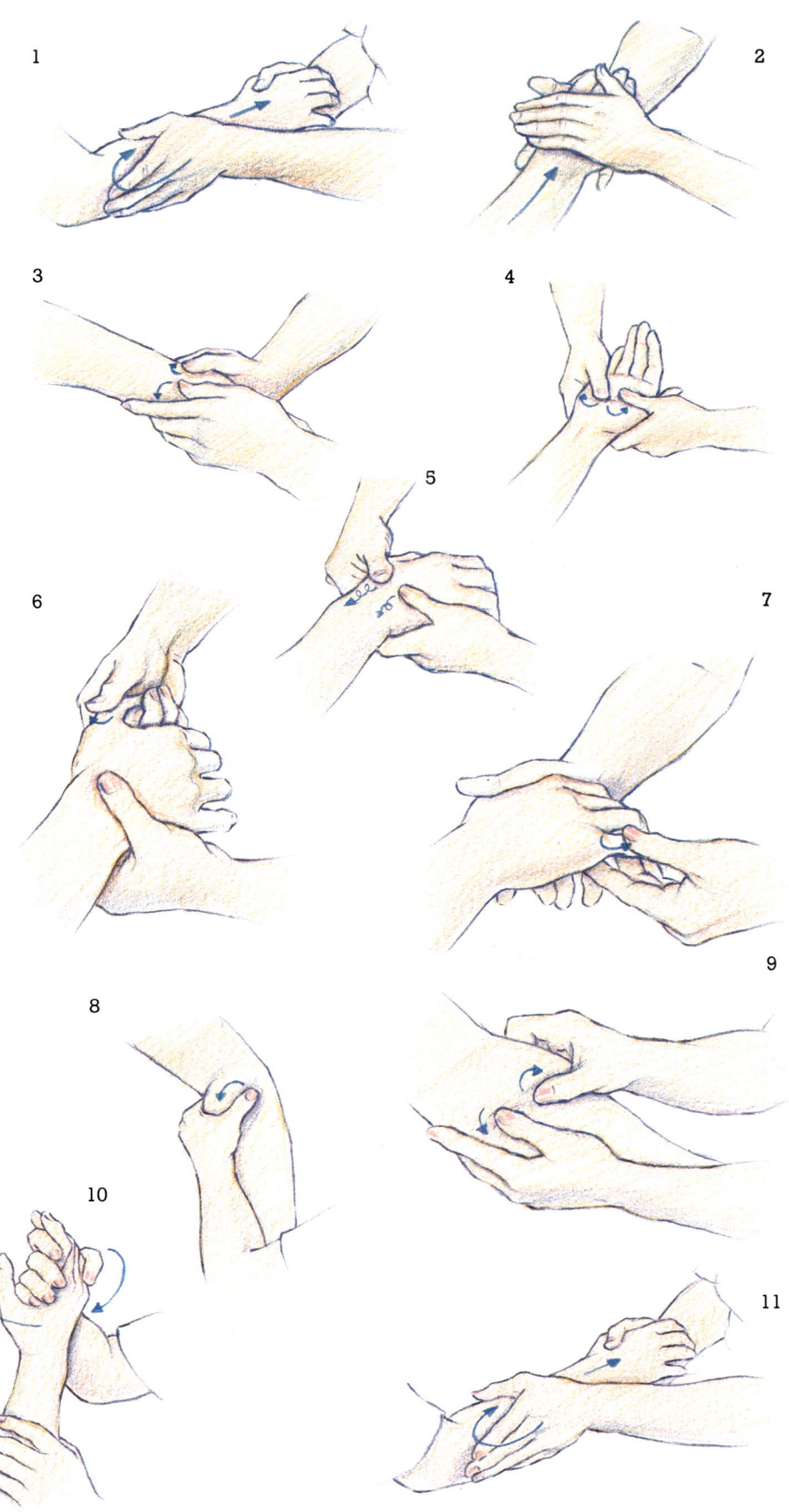

Foot and leg massage

1 Apply oil (see Arm massage).

2 Holding the foot firmly – one hand under the heel and the other on the top of the foot – lift the left leg off the bed and shake vigorously. This helps relax the whole leg.

3 Stroke lightly and evenly over the calf and foot until the muscles become relaxed (1 and 2).

4 Knead the arch of the foot with firm, circular movements (3).

5 Apply firm, outward strokes to the top of the foot (4 and 5).

6 Press the toes firmly, but smoothly, downward to their fullest extension (6).

7 Using the fingers, lightly but rapidly snatch at the toes (7 and 8).

8 Apply a whipping movement over the toes. This increases circulation (9 and 10).

9 Using circular movements, knead and stroke the Achilles tendon (11).

10 Apply short, outward movements to the calf (12).

11 Firmly knead the calf (13 and 14).

12 Cup your hands and briskly but gently smack the calf (15 and 16). This stimulates circulation.

13 Apply gentle, circular movements around the knee.

14 Stroke lightly and evenly over the thigh in a rhythmical fashion. Stroke inwards as well as upwards.

15 Using circular movements, knead the thigh, lifting and pinching the flesh at the same time.

16 Stroke gently and evenly over the entire foot and leg, finishing at the toes (17).

17 Repeat on the right leg and foot.

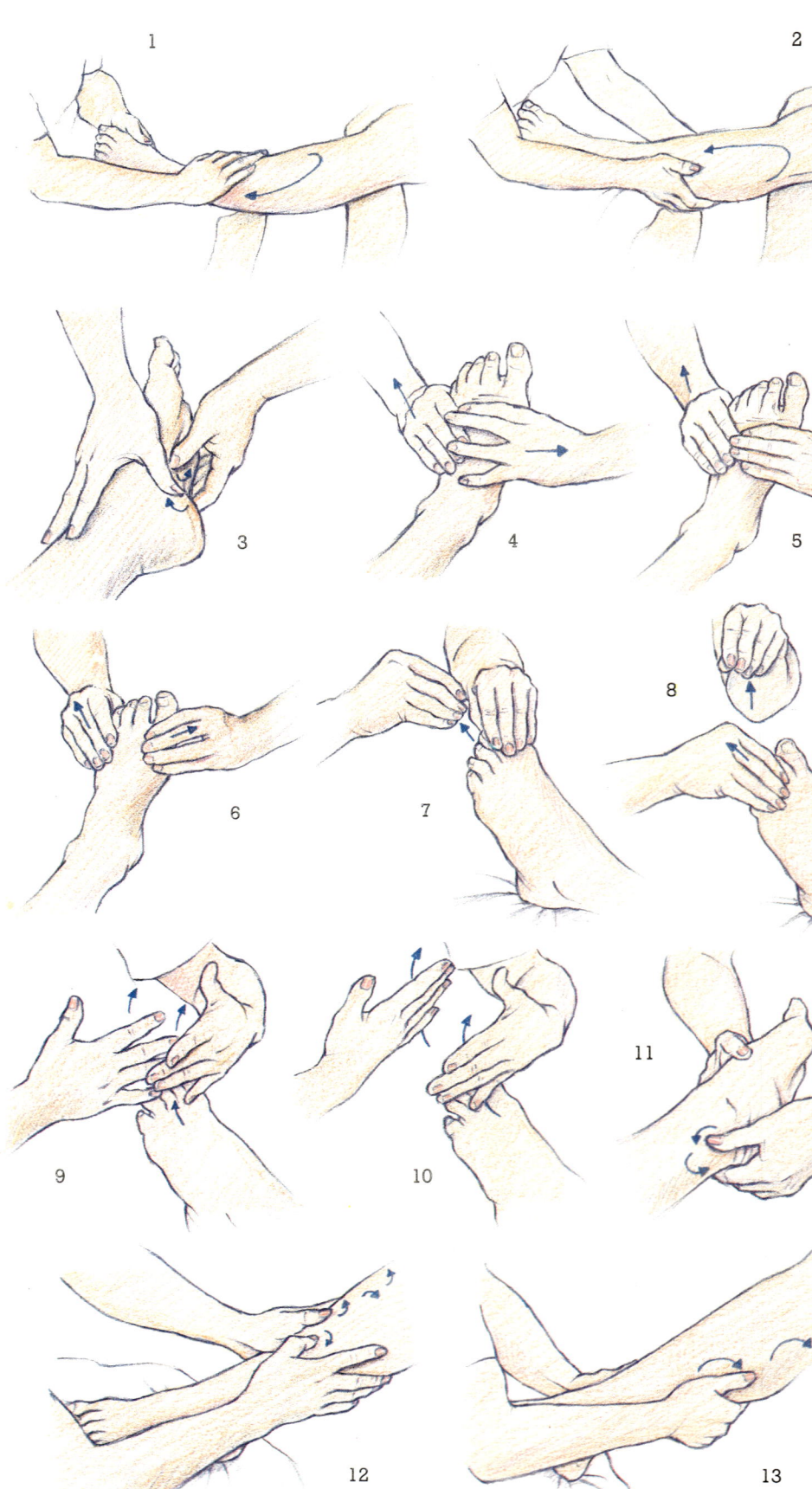

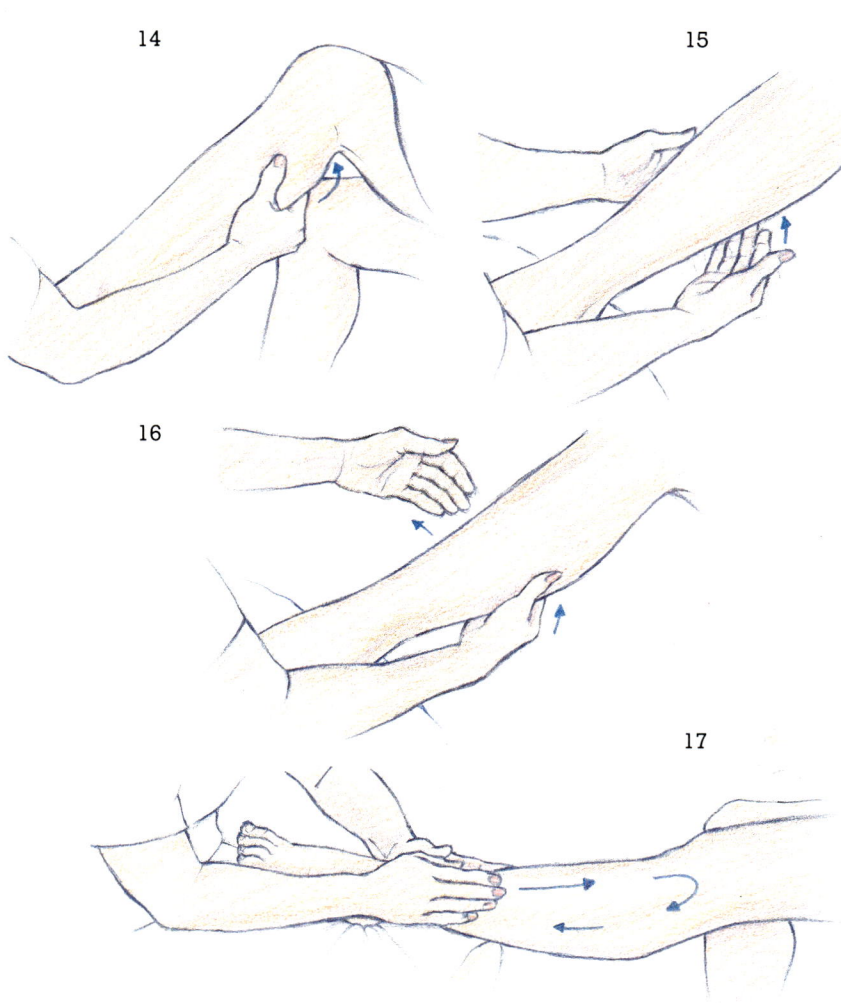

Back massage

1 Turn the person being massaged onto their stomach and apply oil (see Arm massage).

2 Stroke gently over the whole back moving up and away from the spine.

3 Firmly knead the back with circular movements, slowly working round the shoulder blades and sides of the spine.

4 Cup your hands and briskly smack the back.

5 Stroke gently over the whole back.

To complete the massage

Remove any remaining oil from the body with a pad of cotton wool dampened with skin tonic, freshener or astringent. Pat dry with tissues or a towel and dust over with talcum powder.

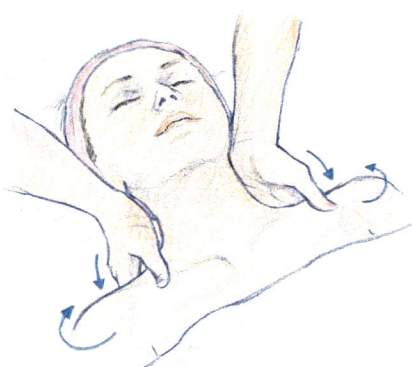

Stomach massage

Apply oil (see Arm massage). Using circular movements in a clockwise direction (this follows the path of the intestine), stroke *very* gently downwards towards the centre of the stomach, gently lifting the flesh as you do so. Never use heavy movements on the stomach.

Neck massage

1 Apply oil (see Arm massage).

2 Stroke gently and evenly over the shoulders and neck (1).

3 Using circular movements with the thumbs, firmly knead around the neck (2) and out across the shoulders (3). (A lot of tension builds up here.)

4 Stroke gently over the whole area.

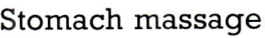
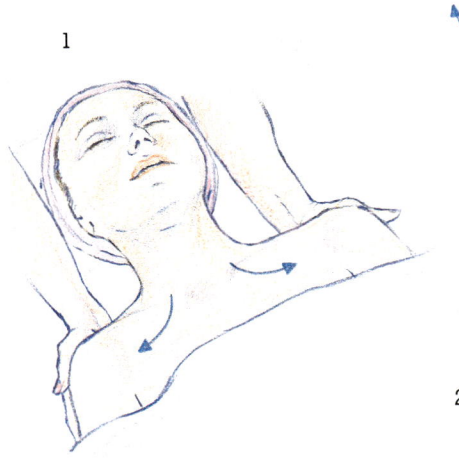

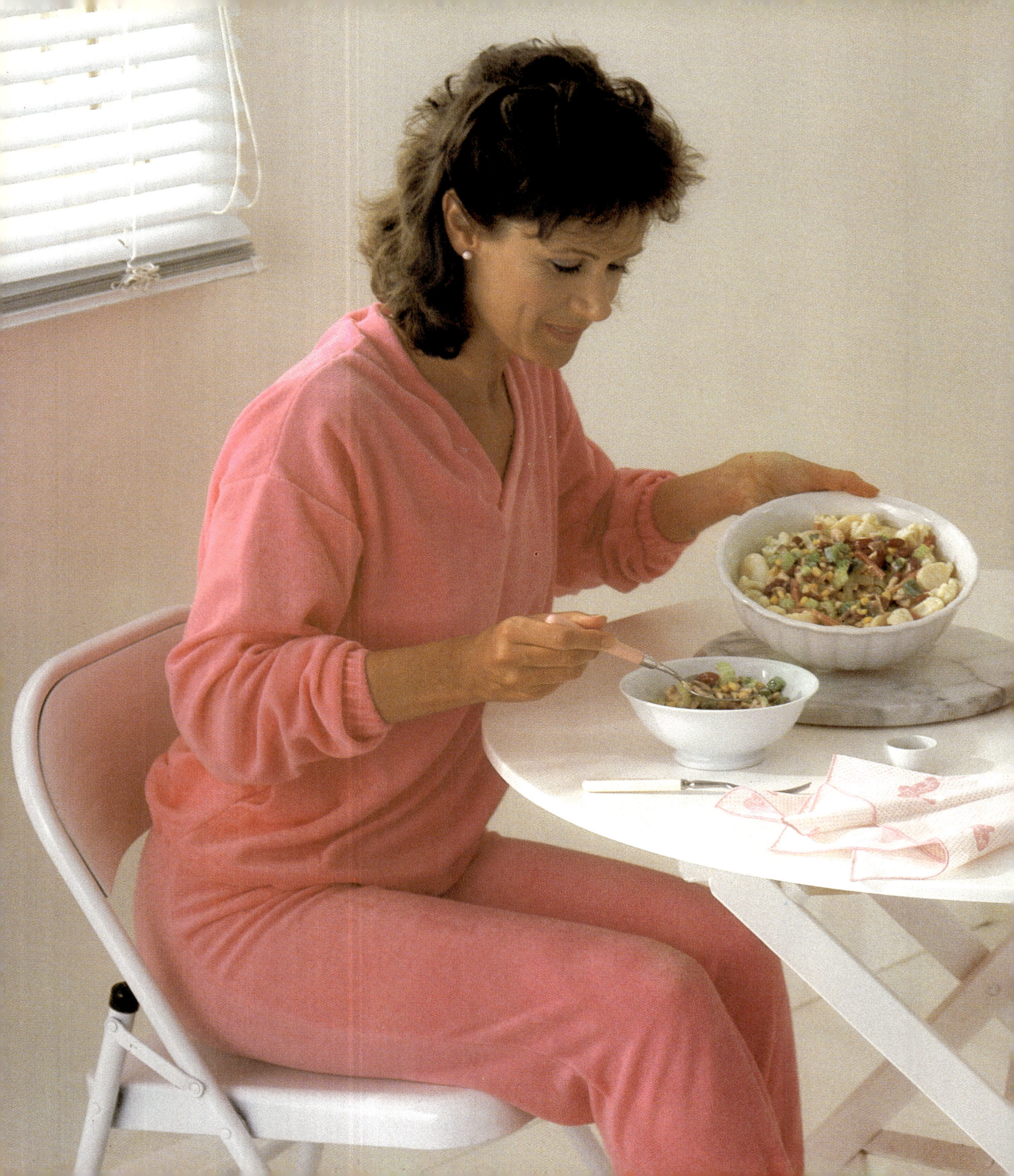

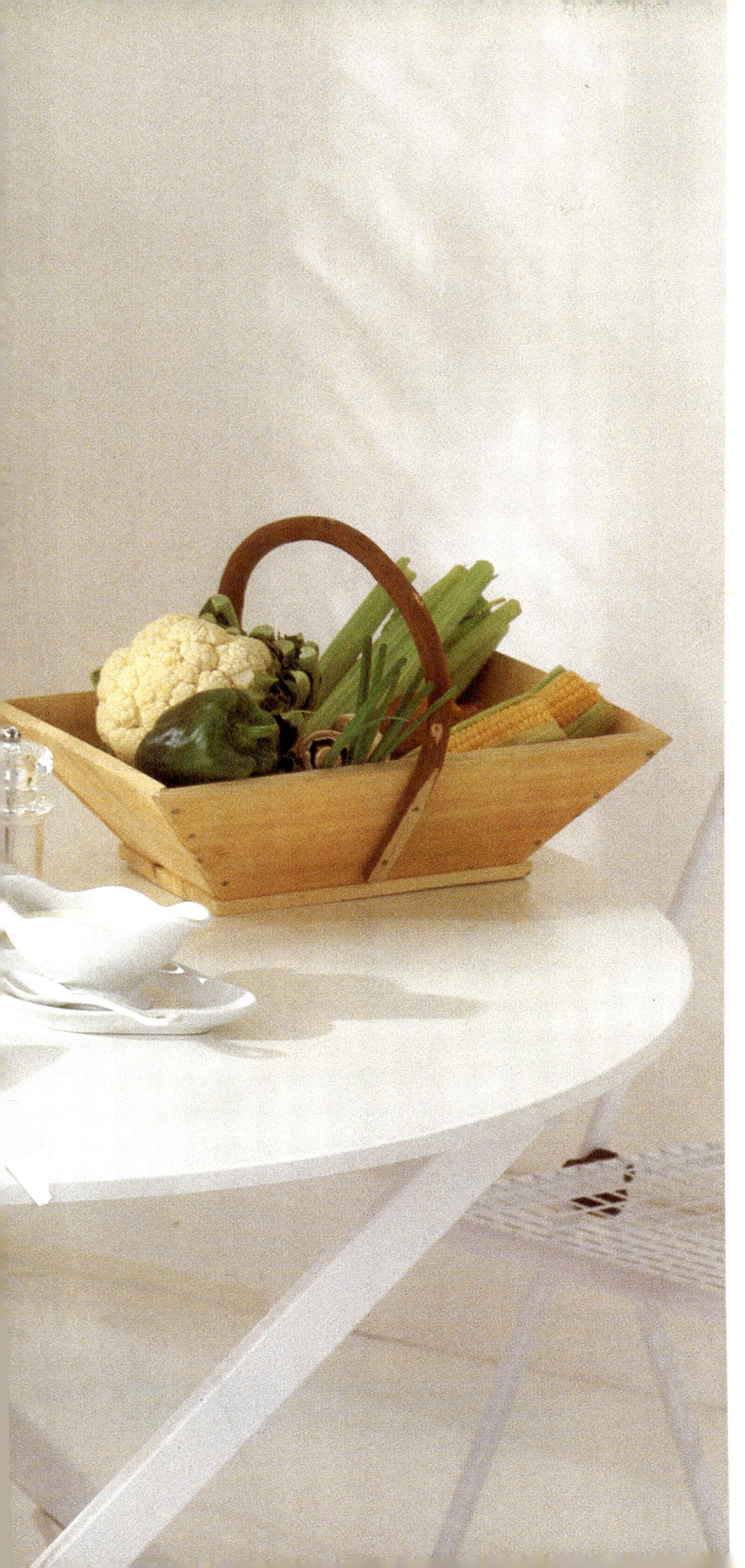

DIET

The Home Health Farm Questionnaire on page 14 will lead you to the diet that is right for you. All you then have to do is follow the diet faithfully for as long as it takes you to reach your target weight.

Turn to the Super-speedy Health Farm Diet on page 150 if you simply want to lose a pound or two during your Home Health Farm days; have chosen to get a long-term diet off to a sprinting start; or if you have strayed from your long-term diet for a day or two and want to undo the damage. A few days on this strict regime will work wonders but remember that you should not continue the Super-speedy diet for more than four days because it is too low in calories for a longer-term dieting plan.

Carefully follow the diet of your choice and we guarantee that you will soon see results, slimming at your personal fastest rate.

The Extra Fibre Formula

Your health as well as your weight will benefit by increasing the amount of fibre in your diet. Dietary fibre occurs naturally in wholegrain cereals, vegetables and fruits, and from high bran products.

But how much fibre do you need? From a purely healthy eating point of view, scientific researchers who have analysed the amount of dietary fibre necessary to get the desirable effects believe that the daily 'ration' should be around 30 grams. If you follow the Extra Fibre Formula you will be getting at least this amount each day and still be keeping to a slimming 1,500 Calories.

This diet is not only high in fibre, it is also low in fat. The world's top health authorities tell us to cut down on all fats, especially the cholesterol-raising 'saturated' sort from animal sources. This is very good news for dieters because fats are the highest calorie foods of all and by cutting fats you will automatically cut your Calories.

Most women and all men will lose weight on 1,500 Calories a day. But if you have under 3 stone (19 kg/42 lb) to lose you could find that the pounds will disappear disappointingly slowly. Start with The Extra Fibre Formula if you have over 3 stone (19 kg/42 lb) to lose and then switch to one of the stricter diets as you near your target. As long as you continue to choose bran cereals, wholemeal bread and lots of fruit and vegetables you should still be getting a healthy amount of fibre in your diet. If you wish you can continue on The Extra Fibre Formula and cut down on the number of snacks you allow yourself each day. Some of the snacks have been chosen mainly to give you pleasure rather than add a great deal of fibre to your day and – sorry – these should be the ones you cut out.

Some of the menus that follow include packed lunches, some include light meals that can be eaten at home and some are completely meatless giving you a choice of vegetarian days. Just select your day's menu and follow it to the letter. The Extra Fibre Formula couldn't be simpler – or more effective.

Diet Rules

1 Choose a selection of the daily menus that follow. You may repeat a menu if you wish, but make sure that you choose at least four different daily menus within each fortnight.

2 Follow each day's menu precisely. You may eat the meals and snacks at any time you like, but do not swap meals with other days. If you do not wish to eat breakfast, you may save that meal to eat later. Each menu gives you 1,500 Calories a day.

3 You may have 275 ml/½ pint/1¼ cups skimmed milk or 190 ml/⅓ pint/⅞ cup semi-skimmed milk each day *in addition* to any milk given in the menus.

4 You can drink as much tea and coffee as you wish, using milk from the above allowance and using artificial sweeteners only. You can also drink unlimited amounts of water or low-calorie soft drinks.

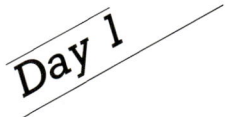

Day 1

Breakfast
Light Meal

BRAN FLAKES AND BANANA
(6.4 grams fibre)
Slice 1 small banana. Serve with 25 g/1 oz/1 cup Bran Flakes (bran breakfast cereal) and 150 ml/¼ pint/⅔ cup skimmed milk.

Peanut Butter and Jam Sandwich (8 grams fibre)

Metric/Imperial	*American*
2 x 40 g/1½ oz slices wholemeal bread	2 x 1½ oz slices wholemeal bread
10 ml/2 level teaspoons peanut butter	2 level teaspoons peanut butter
10 ml/2 level teaspoons jam	2 level teaspoons jam

Spread 1 slice of bread with peanut butter and the other with jam. Sandwich together.

Main Meal

Ham Steak with Pineapple, and Apricot Yogurt
(20.1 grams fibre)

Metric/Imperial	*American*
4 dried apricots, chopped	4 dried apricots, chopped
1 x 100 g/3½ oz bacon or ham steak	1 x 3½ oz ham steak
1 ring pineapple, canned in natural juice	1 ring pineapple, canned in natural juice
125 g/4 oz carrots, sliced	¾ cup sliced carrots
125 g/4 oz canned broad beans	¾ cup drained canned fava beans
125 g/4 oz canned sweetcorn	¾ cup drained canned whole kernel corn
To follow	*To follow*
1 x 150 g/5 oz carton low-fat natural yogurt	⅔ cup low-fat natural yogurt

Place the apricots in a saucepan with water to cover. Simmer for 5 minutes. Leave to cool. Grill (broil) the bacon or ham steak. Heat the pineapple under the grill (broiler). Boil the carrots, and in separate saucepans heat the broad beans (fava beans) and sweetcorn (whole kernel corn). Drain and serve with the meat and pineapple. Drain the apricots, mix with the yogurt and serve for dessert.

Snack 1

NUTTY CHEESE SANDWICH, AND FRUIT
(12.9 grams fibre)
Chop 6 toasted hazelnuts and mix with 75 g/3 oz/3 tablespoons cottage cheese with pineapple. Make into a sandwich with 2 x 40 g/1½ oz slices wholemeal bread. Follow with 1 medium pear.

Snack 2

FISH SPREAD CRISPBREADS
(4.9 grams fibre)
Spread 4 calorie-reduced bran crispbreads with the contents of 1 x 53 g/1⅞ oz pot fish spread (any flavour) and top each crispbread with 3 slices of cucumber.

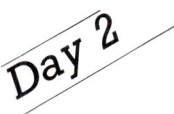

Day 2

Breakfast

ORANGE, TOAST AND MARMALADE OR HONEY
(8.2 grams fibre)
Start with 1 medium orange. Follow with 2 × 25 g/1 oz slices wholemeal toast with 10 ml/2 level teaspoons low-fat spread and 10 ml/2 level teaspoons honey, marmalade or jam.

Light Meal

Garlic Sausage and Butter Bean Salad (8.6 grams fibre)

Metric/Imperial	American
40 g/1½ oz garlic sausage, cubed	1½ oz garlic sausage, cubed
1 x 213 g/7½ oz can butter beans, drained	¼ cup drained canned butter beans
1 tomato, chopped	1 tomato, chopped
1 spring onion, chopped	1 scallion, chopped
¼ green pepper, cored, seeded and diced	¼ green pepper, cored, seeded and diced
30 ml/2 tablespoons oil-free French dressing	2 tablespoons oil-free French dressing
4 black or green olives, stoned	4 ripe or green olives, pitted

Combine the garlic sausage, butter beans, tomato, spring onion (scallion) and green pepper in an individual serving bowl. Toss with oil-free French dressing and serve topped with the olives.

Main Meal

Prawn and Corn Chowder with Bread and Fruit
(20.4 grams fibre)

Metric/Imperial	American
25 g/1 oz diced onion	¼ cup diced onion
1 x 75 g/3 oz potato, peeled weight, diced	½ cup diced potato
115 ml/4 fl oz water	½ cup water
¼ chicken stock cube	½ chicken bouillon cube
50 g/2 oz peeled prawns	⅓ cup shelled shrimp
150 g/5 oz canned sweetcorn, drained	scant 1 cup drained canned whole kernel corn
150 ml/¼ pint skimmed milk	⅔ cup skimmed milk
10 ml/2 level teaspoons cornflour	2 level teaspoons cornstarch
salt and pepper	salt and pepper
2 x 25 g/1 oz slices wholemeal bread	2 x 1 oz slices wholemeal bread
parsley to garnish	parsley to garnish
To follow	To follow
1 medium pear	1 medium pear

Place the onion and the potato in a saucepan with the water and stock cube (bouillon cube). Bring to the boil, cover and simmer for 10 minutes. Add the prawns (shrimp), sweetcorn (whole kernel corn) and skimmed milk. Simmer gently for 5 minutes. Blend the cornflour (cornstarch) with a little cold water in a cup. Add to the pan, stirring all the time. Simmer for 2 minutes. Season with salt and pepper, top with parsley and serve with the bread. Follow with the pear.

Snack 1

MUESLI AND YOGURT
(3.1 grams fibre)
Mix 1 × 150 g/5 oz carton low-fat natural yogurt with 25 g/1 oz muesli (Swiss style cereal). Stir in 15 ml/1 level tablespoon sultanas (golden raisins) or raisins and 5 hazelnuts.

Snack 2

BANANA SANDWICH
(7.0 grams fibre)
Mash 1 small banana and mix with 5 ml/1 level teaspoon raisins or sultanas (golden raisins). Use as a filling between 2 × 25 g/1 oz slices wholemeal bread.

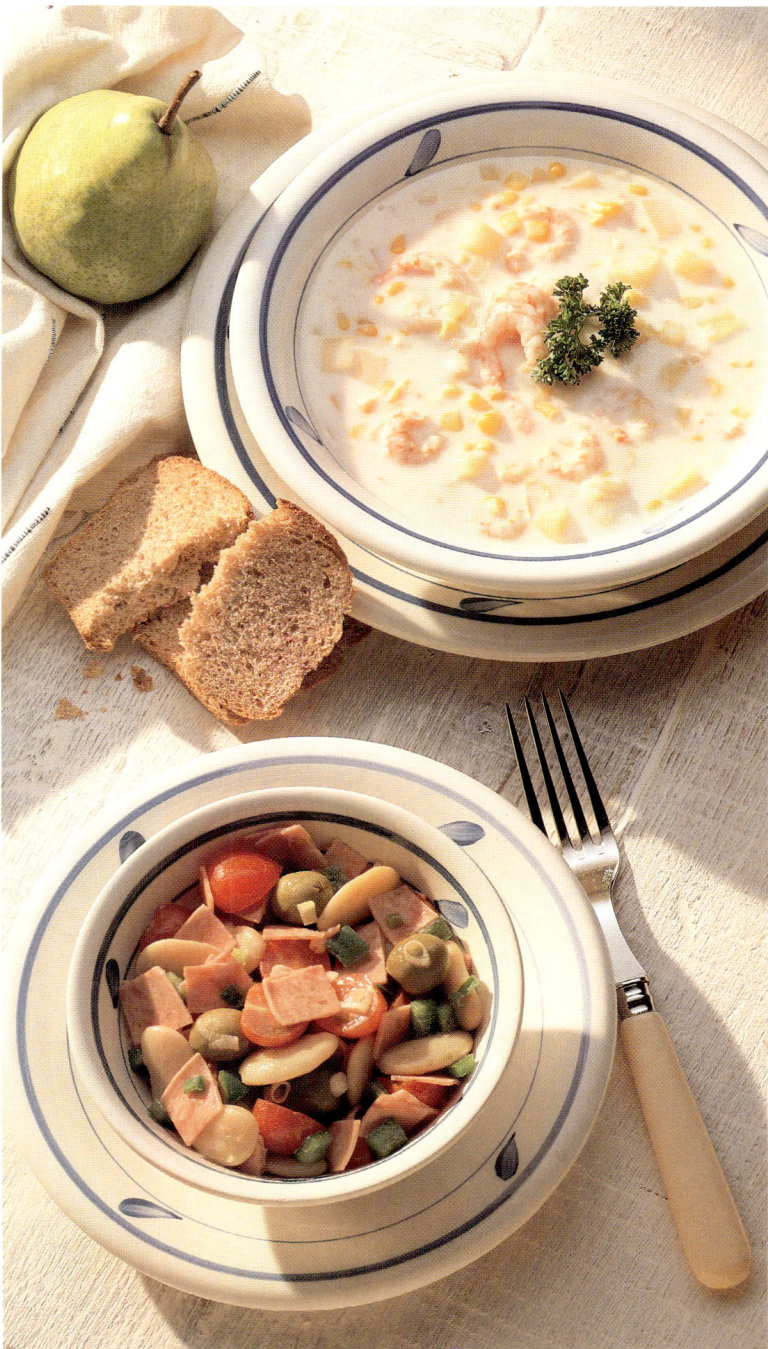

DAY 2: Prawn and Corn Chowder; Garlic Sausage and Butter Bean Salad

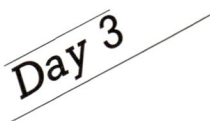

Day 3

Breakfast
Light Meal

GRAPEFRUIT AND POACHED EGG ON TOAST (4.1 grams fibre)
Start with ½ grapefruit, sprinkled with 5 ml/1 level teaspoon fructose. To follow poach 1 size 3 (medium) egg. Serve on 1 × 40 g/1½ oz slice wholemeal toast

Red Bean and Tuna Salad, and Fruit (15.2 grams fibre)

Metric/Imperial	American
1 x 225 g/8 oz can red kidney beans, drained	1⅓ cups canned red kidney beans, drained
1 x 100 g/3½ oz can tuna in brine, drained and flaked	1 x 3½ oz can tuna in brine, drained and flaked
1 spring onion, chopped	1 scallion, chopped
15 ml/1 level tablespoon chutney	1 level tablespoon chutney
15 ml/1 level tablespoon oil-free French dressing	1 tablespoon oil-free French dressing
To follow	*To follow*
1 medium pear	1 medium pear

Mix the salad ingredients. Follow with the pear.

Main Meal

Hawaiian Chicken, and Fruit (6.1 grams fibre)

Metric/Imperial	American
40 g/1½ oz long-grain brown rice	3 tablespoons long-grain brown rice
50 g/2 oz cooked chicken	2 oz cooked chicken
¼ red or green pepper, cored, seeded and diced	¼ red or green pepper, cored, seeded and diced
2 rings canned pineapple in natural juice, chopped	2 rings canned pineapple in natural juice, chopped
30 ml/2 tablespoons pineapple juice from can	2 tablespoons pineapple juice from can
2.5 ml/½ teaspoon soy sauce	½ teaspoon soy sauce
15 ml/1 level tablespoon flaked almonds	1 level tablespoon slivered almonds
To follow	*To follow*
1 small banana	1 small banana

Cook the rice in plenty of boiling water for about 25 minutes or until tender, and drain. Discard skin from chicken and dice the flesh. Heat the rice with the pepper, chicken, pineapple, juice and soy sauce. Toast the almonds and sprinkle on top. Follow with the banana.

Snack 1

SALAD SANDWICH, AND FRUIT (11.6 grams fibre)
Spread 15 ml/1 level tablespoon low-calorie salad dressing on 2 × 40 g/1½ oz slices of wholemeal bread. Make into a sandwich with 1 sliced tomato, a few slices cucumber and mustard and cress. Follow with 1 orange.

Snack 2

SOUP AND WHOLEMEAL ROLL (4.2 grams fibre)
Heat 1 × 275 g/10 oz can low-calorie beef and vegetable or vegetable soup. Serve with 1 × 45 g/1¾ oz wholemeal roll.

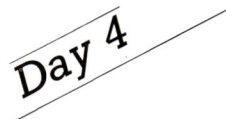

Day 4

Breakfast
Light Meal

GRAPEFRUIT, AND POACHED EGG ON TOAST (4.1 grams fibre)
Start with ½ grapefruit sprinkled with 5 ml/1 level teaspoon fructose. To follow, poach 1 size 3 (medium) egg and serve on 1 × 40 g/1½ oz slice unbuttered wholemeal toast.

Tuna Brown Rice Salad, and Fruit (7.3 grams fibre)

Metric/Imperial	American
25 g/1 oz long-grain brown rice	2 tablespoons long-grain brown rice
125 g/4 oz fresh or frozen French beans or haricots verts	1 cup fresh or frozen green beans
1 x 100 g/3½ oz can tuna in brine, drained	1 x 3½ oz can tuna in brine, drained
¼ red or green pepper, cored, seeded and diced	¼ red or green pepper, seeded and diced
40 g/1½ oz cucumber, diced	⅓ cup diced cucumber
30 ml/2 tablespoons oil-free French dressing	2 tablespoons oil-free French dressing
To follow	*To follow*
1 small orange	1 small orange

Boil the rice and beans separately in salted water. Drain and rinse in cold water. Drain again. Mix rice, beans, tuna, pepper and cucumber in an individual salad bowl. Toss with dressing and serve. Follow with the orange.

Main Meal

Boston Beans, and Fruit (28 grams fibre)

Metric/Imperial	American
2 x 150 g/5 oz cans baked beans in tomato sauce	2 x 5 oz cans baked beans in tomato sauce
125 g/4 oz canned tomatoes, drained	½ cup drained canned tomatoes
1.25 ml/¼ teaspoon French mustard	¼ teaspoon Dijon mustard
1.25 ml/¼ teaspoon Worcestershire sauce	¼ teaspoon Worcestershire sauce
10 ml/2 level teaspoons black treacle	2 level teaspoons molasses
2 rashers streaky bacon	2 slices bacon
1 x 40 g/1½ oz slice wholemeal bread	1 x 1½ oz slice wholemeal bread
5 ml/1 level teaspoon low-fat spread	1 level teaspoon low-fat spread
To follow	*To follow*
1 medium peach	1 medium peach

Place the baked beans, tomatoes, mustard, Worcestershire sauce and treacle (molasses) in a saucepan. Bring to the boil, reduce heat and simmer until the liquid has reduced – about 10 minutes. Stir occasionally while cooking to prevent sticking. Grill (broil) the bacon until crisp, then break into small pieces. Add to the beans. Toast bread, spread with low-fat spread and serve with the beans. Follow with the medium peach.

Snack 1

YEAST EXTRACT OPEN SANDWICH
(3.6 grams fibre)
Spread a 40 g/1½ oz slice wholemeal bread with 10 ml/2 level teaspoons low-fat spread and 10 ml/2 level teaspoons yeast extract.

Snack 2

DRINKING CHOCOLATE AND BISCUITS
(1.6 grams fibre)
Heat 225 ml/8 fl oz/1 cup skimmed milk until boiling. Stir into a mug containing 20 ml/2 rounded teaspoons drinking chocolate (sweetened cocoa). Serve with 2 digestive biscuits (graham crackers).

ALL BRAN AND RAISINS
(13.4 grams fibre)
Mix 40 g/1½ oz/10 level tablespoons All Bran (bran breakfast cereal) with 30 ml/2 level tablespoons raisins in a serving bowl. Serve with 150 ml/¼ pint/⅔ cup skimmed milk.

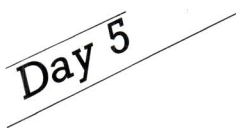
Day 5

Breakfast

Light Meal

Pizza Toast (4.6 grams fibre)

Metric/Imperial	American
2 rashers streaky bacon	2 slices bacon
1 x 40 g/1½ oz slice wholemeal bread	1 x 1½ oz slice wholemeal bread
5 ml/1 level teaspoon yeast extract	1 level teaspoon yeast extract
1 tomato, sliced	1 tomato, sliced
25 g/1 oz Edam cheese, grated	¼ cup grated Dutch cheese
1 olive, stoned and sliced	1 olive, pitted and sliced

Cut the bacon rashers (slices) in half lengthways and grill (broil) until crisp. Toast the bread on one side only. Spread the untoasted side with yeast extract. Top with the sliced tomato and sprinkle with the cheese. Grill (broil) until the cheese has melted. Arrange the bacon rashers (slices) on top, criss-cross fashion and decorate with the sliced olive.

Main Meal

Tuna and Tomato Bake, and Fruit (14.4 grams fibre)

Metric/Imperial	American
1 x 150 g/5 oz potato	1 x 5 oz potato
1 spring onion, chopped	1 scallion, chopped
40 g/1½ oz fresh wholemeal breadcrumbs	¾ cup fresh wholemeal breadcrumbs
1.25 ml/¼ level teaspoon dried mixed herbs	¼ level teaspoon dried mixed herbs
salt and pepper	salt and pepper
2 tomatoes, sliced	2 tomatoes, sliced
1 x 100 g/3½ oz can tuna in brine, drained and flaked	1 x 3½ oz can tuna in brine, drained and flaked
25 g/1 oz Edam cheese, grated	¼ cup grated Dutch cheese
125 g/4 oz green beans	1 cup green beans
To follow	*To follow*
1 medium apple	1 medium apple

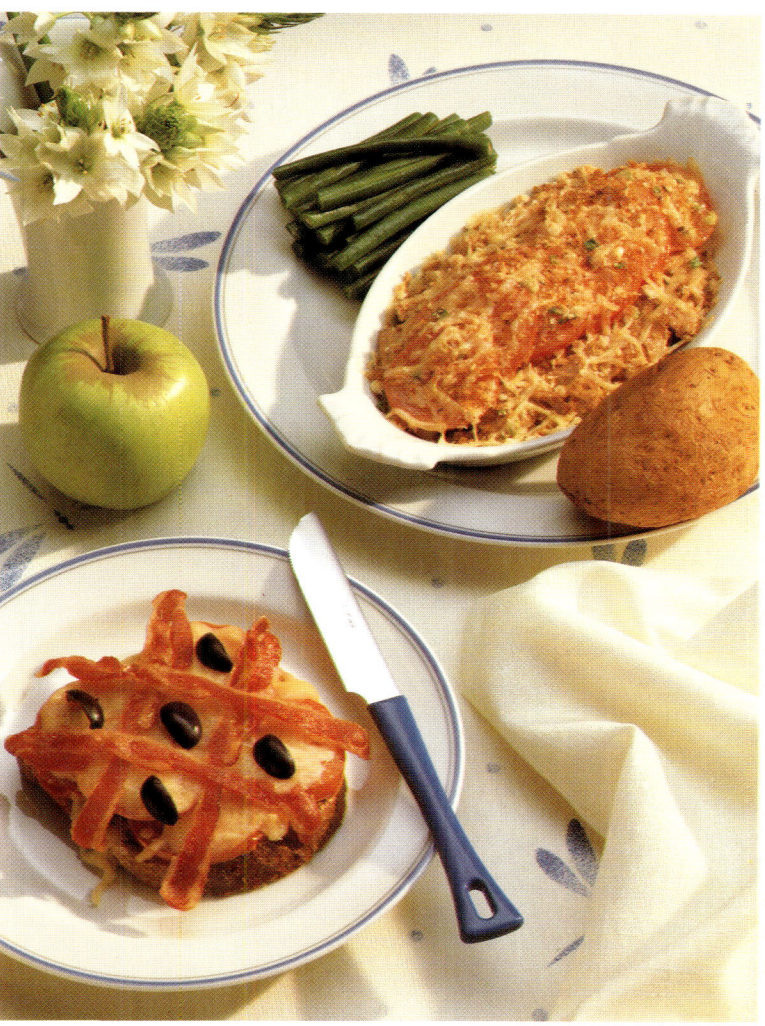
DAY 5: Pizza Toast; Tuna and Tomato Bake

Bake the potato in a preheated moderate oven (190°C/375°F/Gas Mark 5) for 45 minutes or until soft when pinched. Mix the spring onion (scallion) with the breadcrumbs and herbs. Season with salt and pepper. Spread half the crumb mixture over the base of a small ovenproof dish. Cover with half the tomatoes and all the tuna. Arrange the remaining tomato slices on top. Mix the cheese with the remaining crumbs and sprinkle over the tomato. Bake alongside the potato for the last 20 minutes. Boil the beans, drain and serve with the tuna bake and baked potato. Follow with the apple.

Snack 1

BANANA AND COTTAGE CHEESE OPEN SANDWICH
(6 grams fibre)
Spread 1 × 40 g/1½ oz slice wholemeal bread with 50 g/2 oz/¼ cup natural cottage cheese. Top with 1 small sliced banana and 5 ml/1 level teaspoon sultanas (golden raisins).

Snack 2

SOUP AND WHOLEWHEAT ROLL
(4.2 grams fibre)
Heat 1 × 290 g/10 oz can low-calorie beef and vegetable, vegetable or tomato soup. Serve with 1 × 45 g/1¾ oz unbuttered wholemeal roll.

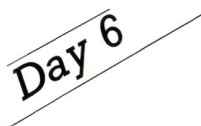

Day 6

Breakfast

Light Meal

SULTANA BRAN
(7.3 grams fibre)
Place 50 g/2 oz/½ cup Sultana Bran
(bran breakfast cereal with
golden raisins) in a bowl. Serve
with 115 ml/4 fl oz/½ cup skimmed
milk.

Banana and Cottage Cheese Open Sandwiches, and Fruit (10.4 grams fibre)

Metric/Imperial	American
2 x 25 g/1 oz slices wholemeal bread	2 x 1 oz slices wholemeal bread
lettuce leaves	lettuce leaves
125 g/4 oz cottage cheese with pineapple	½ cup cottage cheese with pineapple
1 small banana, sliced	1 small banana, sliced
To follow	*To follow*
1 medium orange	1 medium orange

Arrange lettuce leaves on both slices of bread. Top each with cottage
cheese then sliced banana. Follow with the orange.

Main Meal

Yogurt-baked Chicken with Vegetables, and Fruit
(14.5 grams fibre)

Metric/Imperial	American
1 x 225 g/8 oz potato	1 x 8 oz potato
1 x 175 g/6 oz chicken breast, skinned	1 x 6 oz chicken breast, skinned
30 ml/2 level tablespoons low-fat natural yogurt	2 tablespoons low-fat natural yogurt
15 ml/1 level tablespoon tomato purée	1 level tablespoon tomato paste
5 ml/1 level teaspoon paprika	1 level teaspoon paprika
salt and pepper	salt and pepper
175 g/6 oz broccoli	1 cup broccoli
To follow	*To follow*
1 medium apple	1 medium apple

Bake the potato in a preheated moderate oven (180°C/350°F/Gas Mark
4) for 1 hour or until soft when pinched. Place the chicken breast in a
small ovenproof dish. Mix the yogurt, tomato purée (paste), paprika,
salt and pepper and spoon over the chicken. Cover and bake alongside
the potato for the final 45 minutes of the cooking time. Sprinkle with a
little extra paprika and serve with the lightly boiled broccoli and the
potato. Follow with the apple.

Snack 1

BAKED BEANS ON TOAST
(14.6 grams fibre)
Heat 1 × 150 g/5 oz can baked
beans in tomato sauce in a
saucepan. Serve on a 1 × 40 g/
1½ oz slice wholemeal toast.

Snack 2

ICE CREAM AND FRUIT
(2.4 grams fibre)
Serve 1 × 220 g/7½ oz can fruit
salad in low-calorie syrup with a
75 g/3 oz scoop of vanilla ice
cream.

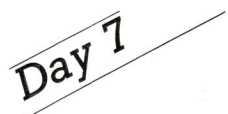

Day 7

Breakfast

**BRAN FLAKES AND
BANANA**
(6.4 grams fibre)
Serve 25 g/1 oz/1 cup Bran Flakes
(bran breakfast cereal) with 1
small sliced banana and 150 ml/¼
pint/⅔ cup skimmed milk.

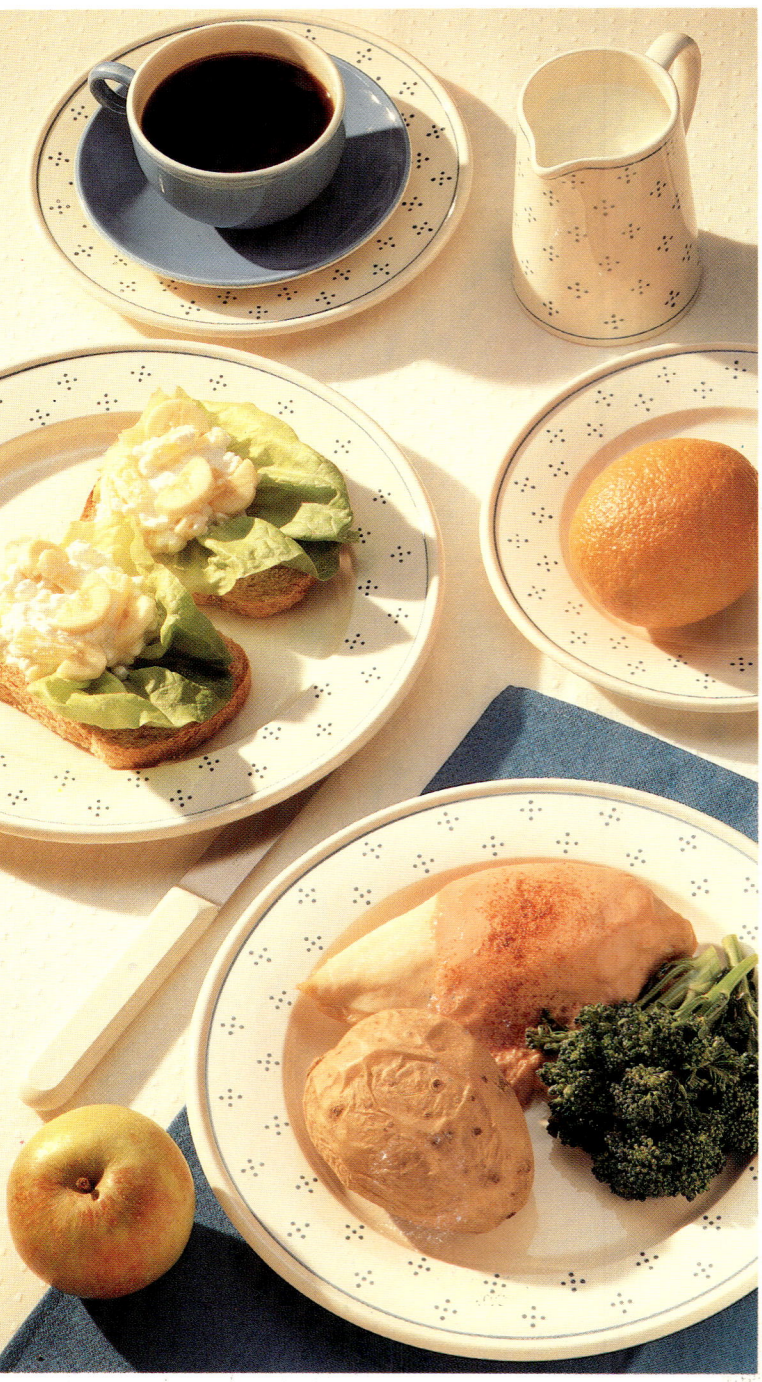

*DAY 6: Banana and Cottage Cheese Open Sandwiches; Yogurt-baked
Chicken with Vegetables*

Light Meal

Oriental Prawn Salad, and Yogurt (7.9 grams fibre)

Metric/Imperial	American
125 g/4 oz canned sweetcorn,	⅔ cup drained canned whole kernel corn
¼ red or green pepper, cored, seeded and sliced	¼ red or green pepper, seeded and sliced
125 g/4 oz bean sprouts	2 cups bean sprouts
75 g/3 oz peeled prawns	½ cup shelled shrimp
15 ml/1 tablespoon white wine or cider vinegar	1 tablespoon white wine or cider vinegar
5 ml/1 teaspoon soy sauce	1 teaspoon soy sauce
2.5 ml/½ level teaspoon runny honey	½ level teaspoon runny honey
To follow	*To follow*
1 x 150 g/5 oz carton low-fat natural yogurt	⅔ cup low-fat natural yogurt

Place the sweetcorn, pepper, beansprouts and prawns in a bowl. Mix the vinegar, soy sauce and honey together. Add to the salad and toss to mix. Serve. Follow with yogurt.

Main Meal

Bacon and Bean Risotto, and Fruit (18.1 grams fibre)

Metric/Imperial	American
1 small onion, chopped	1 small onion, chopped
1 tomato, chopped	1 tomato, chopped
¼ green or red pepper, cored, seeded, and diced	¼ green or red pepper, seeded, and chopped
25 g/1 oz mushrooms, sliced	¼ cup sliced mushrooms
25 g/1 oz long-grain brown rice	2 level tablespoons long-grain brown rice
150 ml/¼ pint water	⅔ cup water
¼ beef stock cube	½ beef bouillon cube
1 x 100 g/3½ oz bacon or ham steak	1 x 3½ oz bacon or ham steak
1 x 225 g/8 oz can red kidney beans, drained	1 x 8 oz can red kidney beans, drained
To follow	*To follow*
1 medium pear	1 medium pear

Place the prepared vegetables in a small saucepan with the rice, water and stock cube (bouillon cube). Cover the pan, bring to the boil and stir once. Cover the pan again, reduce heat and simmer gently for 30 minutes. Check occasionally while cooking, and if water has evaporated add a little more to prevent the rice from sticking. Grill (broil) the bacon or ham steak well. Discard any visible fat and cut the lean meat into small pieces. Add to the pan and cook for a further 5–10 minutes until rice is tender and the water absorbed. Add the beans, heat through and serve. Follow with the pear.

Snack 1

HAM AND TOMATO SANDWICH (5.6 grams fibre)
Discard all visible fat from 25 g/1 oz lean cooked ham. Slice 1 small tomato. Make into a sandwich with 2 × 25 g/1 oz slices wholemeal bread and 10 ml/2 level teaspoons low-fat spread.

Snack 2

COTTAGE CHEESE, APPLE AND SULTANAS (7 grams fibre)
Core and chop 1 medium apple, mix with 125 g/4 oz/½ cup natural cottage cheese and 10 ml/1 level tablespoon sultanas (golden raisins). Serve with 2 calorie-reduced bran crispbreads.

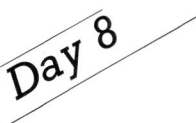
Day 8

Breakfast
Light Meal

BRAN FLAKES AND BANANA
(6.4 grams fibre)
Slice 1 small banana. Serve with 25 g/1 oz/1 cup Bran Flakes (bran breakfast cereal) and 150 ml/¼ pint/⅔ cup skimmed milk.

Cheese and Chutney Toast, and Fruit (7.6 grams fibre)

Metric/Imperial	American
1 x 40 g/1½ oz slice wholemeal bread	1 x 1½ oz slice wholemeal bread
5 ml/1 level teaspoon chutney	1 level teaspoon chutney
1 ring canned pineapple in natural juice, drained	1 ring canned pineapple in natural juice, drained
40 g/1½ oz Lancashire or Edam cheese, grated	½ cup grated Lancashire or Dutch cheese
To follow	*To follow*
1 medium orange	1 medium orange

Toast the bread on one side only. Spread the untoasted side with chutney and place pineapple on top. Sprinkle with cheese and grill (broil) until cheese has melted. Follow with the orange.

Main Meal

Chicken, Peas and Sweetcorn, and Raspberry Yogurt (33 grams fibre)

Metric/Imperial	American
1 x 175 g/6 oz chicken breast	1 x 6 oz chicken breast
75 g/3 oz frozen peas	½ cup frozen peas
1 x 193 g/7 oz can sweetcorn	1 x 7 oz can whole kernel corn
To follow	*To follow*
1 x 150 g/5 oz carton low-fat natural yogurt	⅔ cup low-fat natural yogurt
125 g/4 oz fresh or frozen and thawed raspberries	1 scant cup fresh or frozen and thawed raspberries

Grill (broil) the chicken and discard the skin. Boil the peas, and drain. Heat the sweetcorn (whole kernel corn) in a small saucepan. Serve the vegetables with the chicken. Follow with the yogurt, mixed with the raspberries.

Snack 1

EGG AND SAUCY BEANS
(11 grams fibre)
Place 1 × 150 g/5 oz can baked beans in tomato sauce in a saucepan. Add 5 ml/1 level teaspoon sweet pickle and 5 ml/1 teaspoon Worcestershire sauce. Poach 1 size 3 (medium) egg and serve on the beans.

Snack 2

PÂTÉ AND TOAST
(4.5 grams fibre)
Toast 1 × 40 g/1½ oz slice wholemeal bread. Spread with 40 g/1½ oz ham and tongue pâté. Arrange 1 medium sliced tomato and 25 g/1 oz sliced cucumber on top.

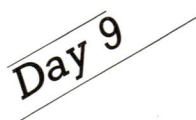

Day 9

Breakfast

ALL BRAN AND RAISINS
(13.4 grams fibre)
Mix 40 g/1½ oz/10 level tablespoons All Bran (bran cereal) with 30 ml/2 level tablespoons raisins in a serving bowl. Serve with 115 ml/4 fl oz/½ cup skimmed milk.

Light Meal

Cheese Salad Sandwich, and Fruit (10.8 grams fibre)

Metric/Imperial	American
2 x 40 g/1½ oz slices wholemeal bread	2 x 1½ oz slices wholemeal bread
15 ml/1 level tablespoon cheese spread, plain or flavoured	1 level tablespoon cheese spread, plain or flavored
1 small tomato, sliced	1 small tomato, sliced
1 spring onion, chopped	1 scallion, chopped
1 lettuce leaf	1 lettuce leaf
a few slices of cucumber	a few slices of cucumber
To follow	To follow
1 medium apple	1 medium apple

Spread bread with cheese spread. Make into a sandwich with the salad vegetables. Follow with the apple.

Main Meal

Vegetable Pie, and Fruit (20.1 grams fibre)

Metric/Imperial	American
1 x 175 g/6 oz potato	1 x 6 oz potato
75 g/3 oz carrots, sliced	½ cup sliced carrots
125 g/4 oz frozen broad beans	⅔ cup frozen fava beans
50 g/2 oz button mushrooms	½ cup button mushrooms
15 ml/1 level tablespoon cornflour	1 level tablespoon cornstarch
30 ml/2 level tablespoons skimmed milk powder	2 level tablespoons skimmed milk powder
15 ml/1 level tablespoon chopped fresh parsley	1 tablespoon chopped fresh parsley
salt and pepper	salt and pepper
25 g/1 oz Edam cheese, grated	¼ cup grated Dutch cheese
15 g/½ oz fresh wholemeal breadcrumbs	¾ cup fresh wholemeal breadcrumbs
To follow	To follow
1 medium orange	1 medium orange

Bake the potato in a preheated moderately hot oven (200°C/400°F/Gas Mark 6) until soft when pinched (about 45 minutes). Boil the carrots in salted water for 15 minutes. Add broad beans (fava beans) and mushrooms and cook for a further 5 minutes. Drain, reserving 115 ml/ 4 fl oz/½ cup water. In a small bowl blend cornflour (cornstarch) and skimmed milk powder with 45 ml/3 tablespoons cold water. Stir in the reserved vegetable water and return to the pan. Bring to the boil, stirring all the time. Reduce heat and simmer for 2 minutes. Add the vegetables and parsley and heat through. Season with salt and pepper and turn into an ovenproof dish. Sprinkle the grated cheese on top with the breadcrumbs. Grill (broil) until the cheese melts, and serve. Follow with the orange.

Snack 1

MUSHROOM OMELETTE
(2.1 grams fibre)
Slice 75 g/3 oz/¾ cup mushrooms and cook in a little water to cover for 3–5 minutes. Melt 7 g/¼ oz/1½ level teaspoons low-fat spread in a non-stick omelette pan. Beat 2 size 3 (medium) eggs, pour into the pan and make an omelette. Add the drained mushrooms. Slide the omelette on to a serving dish, fold over and serve.

Snack 2

SOUP AND WHOLEMEAL ROLL
(4.2 grams fibre)
Heat 1 × 275 g/10 oz can low-calorie tomato or vegetable soup. Serve with 1 × 45 g/1¾ oz wholemeal roll.

Day 10

Breakfast

SULTANA BRAN
(7.3 grams fibre)
Serve 50 g/2 oz/½ cup Sultana Bran (bran breakfast cereal with golden raisins) with 150 ml/¼ pint/ ⅔ cup skimmed milk.

Light Meal

Egg Florentine, and Fruit (7.4 grams fibre)

Metric/Imperial	American
25 g/1 oz wholewheat spaghetti	⅓ cup wholewheat spaghetti
75 g/3 oz fresh or frozen spinach	3 oz fresh or frozen spinach
1 egg, size 3	1 medium egg
salt and pepper	salt and pepper
To follow	To follow
1 medium apple	1 medium apple

Cook the spaghetti in plenty of salted water until tender. Cook the spinach, drain well and chop. Poach the egg in water. Arrange the spaghetti on a hot serving dish, and top with spinach, seasoned with salt and pepper. Place the egg on top and serve. Follow with the apple.

Main Meal

Walnut Stuffed Potato, and Fruit (6.8 grams fibre)

Metric/Imperial	American
1 x 225 g/8 oz potato	1 x 8 oz potato
125 g/4 oz cottage cheese with chives	½ cup cottage cheese with chives
4 walnut halves, chopped	4 walnut halves, chopped
salt and pepper	salt and pepper
To follow	To follow
1 medium orange	1 medium orange

Bake the potato in its jacket in a preheated moderately hot oven (200°C/ 400°F/Gas Mark 6) for 1 hour or until soft. Cut in half lengthways and scoop out the flesh. Retain the shells. Mash the flesh with the cottage cheese. Add the walnuts, salt and pepper and then pile back into the potato shells. Reheat for about 10 minutes. Follow with the orange.

Snack 1

BAKED BEANS ON TOAST
(20.2 grams fibre)
Heat 1 × 225 g/8 oz can baked beans in tomato sauce in a saucepan. Serve with 1 × 40 g/1½ oz slice wholemeal toast.

Snack 2

DRINKING CHOCOLATE AND BISCUITS
(2.1 grams fibre)
Heat 225 ml/8 fl oz/1 cup skimmed milk until boiling. Stir into a mug containing 20 ml/2 rounded teaspoons drinking chocolate (sweetened cocoa). Serve with 3 fig rolls (cookies) or 2 digestive biscuits.

Light Meal

Prawn Sandwich, and Fruity Yogurt (8.3 grams fibre)

Metric/Imperial
2 x 25 g/1 oz slices wholemeal bread
50 g/2 oz peeled prawns
15 ml/1 level tablespoor. low-calorie seafood dressing
To follow
1 x 150 g/5 oz carton low-fat natural yogurt
1 small banana
15 ml/1 level tablespoon sultanas

American
2 x 1 oz slices wholemeal bread
⅓ cup shelled shrimp
1 level tablespoon low-calorie seafood dressing
To follow
⅔ cup low-fat natural yogurt
1 small banana
1 level tablespoon golden raisins

Mix the prawns (shrimp) with the dressing. Make into a sandwich with the bread. Peel and slice the banana. Mix into the yogurt with the sultanas (golden raisins) and serve.

Main Meal

Fish and Tomato Wholemeal Pie (15.1 grams fibre)

Metric/Imperial
1 x 175 g/6 oz potato
175 g/6 oz cod or haddock fillet
125 g/4 oz canned tomatoes, drained and roughly chopped
50 g/2 oz mushrooms, roughly chopped
a pinch of mixed herbs
salt and pepper
25 g/1 oz wholemeal breadcrumbs
25 g/1 oz Edam cheese, grated
175 g/6 oz broccoli

American
1 x 6 oz potato
6 oz cod or haddock fillet
½ cup drained canned tomatoes, roughly chopped
½ cup chopped mushrooms
a pinch of mixed herbs
salt and pepper
½ cup wholemeal bread crumbs
¼ cup grated Dutch cheese
1 cup broccoli

Bake the potato in a preheated moderate oven (180°C/350°F, Gas Mark 4) for 45 minutes or until soft when pinched. Meanwhile, place the fish in an ovenproof dish. Season the tomatoes and mushrooms with herbs, salt and pepper and spread over the fish. Cover the dish with foil. When the potato has been baking for 15 minutes, place the fish dish beside it and bake for 15 minutes more. Remove the fish from the oven and top with the breadcrumbs and grated cheese. Return to the oven for 10–15 minutes, by which time the potato should be cooked. Cook the broccoli in boiling, salted water, drain and serve with the pie and the baked potato.

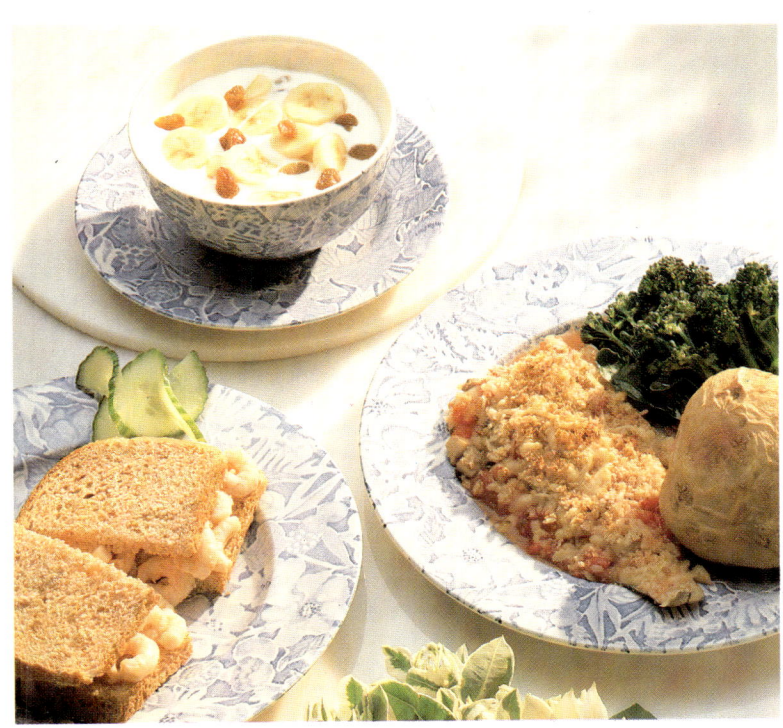

DAY 11: Prawn Sandwich and Fruity Yogurt; Fish and Tomato Wholemeal Pie

Day 11

Snack 1

SOUP AND WHOLEMEAL ROLL
(4.2 grams fibre)
Heat 1 × 275 g/10 oz can low-calorie tomato, beef and vegetable or vegetable soup and serve with 1 × 45 g/1¾ oz wholemeal roll.

Snack 2

MUSHROOMS ON TOAST
(2.4 grams fibre)
Toast 1 × 25 g/1 oz slice wholemeal bread. Spread with 5 ml/1 level teaspoon low-fat spread and 5 ml/1 level teaspoon yeast extract. Heat 1 × 213 g/7½ oz can mushrooms in brine; drain and serve on the toast.

Breakfast

ALL BRAN AND DRIED APRICOTS
(21.4 grams fibre)
Mix 50 g/2 oz/1 cup All Bran (bran breakfast cereal) with 4 dried apricots in an individual serving bowl. Serve with 150 ml/¼ pint/⅔ cup skimmed milk.

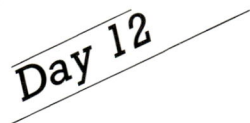

Day 12

Breakfast
Light Meal

Smoked Haddock with Vegetables (11 grams fibre)

Metric/Imperial
150 g/5 oz smoked haddock
75 g/3 oz frozen peas
1 x 40 g/1½ oz slice wholemeal
  bread
5 ml/1 level teaspoon low-fat
  spread
1 tomato, sliced
parsley to garnish

American
5 oz finnan haddie
½ cup frozen peas
1 x 1½ oz slice wholemeal bread
1 level teaspoon low-fat spread
1 tomato, sliced
parsley to garnish

Poach the haddock (finnan haddie) in water. Cook the peas. Spread the bread with low-fat spread. Top the haddock (finnan haddie) with parsley and serve with sliced tomato, peas and bread.

ORANGE, WHOLEMEAL TOAST AND MARMALADE OR HONEY
(5.7 grams fibre)
Start with 1 small orange. To follow, spread 1 × 40 g/1½ oz slice wholemeal toast with 10 ml/2 level teaspoons low-fat spread and 10 ml/2 level teaspoons honey, marmalade or jam.

Main Meal

Chicken in Mushroom Sauce with Vegetables
(16.4 grams fibre)

Metric/Imperial
1 x 175 g/6 oz potato
175 ml/6 fl oz skimmed milk
15 ml/1 level tablespoon
  cornflour
50 g/2 oz mushrooms, chopped
salt and pepper
a pinch of nutmeg
175 g/6 oz chicken breast
125 g/4 oz French beans
125 g/4 oz canned sweetcorn,
  drained
chopped parsley to garnish

American
1 x 6 oz potato
¾ cup skimmed milk
1 level tablespoon cornstarch
½ cup finely chopped mushrooms
salt and pepper
a pinch of nutmeg
6 oz chicken breast
1 cup green beans
⅔ cup drained canned whole
  kernel corn
chopped parsley to garnish

Bake the potato in its jacket in a moderately hot oven (200°C/400°F/Gas Mark 6) for about 45 minutes or until soft when pinched. In a cup blend a little skimmed milk with the cornflour (cornstarch) then pour the remainder into a saucepan and heat. Stir the cornflour (cornstarch) mixture into the hot milk. Add the mushrooms and season with salt, pepper and nutmeg. Bring to the boil, reduce heat and simmer for 2 minutes, stirring constantly. Grill (broil) the chicken, remove and discard the skin. Cook the vegetables and drain. Pour the sauce over the chicken, sprinkle with parsley and serve with the beans and corn.

Snack 1

MUESLI YOGURT
(4.5 grams fibre)
Chop 2 dried apricots. Place 1 × 150 g/5 oz carton low-fat natural yogurt in an individual serving bowl. Stir in the apricots with 15 ml/1 level tablespoon sultanas (golden raisins) and 30 ml/2 level tablespoons muesli (Swiss-style cereal) and serve.

Snack 2

CHEESE AND FRUIT
(3.5 grams fibre)
Cube 25 g/1 oz Edam cheese. Core and slice 1 apple. Halve and remove pips from 75 g/3 oz green grapes. Serve the cheese with the fruit.

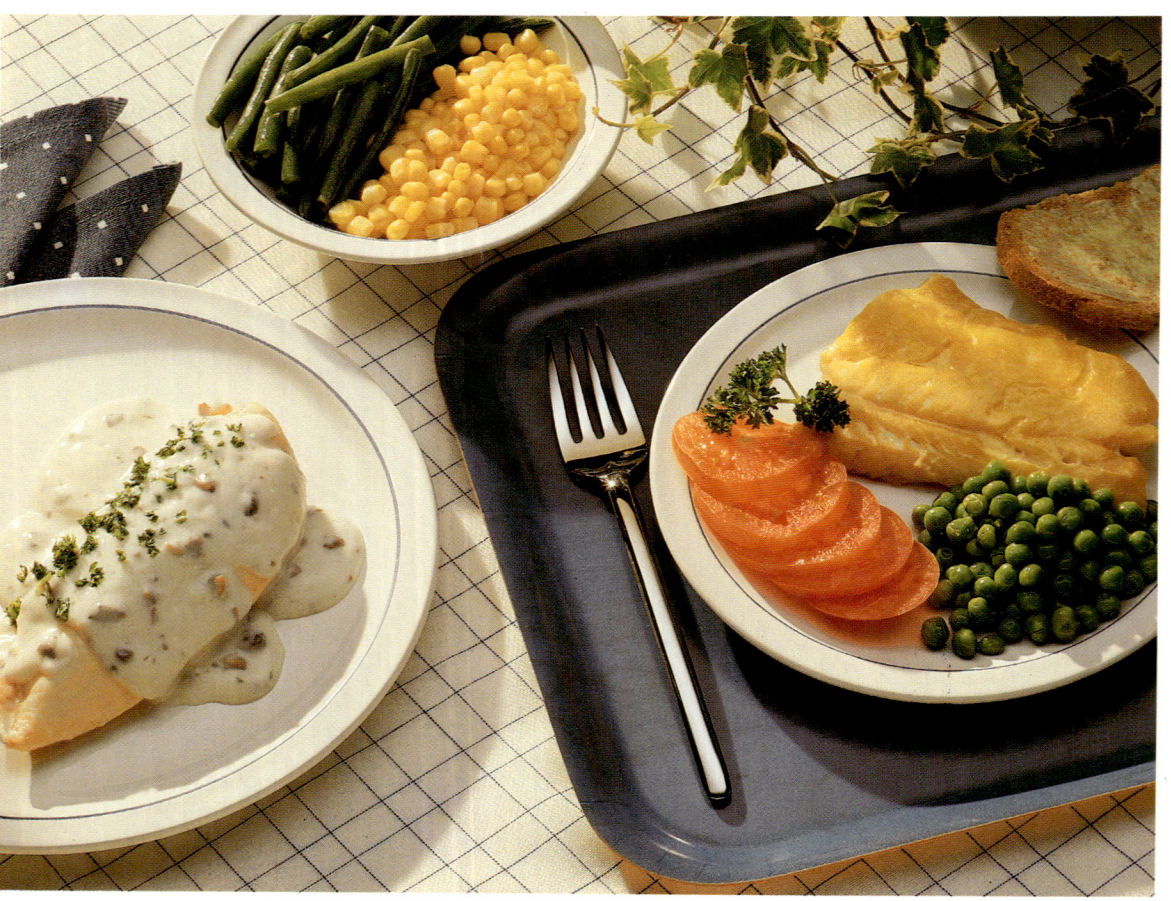

DAY 12: Smoked Haddock with Vegetables; Chicken in Mushroom Sauce with Vegetables

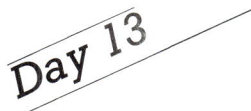

Day 13

Breakfast

Light Meal

GRAPEFRUIT, AND POACHED EGG ON TOAST
(4.1 grams fibre)
Start with ½ grapefruit, sprinkled with 5 ml/1 level teaspoon fructose. Poach 1 size 3 (medium) egg. Serve on 1 × 40 g/1½ oz slice wholemeal toast.

Saucy Beans on Toast, and Fruit with Ice Cream
(25.1 grams fibre)

Metric/Imperial	American
1 x 150 g/5 oz can baked beans in tomato sauce	1 x 5 oz can baked beans in tomato sauce
5 ml/1 level teaspoon sweet pickle	1 level teaspoon sweet pickle
5 ml/1 teaspoon Worcestershire sauce	1 teaspoon Worcestershire sauce
1 x 40 g/1½ oz slice wholemeal bread	1 x 1½ oz slice wholemeal bread
To follow	*To follow*
150 g/5 oz raspberries	1 cup raspberries
50 g/2 oz vanilla ice cream	2 small scoops vanilla ice cream

Heat the beans, pickle and Worcestershire sauce together in a saucepan. Toast the bread, top with the beans and serve. Follow with raspberries and ice cream.

Main Meal

Mixed Grill with Vegetables, and Fruit
(20.9 grams fibre)

Metric/Imperial	American
125 g/4 oz lamb's liver	4 oz lamb's liver
1 lamb's kidney	1 lamb's kidney
2 rashers streaky bacon	2 slices bacon
1 tomato, halved	1 tomato, halved
125 g/4 oz mushrooms	1 cup mushrooms
125 g/4 oz carrots, sliced	⅔ cup carrots, sliced
125 g/4 oz frozen peas	⅔ cup frozen peas
To follow	*To follow*
1 medium pear	1 medium pear

Wash and dry the liver, and halve and core the kidney. Grill (broil) the liver, kidney, bacon and tomato until well cooked. Poach the mushrooms in a little stock or water. Boil the other vegetables, and drain. Serve the mixed grill with the vegetables. Follow with the pear.

Snack 1

NUTTY CHEESE OPEN SANDWICH
(3.6 grams fibre)
Chop 6 toasted hazelnuts and mix with 75 g/3 oz/3 level tablespoons cottage cheese. Spread on 1 × 40 g/1½ oz slice of wholemeal bread and serve.

Snack 2

ALL BRAN AND RAISINS
(15.4 grams fibre)
Serve 25 g/1 oz/8 tablespoons All Bran (bran breakfast cereal) with 15 ml/1 level tablespoon sultanas (golden raisins) or raisins and 150 ml/¼ pint/⅔ cup skimmed milk.

Day 14

Breakfast

Light Meal

ALL BRAN AND FRUIT
(16 grams fibre)
Place 25 g/1 oz/½ cup All Bran (bran breakfast cereal) in a bowl. Stir in 1 small sliced banana and 2 chopped dried figs. Serve with 150 ml/¼ pint/⅔ cup skimmed milk.

Salmon Salad and Wholemeal Roll (5.5 grams fibre)

Metric/Imperial	American
1 x 100 g/3½ oz can pink or red salmon, drained and flaked	1 x 3½ oz can pink or red salmon, drained and flaked
green salad (no avocado)	green salad (no avocado)
1 tomato, sliced	1 tomato, sliced
15 ml/1 tablespoon oil-free French dressing	1 tablespoon oil-free French dressing
1 x 45 g/1¾ oz wholemeal roll	1 x 1¾ oz wholemeal roll
10 ml/2 level teaspoons low-fat spread	2 level teaspoons low-fat spread

Arrange the salmon, salad and tomato on a plate (or in a container if it is to be a packed lunch). At serving time, toss the salad with the dressing and serve with the wholemeal roll spread with the low-fat spread.

Main Meal

Liver Casserole with Brown Rice (16.0 grams fibre)

Metric/Imperial	American
125 g/4 oz lamb's liver, sliced	4 oz lamb's liver, sliced
10 ml/2 level teaspoons flour	2 level teaspoons flour
50 g/2 oz mushrooms, sliced	½ cup sliced mushrooms
15 g/½ oz onion, chopped	1 level tablespoon chopped onion
1 large tomato, chopped	1 large tomato, chopped
salt and pepper	salt and pepper
a pinch of mixed herbs	a pinch of mixed herbs
½ beef stock cube	1 beef bouillon cube
75 ml/3 fl oz water	6 tablespoons water
25 g/1 oz brown rice	2 level tablespoons brown rice
125 g/4 oz frozen peas	⅔ cup frozen peas
125 g/4 oz carrots, sliced	⅔ cup sliced carrots

Toss the liver in flour. Place in a casserole with the mushrooms, onion, tomato, seasoning and herbs. Dissolve the stock cube in the water and add. Cover and place in a preheated oven (180°C/350°F/Gas Mark 4) for 45 minutes. Serve with the cooked rice and vegetables.

Snack 1

HAM SANDWICH
(5.6 grams fibre)
Discard all visible fat from 25 g/1 oz lean ham. Spread 15 ml/1 level tablespoon low-calorie salad dressing on 2 × 25 g/1 oz slices of wholemeal bread. Make a sandwich with lettuce, 1 sliced tomato and the ham.

Snack 2

COTTAGE CHEESE AND CRISPBREADS
(4.8 grams fibre)
Season 125 g/4 oz/½ cup natural cottage cheese with freshly ground black pepper. Spread on 4 calorie-reduced bran crispbreads and top with slices of cucumber.

The Flexible Solution

Do you lead a rather erratic life and find you can't stick to a set diet plan? Or do you just want to eat more some days than others? If your weight problem consists of more than a couple of excess stone, you'll need a diet you can follow for just as long as it takes you to get right down to target. The Flexible Solution will do just that and will allow you to lose weight at exactly the rate you wish.

If you are feeling really determined and your willpower is at its highest peak you can keep to a strict 1,000 Calories a day total. Just choose any of the meals and snacks which add up to that amount. However, one morning your resolve may be lion-strong but by the evening of the same day you may lack the backbone of a jelly fish. The Flexible Solution will take care of these fluctuating moods. On days when your willpower wavers you could eat up to 2,000 Calories' worth of meals and still continue to lose weight. The Flexible Solution allows you the freedom to choose from snacks that start at 50 Calories and meals that go up to 500 Calories (all nicely rounded for easy counting).

There are lots of low-calorie meals from which you can choose to start the day – willpower is usually at its strongest in the morning – or to eat as a suppertime snack. If you prefer to eat vegetarian there are meals to suit you, and there are four-portion meals to share with family or friends (non-dieters can be served with extra rice, pasta or vegetables if you wish). There are drinks which you can count into your allowance on a social occasion, although if you eat out regularly the Dine and Diet Plan will be the better diet for you to follow.

It really doesn't matter in what order you eat your meals or exactly what items you choose (although you should vary your choice for good nutrition and eat some higher calorie meals, not just snacks). As long as your weekly total is no more than 10,500 Calories you will lose weight. You'll find milk listed in the snacks sections and you'll benefit in a healthy way by allowing yourself 275 ml/½ pint each day. Alcohol and sugary foods add little of nutritional value to your diet, so keep these to a minimum.

Recheck the chart at the beginning of the book as you shed each stone, for as you get lighter it may be best for you to swap to another diet plan. Or if you are continuing to lose weight at a steady rate you may keep to the Flexible Solution – it lets you live your life and lose weight the way you choose.

Diet Rules

1 Decide on your day's calorie allowance and choose foods from any of the groups to add up to your total. Remember, that your weekly total should not exceed 10,500 Calories, an average of 1500 Calories a day.

2 Milk is given in the 100-Calorie snack section and if you wish to add it to tea and coffee you must

count this into your day's total.

3 Black tea and coffee can be drunk freely, with artificial sweetener if you wish. You are also allowed unlimited amounts of water, yeast extract drinks and low-calorie squashes and mixers.

4 For good nutrition, make your meal choices as varied as possible and try to include at least one liver meal once a week.

50-Calorie Snacks and Drinks

FRUIT
Choose any one of the following:
1 medium apple
1 medium pear
1 medium nectarine
1 medium orange
1 small banana
1 large grapefruit
1 large peach
2 kiwifruit
1 pomegranate
2 tangerines or mandarin oranges, each weighing 75 g/3 oz
350 g/12 oz slice melon, weighed with skin
125 g/4 oz/1 cup cherries
150 g/5 oz dessert plums, weighed with stones
75 g/3 oz/¾ cup grapes
225 g/8 oz/1⅔ cups raspberries, fresh or frozen
225 g/8 oz/1⅔ cups strawberries, fresh or frozen
225 g/8 oz/1⅔ cups blackberries, fresh or frozen
5 dried apricots
3 fresh dates
5 dried prunes

BISCUITS
Choose any one of the following:
2 rich tea fingers
2 morning coffee biscuits
2 sponge fingers (lady fingers)
1 medium digestive biscuit (graham cracker)
2 chocolate finger biscuits

DRINKS
Choose any one of the following:
Tomato juice
2 small bottles tomato juice or tomato cocktail, 120 ml/4 fl oz/½ cup each

Whisky and water
25 ml/1 fl oz/2 tablespoons whisky
water, ice or soda (carbonated water)

Brandy and American
25 ml/1 fl oz/2 tablespoons brandy
1 small bottle low-calorie American ginger ale

Rum and Cola
25 ml/1 fl oz/2 tablespoons white or dark rum
1 small bottle low-calorie cola

Whisky and dry
25 ml/1 fl oz/2 tablespoons whisky or bourbon
1 small bottle low-calorie dry ginger ale

Gin and bitter lemon
25 ml/1 fl oz/2 tablespoons gin
1 small bottle low-calorie bitter lemon

Sherry
50 ml/2 fl oz/¼ cup sherry

Vermouth
50 ml/2 fl oz/¼ cup dry white vermouth
ice and lemon

Kirsch
25 ml/1 fl oz/2 tablespoons Kirsch

Vodka and tonic
25 ml/1 fl oz/2 tablespoons vodka
1 small bottle low-calorie tonic

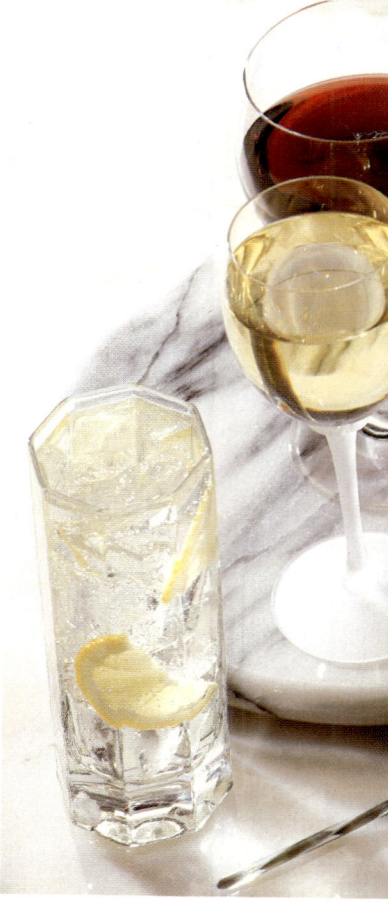

100-Calorie Snacks and Drinks

MILK
275 ml/½ pint/1¼ cups skimmed milk *or* 190 ml/⅓ pint/⅞ cup semi-skimmed milk *or* 150 ml/¼ pint/⅝ cup whole milk

FRUIT JUICE
275 ml/½ pint/1¼ cups unsweetened apple, grapefruit or orange juice

DRINKING CHOCOLATE
20 ml/2 rounded teaspoons drinking chocolate powder (sweetened cocoa), mixed with 150 ml/¼ pint/⅝ cup hot skimmed milk and artificial sweetener (optional). Top up with hot water (optional).

FRUIT
Choose any one of the following:
1 large apple
1 large orange
1 large banana
1 medium mango
40 g/1½ oz currants
40 g/1½ oz dried stoned dates
40 g/1½ oz dried figs
40 g/1½ oz raisins
40 g/1½ oz sultanas (golden raisins)

TOAST AND MARMALADE, JAM OR HONEY
1 × 25 g/1 oz slice wholemeal toast spread with 5 ml/1 level teaspoon low-fat spread and 5 ml/1 level teaspoon marmalade, jam or honey.

TOAST WITH CHEESE SPREAD
1 × 25 g/1 oz slice wholemeal toast spread with 15 ml/1 level tablespoon cheese spread.

ICE CREAM
50 g/2 oz/2 scoops vanilla or strawberry ice cream.

CRISPBREADS WITH CHEESE SPREAD AND TOMATO
Spread 15 ml/1 level tablespoon cheese spread over 2 calorie-reduced crispbreads. Top with 1 thinly sliced tomato.

CRISPBREADS WITH COTTAGE CHEESE AND GRAPES
Spread 30 ml/2 level tablespoons cottage cheese over 2 calorie-reduced crispbreads. Halve and de-pip 50 g/2 oz/⅓ cup grapes. Arrange on top, cut side down.

CRISPBREADS WITH BANANA
Mash one small banana and spread over 2 calorie-reduced crispbreads.

ALL BRAN
Place 25 g/1 oz/¼ cup All Bran cereal in a bowl and pour over 75 ml/3 fl oz/⅓ cup skimmed milk to serve.

HONEY YOGURT
Stir 5 ml/1 level teaspoon honey into 1 × 150 g/5 oz carton/⅔ cup low-fat natural yogurt.

FRUIT YOGURT
Pour 1 × 150 g/5 oz carton/⅔ cup low-fat natural yogurt into an individual serving bowl, stir in 50 g/2 oz/½ cup strawberries or raspberries (fresh or defrosted if frozen) and add a few drops of artificial sweetener if needed.

TOAST AND YEAST EXTRACT
1 × 25 g/1 oz slice wholemeal toast spread with 10 ml/2 level teaspoons low-fat spread and 5 ml/1 level teaspoon yeast extract.

DRINKS
Choose any one of the following:

Wine
150 ml/5 fl oz/⅝ cup dry or medium-dry red, rosé or white wine

Martini and lemonade
50 ml/2 fl oz/4 tablespoons Martini Bianco or Cinzano Bianco
1 small bottle low-calorie lemonade

Liqueurs
25 ml/1 fl oz/2 tablespoons Tia Maria, Grand Marnier, Southern Comfort, Cointreau, Drambuie or Benedictine

Cider
275 ml/½ pint/1¼ cups cider

Ale
275 ml/½ pint/1¼ cups brown ale, pale ale or light ale

Bitter
275 ml/½ pint/1¼ cups bitter (dark beer)

Sherry and nibbles
50 ml/2 fl oz/4 tablespoons sherry
6 cocktail gherkins

Port
50 ml/2 fl oz/4 tablespoons port

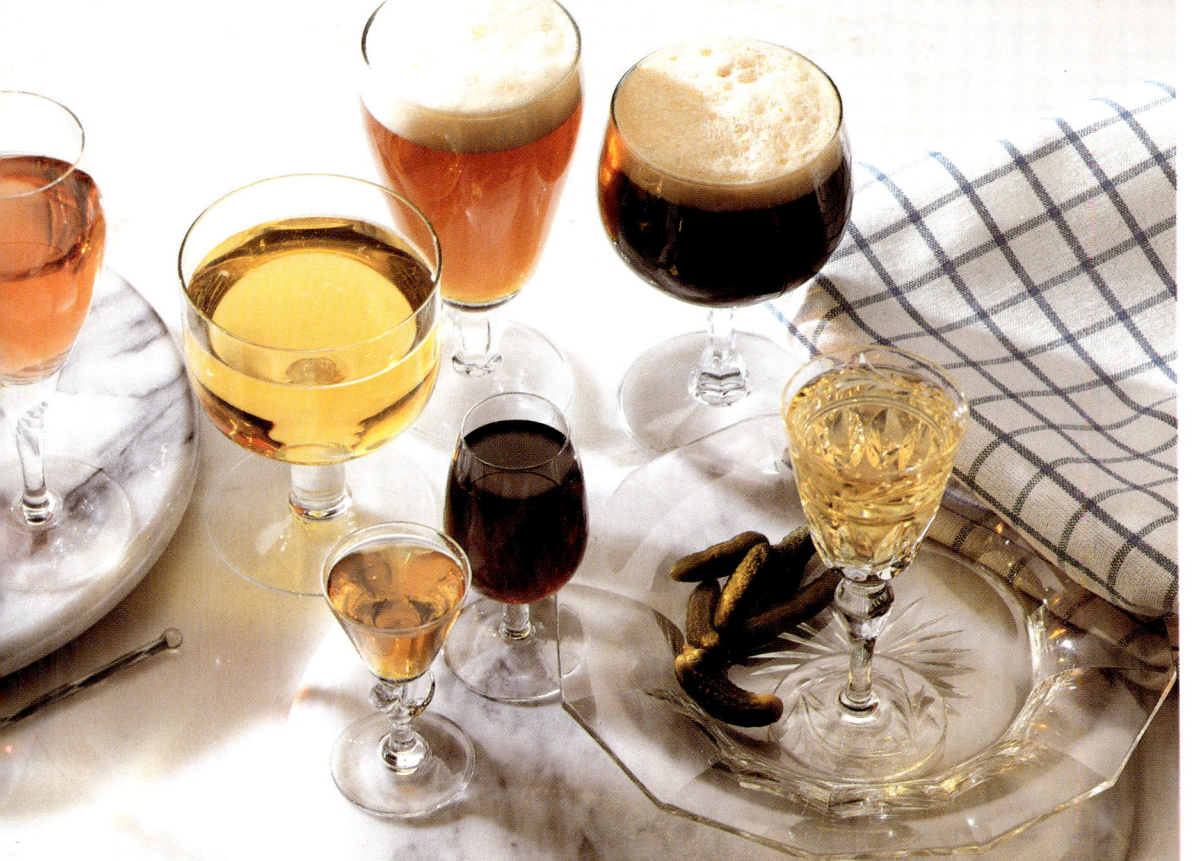

A selection of 100-Calorie Drinks

150-Calorie Snack Meals

CHEESE SPREAD AND PICKLE ON CRISPBREAD
Spread 15 ml/1 level tablespoon cheese spread over 3 calorie-reduced crispbreads and top with 15 ml/1 level tablespoon sweet pickle.

FISH PASTE AND CUCUMBER CRISPBREADS
Spread a 35 g/1¼ oz pot of fish paste over 4 calorie-reduced crispbreads and top with a few cucumber slices.

YOGURT WITH BANANA
Pour 1 × 150 g/5 oz carton/⅔ cup low-fat natural yogurt into a bowl and stir in 1 small peeled and sliced banana.

FRUIT YOGURT
1 × 150 g/5 oz carton/⅔ cup low-fat fruit yogurt.

MUESLI
Put 25 g/1 oz/⅓ cup muesli (Swiss-style cereal) into an individual serving bowl and stir in 120 ml/4 fl oz/½ cup skimmed milk to serve.

CEREAL
Put 25 g/1 oz/1 cup cornflakes or Rice Krispies into an individual serving bowl and pour over 150 ml/¼ pint/⅔ cup skimmed milk.

MUESLI YOGURT
Put 30 ml/2 level tablespoons muesli (Swiss-style cereal) into an individual serving bowl and stir in 1 × 150 g/5 oz carton/⅔ cup low-fat natural yogurt to serve.

SOUP AND BREAD
Heat 1 × 275 g/10 oz can low-calorie soup, any flavour, pour into a warmed soup bowl and serve with 1 × 35 g/1¼ oz slice of wholemeal bread.

BUTTERED CRUMPET
Toast 1 crumpet (muffin) and spread with 10 ml/2 level teaspoons butter or margarine.

CRISPS
1 × 25 g/1 oz packet crisps (chips), any flavour.

200-Calorie Meals

WEETABIX WITH DRIED APRICOTS
Put 2 Weetabix (wheat breakfast biscuits) into an individual serving bowl. Sprinkle with 3 chopped dried apricots and pour over 115 ml/4 fl oz/½ cup skimmed milk to serve.

SHREDDED WHEAT WITH BANANAS
Put 1 Shredded Wheat into an individual serving bowl. Top with a small peeled and sliced banana and pour over 150 ml/¼ pint/⅔ cup skimmed milk to serve.

FRUIT JUICE AND ALL BRAN
Serve 150 ml/¼ pint/⅔ cup unsweetened apple, grapefruit or orange juice in a glass, followed by 40 g/1½ oz/⅓ cup All Bran cereal in an individual serving bowl with 120 ml/4 fl oz/½ cup skimmed milk.

CEREAL WITH BANANA
Put 25 g/1 oz/1 cup Cornflakes, Rice Krispies or Ricicles into an individual serving bowl with a small peeled and sliced banana and pour over 120 ml/4 fl oz/½ cup skimmed milk to serve.

FRUIT JUICE AND CEREAL
Serve 150 ml/¼ pint/⅔ cup unsweetened apple, grapefruit or orange juice in a glass, followed by 25 g/1 oz/1 cup Cornflakes or Rice Krispies in an individual serving bowl with 5 ml/1 level teaspoon sugar and 120 ml/4 fl oz/½ cup skimmed milk.

POACHED EGG ON TOAST
Poach 1 size 3 (medium) egg. Toast one 35 g/1¼ oz slice of bread. Spread with 10 ml/2 level teaspoons low-fat spread and serve topped with the poached egg.

RICE PUDDING WITH SULTANAS
Pour 1 × 175 g/6 oz can creamed rice pudding into a small saucepan, stir in 15 ml/1 level tablespoon sultanas (golden raisins) and heat through gently.

SCRAMBLED EGG ON TOAST
Lightly beat 1 size 3 (medium) egg and 15 ml/1 tablespoon skimmed milk together. Season with salt and pepper. Melt 10 ml/2 level teaspoons low-fat spread in a non-stick saucepan, pour in the egg mixture and cook over a low heat, stirring, until the egg is just cooked and creamy. Toast 1 × 35 g/1¼ oz slice of wholemeal bread and pile the egg on top.

BAKED BEANS ON TOAST
Toast 1 × 35 g/1¼ oz slice of wholemeal bread. Heat 150 g/5 oz baked beans in tomato sauce in a saucepan and spoon over the toast to serve.

PEANUT BUTTER SANDWICH
Spread 2 × 25 g/1 oz slices wholemeal bread with 10 ml/2 level teaspoons peanut butter and make into a sandwich.

BANANA AND HONEY SANDWICH
Spread 1 × 25 g/1 oz slice wholemeal bread with 5 ml/1 level teaspoon honey. Spread a small peeled and mashed banana on top. Top with another 25 g/1 oz wholemeal bread slice.

FRUIT JUICE PLUS TOAST AND MARMALADE
Serve 150 ml/¼ pint/⅔ cup unsweetened apple, grapefruit or orange juice in a glass. Toast 1 × 35 g/1¼ oz slice wholemeal bread and spread with 10 ml/2 level teaspoons low-fat spread and 10 ml/2 level teaspoons marmalade.

TOAST WITH CURD CHEESE AND FRUIT
Toast 1 × 25 g/1 oz slice wholemeal bread and spread with 50 g/2 oz/¼ cup curd cheese. Serve 1 satsuma or kiwifruit to follow.

GRAPEFRUIT PLUS BACON AND TOMATOES
Serve ½ grapefruit with artificial sweetener if needed. Cook 2 rashers back bacon under a preheated grill (broiler), until crisp. Grill (broil) 2 tomatoes without added fat and serve with the bacon.

SMOKED HADDOCK
Cook 1 × 175 g/6 oz packet frozen smoked haddock (finnan haddie) with butter according to packet instructions. Serve with 1 calorie-reduced crispbread.

SAUSAGES AND BAKED BEANS
Grill (broil) 2 beef chipolata sausages until well cooked. Heat 1 × 150 g/5 oz can baked beans in tomato sauce in a small saucepan and serve with the sausages.

FISH FINGERS WITH PEAS
Cook 3 fish fingers, without added fat, under a preheated grill (broiler), turning once, until golden brown and crisp. Cook 75 g/3 oz frozen peas in boiling water, then drain and serve with the fish fingers and 15 ml/1 level tablespoon tomato ketchup.

BANANA AND YOGURT TREAT
Pour 1 × 150 g/5 oz carton/⅔ cup low-fat natural yogurt into an individual serving dish. Stir in a small peeled and sliced banana, 15 ml/1 level tablespoon raisins or sultanas and 15 ml/1 level tablespoon muesli (Swiss-style cereal) and serve immediately.

YOGURT WITH APRICOTS AND ALMONDS
Pour 150 g/5 oz carton/⅔ cup low-fat natural yogurt into an individual serving dish and stir in 25 g/1 oz/2 tablespoons chopped dried apricots and 30 ml/2 level tablespoons toasted flaked (slivered) almonds.

CANNED FRUIT WITH ICE CREAM
Put 1 × 227 g/8 oz can sliced peaches or pears in natural juice into an individual serving dish and top with 50 g/2 oz/2 scoops vanilla ice cream to serve.

PORRIDGE
Heat 150 ml/¼ pint/⅔ cup skimmed milk in a saucepan and stir in 25 g/1 oz/⅓ cup instant porridge oats. Simmer gently for 2–3 minutes, then pour into a dish and serve with 10 ml/2 level teaspoons sugar or golden (corn) syrup.

300-Calorie Meals

Curd Cheese Sandwich, and Pear

Metric/Imperial
2 x 35 g/1¼ oz slices wholemeal bread
50 g/2 oz curd cheese
5 ml/1 level teaspoon yeast extract
cucumber slices
To follow
1 medium pear

American
2 x 1¼ oz slices wholemeal bread
¼ cup curd cheese
1 level teaspoon yeast extract
cucumber slices
To follow
1 medium pear

Spread one bread slice with curd cheese and the other with yeast extract. Top one slice with the cucumber and make into a sandwich. Serve the pear to follow.

Cheese, Ham and Tomato Sandwich, and Fruit

Metric/Imperial
2 x 35 g/1¼ oz slices wholemeal bread
15 ml/1 level tablespoon cheese spread
25 g/1 oz cooked lean ham
1 tomato, sliced
To follow
1 small orange or 1 apple

American
2 x 1¼ oz slices wholemeal bread
1 level tablespoon cheese spread
1 oz cooked lean ham
1 tomato, sliced
To follow
1 small orange or 1 apple

Thinly spread both slices of bread with cheese spread. Make into a sandwich with the ham and tomato. Serve the orange to follow.

Tuna and Gherkin Sandwich, and Apple

Metric/Imperial
50 g/2 oz tuna, canned in brine, drained and flaked
15 ml/1 level tablespoon low-calorie seafood sauce
2 small gherkins, chopped
2 x 35 g/1¼ oz slices wholemeal bread
To follow
1 medium apple

American
¼ cup tuna, canned in brine, drained and flaked
1 level tablespoon low-calorie seafood sauce
2 small gherkins, chopped
2 x 1¼ oz slices wholemeal bread
To follow
1 medium apple

In a bowl, combine the tuna with the seafood sauce and the chopped gherkins. Make into a sandwich with the bread. Serve the medium apple to follow.

Egg Sandwich, and Tangerine

Metric/Imperial
1 egg, size 3, hard-boiled and chopped
15 ml/1 level tablespoon low-calorie salad dressing
2 x 35 g/1¼ oz slices wholemeal bread
a little mustard and cress
To follow
1 tangerine

American
1 medium egg, hard-cooked and chopped
1 level tablespoon low-calorie salad dressing
2 x 1¼ oz slices wholemeal bread
a little mustard and cress
To follow
1 tangerine

Combine the egg with the salad dressing. Make into a sandwich with the bread and mustard and cress. Serve the tangerine to follow.

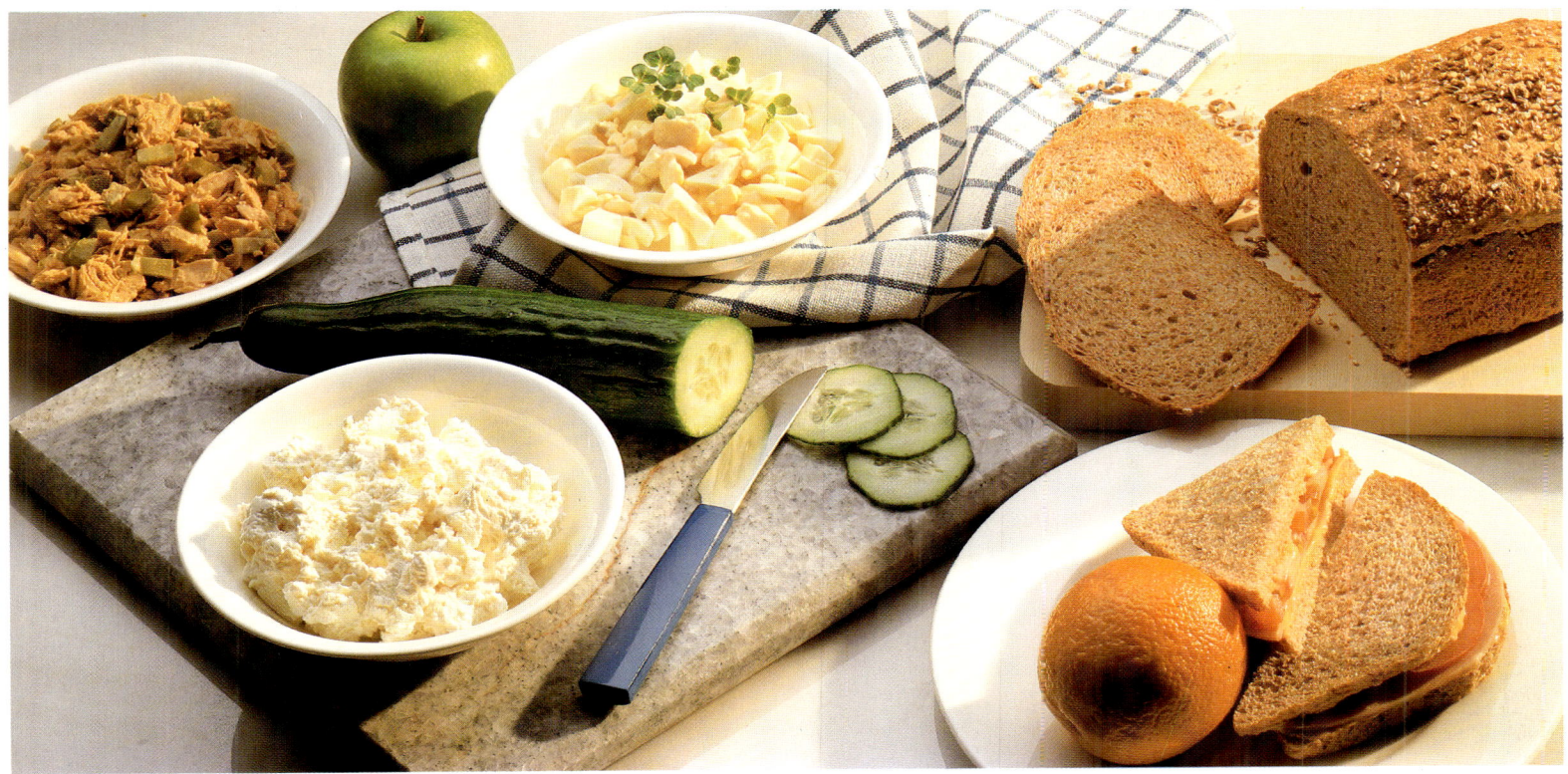

300-CALORIE MEALS: Curd Cheese, Tuna and Gherkin, and Cheese, Ham and Tomato sandwich fillings; Egg Sandwich

Scrambled Eggs with Ham on Toast

Metric/Imperial
2 eggs, size 3
30 ml/2 tablespoons skimmed milk
25 g/1 oz lean cooked ham, fat removed, chopped
salt and pepper
1 x 35 g/1¼ oz slice wholemeal bread

American
2 medium eggs
2 tablespoons skimmed milk
1 oz lean cooked ham, fat removed, chopped
salt and pepper
1 x 1¼ oz slice wholemeal bread

Lightly beat the eggs and milk together. Stir in the ham and season to taste with salt and pepper. Pour the mixture into a non-stick saucepan and cook over a low heat, stirring, until the egg is just cooked and creamy. Toast the bread and pile the scrambled egg on top.

Cod in Sauce

Metric/Imperial
175 g/6 oz packet frozen cod in sauce, any flavour
125 g/4 oz peas, frozen
125 g/4 oz French beans

American
6 oz packet frozen cod in sauce, any flavour
⅔ cup frozen peas
1 cup frozen whole green beans

Cook the cod and vegetables according to packet instructions and serve together.

Fish Cakes with Peas, and Yogurt

Metric/Imperial
2 fish cakes
75 g/3 oz frozen peas
15 ml/1 level tablespoon tomato ketchup
To follow
1 x 150 g/5 oz carton low-fat fruit yogurt

American
2 fish cakes
½ cup frozen peas
1 level tablespoon tomato ketchup
To follow
⅔ cup low-fat fruit yogurt

Grill (broil) the fish cakes without added fat, turning once, until cooked through. Cook the peas in boiling water and serve with the fish cakes and tomato ketchup. Serve the yogurt to follow.

Fish Fingers with Baked Beans

Metric/Imperial
3 fish fingers
1 x 225 g/8 oz can baked beans in tomato sauce

American
3 fish fingers
1 x 8 oz can baked beans in tomato sauce

Grill (broil) the fish fingers without added fat, turning once, until golden-brown. Heat the beans in a saucepan and serve with the fish fingers.

Cheese on Toast

Metric/Imperial
1 x 35 g/1¼ oz slice wholemeal bread
50 g/2 oz mature Cheddar or Lancashire cheese, sliced

American
1 x 1¼ oz slice wholemeal bread
½ cup thinly sliced sharp Cheddar cheese

Toast the bread on one side only. Arrange the cheese slices on the untoasted side and grill (broil) until the cheese is melted.

Tomato Omelette with Mushrooms

Metric/Imperial
125 g/4 oz button mushrooms
150 ml/¼ pint chicken stock
2 eggs, size 3
15 ml/1 tablespoon water
pinch of dried mixed herbs
salt and pepper
7 g/¼ oz butter
1 tomato, chopped
2 calorie-reduced crispbreads
10 ml/2 level teaspoons low-fat spread

American
1 cup button mushrooms
⅔ cup chicken stock
2 medium eggs
1 tablespoon water
pinch of dried mixed herbs
salt and pepper
½ level tablespoon butter
1 tomato, chopped
2 calorie-reduced crispbreads
2 level teaspoons low-fat spread

Poach the mushrooms in the stock for 4–5 minutes, until tender. Meanwhile, make the omelette. Lightly beat the eggs, water and herbs together. Season with salt and pepper. Melt the butter in a small non-stick omelette pan and brush over the surface. Pour in the eggs and cook for 2–3 minutes until just set, tilting the pan and lifting the edges of the omelette so that the uncooked mixture runs underneath. Add the tomato, fold one side of the omelette over and serve with the drained mushrooms and crispbreads spread with low-fat spread.

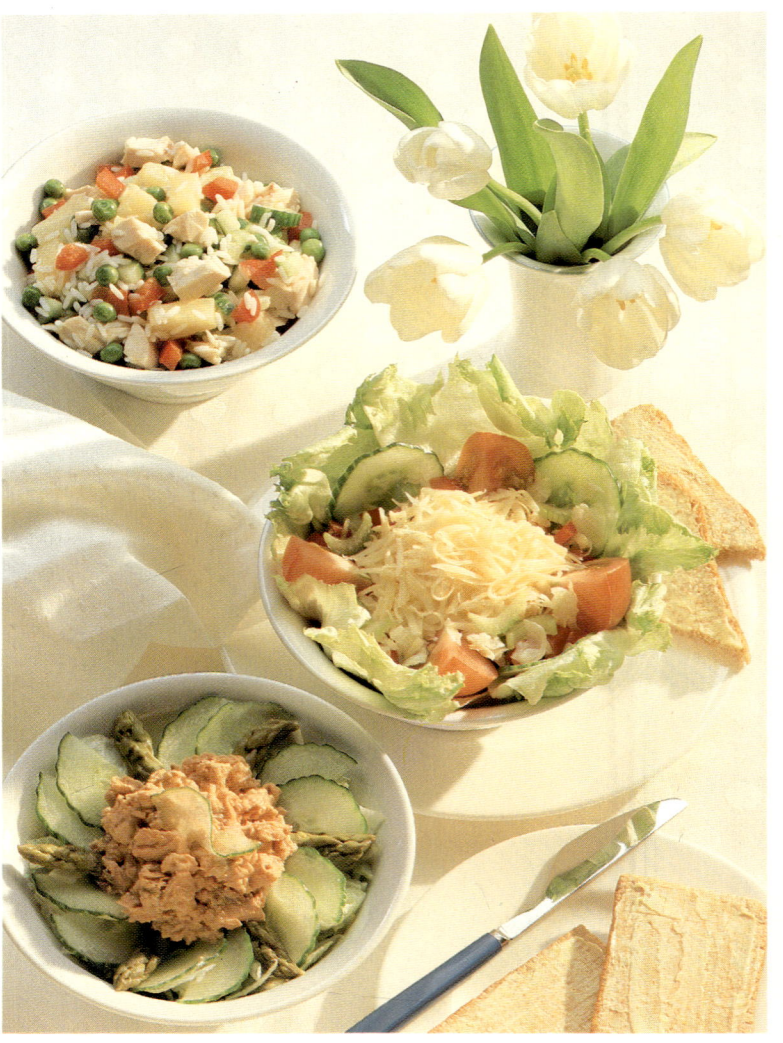

Cheese Salad

Metric/Imperial	American
¼ lettuce, shredded	¼ head lettuce, shredded
¼ small cucumber, sliced	¼ small cucumber, sliced
2 celery sticks, sliced	2 stalks celery, sliced
¼ red pepper, cored, seeded and diced	¼ red pepper, seeded and diced
1 tomato, quartered	1 tomato, quartered
15 ml/1 level tablespoon oil-free French dressing	1 tablespoon oil-free French dressing
50 g/2 oz Edam cheese, grated	½ cup grated Dutch cheese
1 x 25 g/1 oz slice wholemeal bread	1 x 1 oz slice wholemeal bread
5 ml/1 level teaspoon low-fat spread	1 level teaspoon low-fat spread

Arrange the lettuce, cucumber, celery, red pepper and tomato in a bowl. Sprinkle with the dressing and with the cheese. Serve with the bread spread with low-fat spread.

Salmon and Asparagus Salad

Metric/Imperial	American
1 x 100 g/3½ oz can salmon, flaked	½ cup flaked canned salmon
30 ml/2 level tablespoons low-calorie seafood sauce	2 level tablespoons low-calorie seafood sauce
6 canned or cooked asparagus spears, drained	6 canned asparagus spears, drained
¼ lettuce, shredded	¼ head lettuce, shredded
¼ small cucumber, sliced	¼ small cucumber, sliced
2 calorie-reduced crispbreads	2 calorie-reduced crispbreads
10 ml/2 level teaspoons low-fat spread	2 level teaspoons low-fat spread

Mix the salmon with half the seafood sauce. Arrange the asparagus, lettuce, cucumber and salmon in a bowl. Pour over the remaining seafood sauce and serve with the crispbreads spread with low-fat spread.

Chicken and Rice Salad

Metric/Imperial	American
25 g/1 oz long-grain rice	2 level tablespoons long-grain rice
50 g/2 oz frozen peas	⅓ cup frozen peas
75 g/3 oz cooked chicken, skin removed, diced	⅓ cup skinned and diced cooked chicken
¼ small cucumber, diced	¼ cucumber, diced
¼ red or green pepper, cored, seeded and diced	¼ red or green pepper, seeded and diced
1 pineapple ring, canned in natural juice, drained and chopped	1 pineapple ring, canned in natural juice, drained and chopped
30 ml/2 tablespoons oil-free French dressing	2 tablespoons oil-free French dressing
salt and pepper	salt and pepper

Cook the rice in boiling, salted water until tender. Drain, rinse under cold running water and drain again. Cook the peas according to packet instructions. Drain, rinse under cold running water and drain again. Combine all the ingredients and season.

Chicken and Rice Salad; Cheese Salad; Salmon and Asparagus Salad

Cottage Cheese and Egg Salad, and Orange

Metric/Imperial	American
¼ lettuce, shredded	¼ head lettuce, shredded
¼ small cucumber, sliced	¼ small cucumber, sliced
2 celery sticks, sliced	2 stalks celery, sliced
¼ green pepper, cored seeded and diced	¼ green pepper, seeded and diced
2 tomatoes, quartered	2 tomatoes, quartered
1 egg, size 3, hard-boiled and halved	1 medium egg, hard-cooked and halved
125 g/4 oz cottage cheese with onion and Cheddar	½ cup cheese and onion flavored cottage cheese
15 ml/1 level tablespoon low-calorie salad dressing	1 level tablespoon low-calorie salad dressing
To follow	*To follow*
1 small orange	1 small orange

Combine the lettuce, cucumber, celery, green pepper and tomatoes. Serve the salad with the egg, cottage cheese and salad dressing. Serve the orange to follow.

Chicken Drumsticks with Stir-fry Vegetables

Metric/Imperial	American
2 chicken drumsticks	2 chicken drumsticks
7 g/¼ oz butter	½ tablespoon butter
2.5 ml/½ teaspoon oil	½ teaspoon oil
175 g/6 oz frozen stir-fry vegetables	1 cup frozen stir-fry vegetables

Grill (broil) the chicken drumsticks turning often, until cooked through. Discard the skin. Keep hot. Heat the butter and oil in a preheated wok or frying-pan (skillet), add the vegetables and stir-fry according to packet instructions. Serve with the chicken drumsticks.

Lamb Chop with Vegetables, and Fruit

Metric/Imperial	American
1 x 150 g/5 oz lamb chop	1 x 5 oz lamb chop
125 g/4 oz cauliflower, fresh or frozen	⅔ cup cauliflower, fresh or frozen
125 g/4 oz sliced courgettes, fresh or frozen	1 cup sliced courgettes, fresh or frozen
15 ml/1 tablespoon mint sauce	1 tablespoon mint sauce
To follow	*To follow*
1 medium apple or orange	1 medium apple or orange

Grill (broil) the lamb chop without added fat, turning once, until well cooked. Boil the vegetables and serve with the lamb chop and mint sauce. Serve the fruit to follow.

Hamburger

Metric/Imperial	American
50 g/2 oz beefburger	2 oz hamburger
1 bap	1 soft hamburger bun
1 tomato, sliced	1 tomato, sliced
15 ml/1 level tablespoon tomato relish	1 level tablespoon tomato relish

Grill (broil) the burger without added fat until well cooked. Split the bap (hamburger bun) and toast the cut sides only. To serve, fill the toasted bap (hamburger bun) with the burger, tomato slices and relish.

400-Calorie Meals

Chicken, Corn and Baked Potato

Metric/Imperial	American
1 x 175 g/6 oz potato	1 x 6 oz potato
1 x 175 g/6 oz chicken breast portion	1 x 6 oz chicken breast portion
125 g/4 oz sweetcorn kernels, canned or frozen	¾ cup canned or frozen whole kernel corn
15 ml/1 level tablespoon low-fat natural yogurt	1 level tablespoon low-fat natural yogurt

Bake the potato in a preheated moderately hot oven (200°C/400°F/Gas Mark 6) for about 50 minutes, until soft. Cook the chicken without added fat in a covered flameproof dish alongside the potato for the last 30 minutes of cooking time. Remove and discard the chicken skin. Heat the corn if canned, or cook in boiling salted water if frozen, then drain. Top the potato with the yogurt and serve with the chicken and corn.

Gammon and Pineapple with Vegetables

Metric/Imperial	American
1 x 175 g/6 oz gammon rasher	1 x 6 oz ham slice
1 pineapple ring, canned in natural juice, drained	1 pineapple ring, canned in natural juice, drained
150 g/5 oz carrots, diced	⅔ cup diced carrots
150 g/5 oz shelled broad beans	½ cup shelled fava beans
5 ml/1 level teaspoon made mustard	1 level teaspoon mustard

Grill (broil) the gammon (ham) without added fat turning once, until cooked through. Heat the pineapple ring under the grill. Boil the vegetables until tender, then drain. Top the gammon (ham) with the pineapple and serve with the vegetables and mustard.

Liver and Bacon with Baked Beans and Mushrooms

Metric/Imperial	American
125 g/4 oz lamb's liver	4 oz lamb's liver
2.5 ml/½ teaspoon oil	½ teaspoon oil
1 rasher streaky bacon	1 slice streaky bacon
125 g/4 oz button mushrooms	1 cup button mushrooms
1 x 150 g/5 oz can baked beans in tomato sauce	1 x 5 oz can baked beans in tomato sauce

Brush the liver all over with the oil. Grill (broil) with the bacon, turning once, until the liver is cooked through and the bacon is crisp. Meanwhile, poach the mushrooms in a little salted water, then drain. Heat the beans in a saucepan and serve with the liver, bacon and mushrooms.

Shepherd's Pie, and Mousse

Metric/Imperial	American
1 individual frozen shepherd's pie	1 individual frozen shepherd's pie
125 g/4 oz sliced green beans	½ cup sliced green beans
To follow	To follow
1 individual carton frozen mousse, any flavour	1 individual carton frozen mousse, any flavor

Cook the shepherd's pie according to packet instructions and serve with the lightly boiled beans. Serve the mousse to follow.

Eggs and Chips

Metric/Imperial	American
125 g/4 oz oven or grill chips	1 cup oven French fries
2 eggs, size 3	2 medium eggs
a little oil	a little oil
15 ml/1 tablespoon ketchup	1 tablespoon ketchup

Cook the chips according to packet instructions. Fry the eggs in a little oil. Remove the eggs with a fish slice, shaking off all excess oil. Serve the eggs with the chips (French fries) and ketchup.

Pork Chop with Vegetables, and Fruit

Metric/Imperial	American
1 x 175 g/6 oz pork chop	1 x 6 oz pork chop
125 g/4 oz Brussels sprouts	⅔ cup Brussels sprouts
125 g/4 oz carrots, diced	⅔ cup diced carrots
15 ml/1 level tablespoon apple sauce	1 level tablespoon apple sauce
50 ml/2 fl oz gravy, made without added fat	¼ cup gravy, made without added fat
To follow	To follow
125 g/4 oz grapes	1 cup grapes

Grill (broil) the pork chop under a preheated grill, turning once, until cooked well. Serve with the lightly boiled vegetables, apple sauce and gravy. Serve the grapes to follow.

Buttery Cod with Rice, and Cheese Crispbreads

Metric/Imperial	American
1 x 175 g/6 oz packet frozen cod in butter sauce	1 x 6 oz package frozen cod in butter sauce
25 g/1 oz long-grain rice	2 tablespoons long-grain rice
50 g/2 oz frozen peas	⅓ cup frozen peas
50 g/2 oz canned sweetcorn kernels with peppers, drained	⅓ cup canned whole kernel corn with peppers, drained
To follow	To follow
2 calorie-reduced crispbreads	2 calorie-reduced crispbreads
15 ml/1 level tablespoon cheese spread	1 level tablespoon cheese spread

Cook the cod according to packet instructions. Cook the rice and peas in separate saucepans of boiling water until tender, then drain and mix together. Stir in the corn and heat through. Serve with the cod in sauce. Serve the crispbreads spread with cheese spread to follow.

Roast Lamb with Vegetables, and Ice Cream

Metric/Imperial	American
125 g/4 oz cabbage, shredded	1½ cups shredded cabbage
125 g/4 oz carrots, diced	⅔ cup diced carrots
75 g/3 oz lean roast lamb, all visible fat removed	3 oz lean roast lamb, all visible fat removed
15 ml/1 tablespoon mint sauce	1 tablespoon mint sauce
50 ml/2 fl oz gravy, made without added fat	¼ cup gravy, made without added fat
1 x 45 g/1¾ oz roast potato	1 x 1¾ oz roast potato
To follow	To follow
50 g/2 oz vanilla ice cream	2 small scoops vanilla ice cream

Cook the cabbage and carrots separately in boiling, salted water until tender. Drain well and serve with the lamb, mint sauce, gravy and roast potato. Serve the ice cream to follow.

Cheese and Pasta Salad

Metric/Imperial	American
25 g/1 oz pasta shapes	¼ cup pasta shapes
1 medium apple	1 medium apple
squeeze of lemon juice	squeeze of lemon juice
50 g/2 oz Edam cheese, diced	⅓ cup diced Dutch cheese
2 small sticks celery, chopped	2 small celery stalks, chopped
30 ml/2 tablespoons oil-free French dressing	2 tablespoons oil-free French dressing
15 ml/1 tablespoon low-fat natural yogurt	1 tablespoon low-fat natural yogurt
salt and pepper	salt and pepper

Cook the pasta in boiling salted water until tender. Drain, rinse under cold running water and drain again. Core and dice, but do not peel, the apple and toss in the lemon juice. Combine all the ingredients, stir well to mix and season lightly with salt and pepper.

Eggs and Mushrooms in Creamed Sauce

Metric/Imperial	American
1 x 215 g/7½ oz can sliced mushrooms in creamed sauce	1 x 7½ oz can sliced mushrooms in creamed sauce
125 g/4 oz frozen mixed vegetables	½ cup frozen mixed vegetables
2 eggs, size 3, hard-boiled	2 medium eggs, hard-cooked
parsley to garnish	parsley to garnish

Heat the mushrooms in creamed sauce. Cook the mixed vegetables in boiling salted water until tender, then drain. Halve the eggs, place on a warmed plate and spoon over the mushrooms. Surround with the mixed vegetables and garnish with parsley.

500-Calorie Family Menus

Toad-in-the-Hole with Baked Beans, and Fruit
Serves 4 (500 Calories per serving)

Metric/Imperial	American
12 pork chipolata sausages	12 small pork sausages
125 g/4 oz plain flour	1 cup all-purpose flour
2.5 ml/½ teaspoon salt	½ teaspoon salt
1 egg, size 3	1 medium egg
275 ml/½ pint skimmed milk	1¼ cups skimmed milk
15 ml/1 tablespoon oil	1 tablespoon oil
1 x 450 g/16 oz can baked beans in tomato sauce	1 x 16 oz can baked beans in tomato sauce
To follow	To follow
4 medium apples or oranges	4 medium apples or oranges

Grill (broil) the sausages, turning often to brown evenly. Sift the flour and salt into a mixing bowl and make a well in the centre. Break in the egg and add half the milk. Using a wooden spoon, gradually beat the flour to make a thick, smooth batter, then beat in the remaining milk.

Brush the base and sides of a shallow baking dish about 17.5 cm/7 inches square with oil. Arrange the sausages in the dish and heat in a preheated hot oven (220°C/425°F/Gas Mark 7) for 5 minutes. Pour the batter over the sausages and cook in the oven for 35–40 minutes until puffy and golden.

Just before the toad-in-the-hole is cooked, heat the beans in a saucepan and serve with the toad-in-the-hole.

Serve the fruit to follow.

400-CALORIE MEALS: Eggs and Mushrooms in Creamed Sauce; Shepherd's Pie and Mousse; Liver and Bacon with Baked Beans and Mushrooms

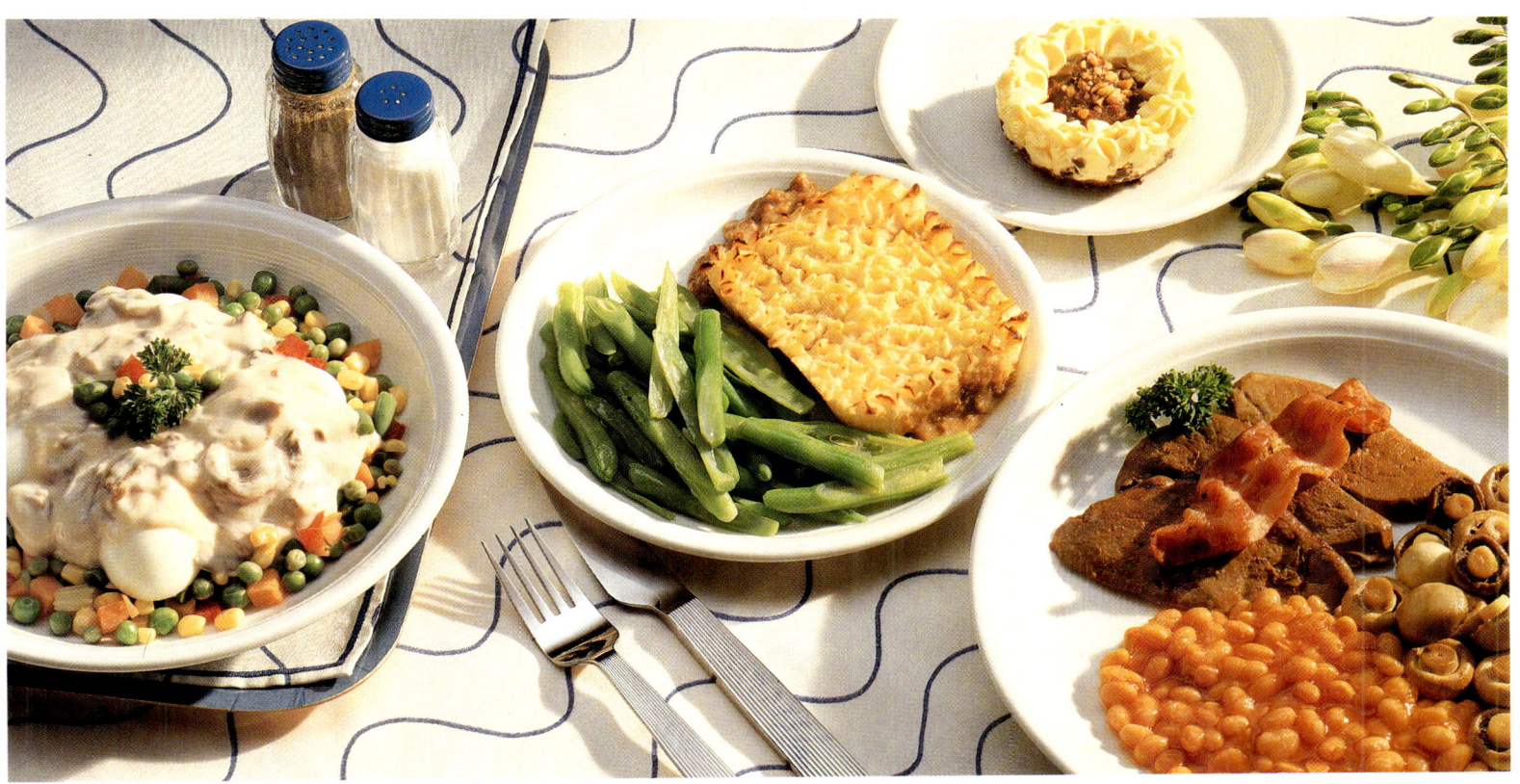

Bobotie with Salad, and Berry Yogurt

Serves 4 (500 Calories per serving)

Metric/Imperial	*American*
1 x 40 g/1½ oz slice of bread	1 x 1½ oz slice of bread
250 ml/9 fl oz skimmed milk	1¼ cups skimmed milk
450 g/1 lb very lean minced beef	2 cups ground beef
1 x 225 g/8 oz cooking apple	1 x 8 oz tart apple
1 medium onion, peeled and finely chopped	1 medium onion, peeled and finely chopped
20 ml/4 level teaspoons curry powder	4 level teaspoons curry powder
10 ml/2 level teaspoons apricot jam	2 level teaspoons apricot jam
30 ml/2 level tablespoons sultanas	2 level tablespoons golden raisins
15 ml/1 tablespoon lemon juice	1 tablespoon lemon juice
salt and pepper	salt and pepper
2 bay leaves	2 bay leaves
2 eggs, size 3	2 medium eggs
1 small lettuce	1 small head of lettuce
1 small cucumber, sliced	1 small cucumber, sliced
1 green pepper, cored, seeded and diced	1 green pepper, seeded and diced
4 celery sticks, chopped	4 stalks celery, chopped
1 bunch watercress	1 bunch watercress
60 ml/4 tablespoons oil-free French dressing	4 tablespoons low-calorie French dressing
To follow	*To follow*
4 x 150 g/5 oz cartons low-fat fruit yogurt	4 x 5 oz cartons low-fat fruit yogurt
450 g/1 lb raspberries or strawberries, fresh or defrosted if frozen	3 cups raspberries or strawberries, fresh or defrosted if frozen

Put the bread into a bowl with 125 ml/4 fl oz/½ cup of the milk. Leave to soak. Put the meat in a large non-stick frying pan (skillet) and fry gently until brown, stirring constantly. Drain off the fat.

Peel, core and chop the apple. Add the apple with the onion, curry powder, jam, sultanas (golden raisins) and lemon juice to the meat. Add the bread and milk and stir well to mix. Season with salt and pepper.

Turn the mixture into an ovenproof dish or foil container and arrange the bay leaves on top. Cover and cook in a preheated moderate oven (180°C/350°F/Gas Mark 4) for 1 hour.

Discard the bay leaves. Lightly beat the eggs with the remaining milk and season with salt and pepper. Pour over the meat and cook in the oven, uncovered, for a further 30 minutes.

Combine the lettuce, cucumber, green pepper, celery and watercress and toss in the French dressing just before serving with the hot Bobotie (removed from the foil container, if used).

Serve the berries to follow, divided equally between four dishes with a carton of yogurt poured over each.

Beefburgers with Spinach, and Fruit

Serves 4 (500 Calories per serving)

Metric/Imperial	*American*
8 x 50 g/2 oz beefburgers	8 x 2 oz hamburgers
450 g/1 lb frozen spinach	1½ cups frozen spinach
pinch of grated nutmeg	pinch of grated nutmeg
salt and black pepper	salt and black pepper
1 x 295 g/10½ oz can condensed tomato soup	1 x 10½ oz can condensed tomato soup
15 ml/1 level tablespoon grated Parmesan cheese	1 level tablespoon grated Parmesan cheese

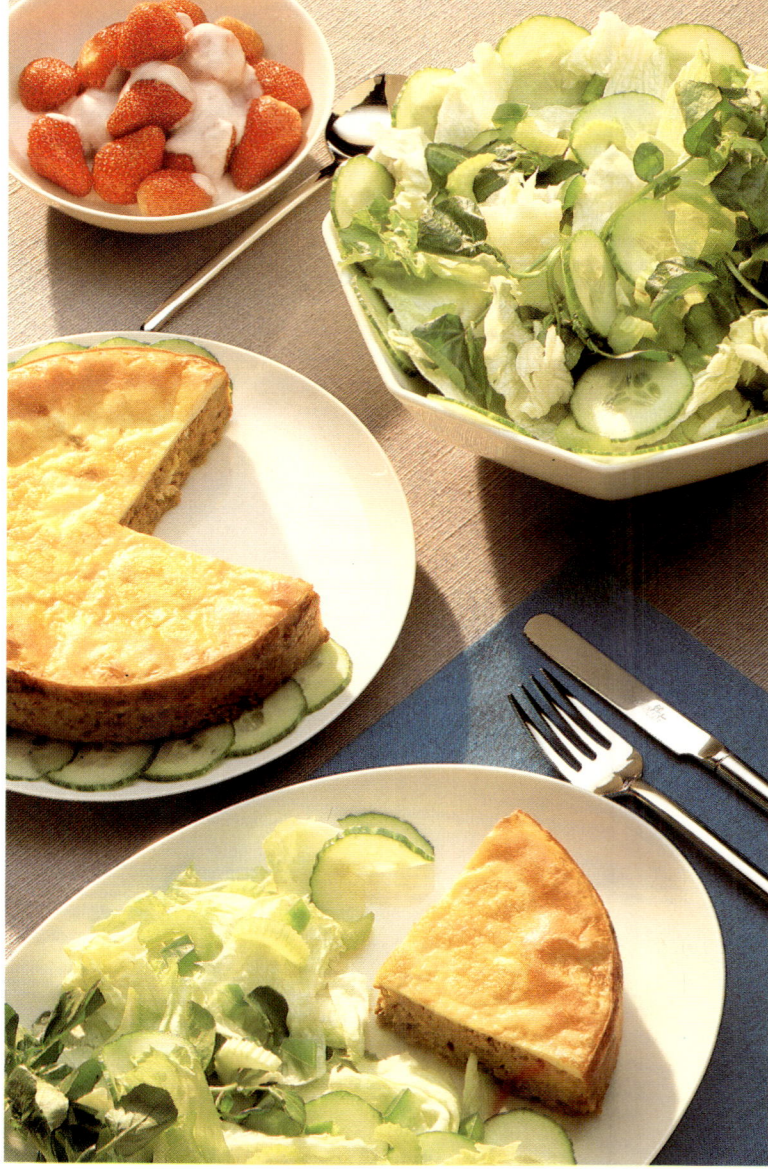

500-CALORIE FAMILY MENU: Bobotie with Salad, and Berry Yogurt

dash of Worcestershire sauce	dash of Worcestershire sauce
150 g/5 oz instant mashed potato powder	1 cup instant mashed potato powder
To follow	*To follow*
4 medium bananas or 4 large oranges	4 medium bananas or 4 large oranges

Grill (broil) the beefburgers under a preheated grill, turning once, until they are well cooked. Meanwhile, cook the spinach according to packet instructions. Drain well and season with the nutmeg and salt and pepper. Spoon the spinach into an ovenproof dish and arrange the beefburgers on top. Keep warm.

Heat the soup in a saucepan to just below boiling point. Stir in the cheese and Worcestershire sauce. Pour the mixture over the beefburgers. Make up the instant potato powder with boiling water according to packet instructions and serve with the beefburgers.

Serve the fruit to follow.

Spaghetti with Chicken Liver Sauce, and Ice Cream with Fruit Serves 4 (500 Calories per serving)

Metric/Imperial	American
450 g/1 lb chicken livers, trimmed and chopped	1 lb chicken livers, trimmed and chopped
50 g/2 oz lean cooked ham, chopped	¼ cup chopped lean cooked ham
225 g/8 oz button mushrooms	2 cups button mushrooms
1 medium onion, chopped	1 medium onion, chopped
60 ml/4 level tablespoons tomato purée	4 level tablespoons tomato paste
2.5 ml/½ teaspoon dried mixed herbs	½ level teaspoon dried mixed herbs
275 ml/½ pint water	1¼ cups water
1 chicken stock cube	2 chicken bouillon cubes
salt and pepper	salt and pepper
15 ml/1 level tablespoon cornflour	1 level tablespoon cornstarch
175 g/6 oz spaghetti	1½ cups spaghetti
To follow	To follow
250 g/9 oz brick of vanilla ice cream	9 oz vanilla ice cream
225 g/8 oz raspberries or strawberries	1½ cups raspberries or strawberries

Put the chicken livers, ham, mushrooms, onion, tomato purée (paste), herbs, water and stock (bouillon) cube into a saucepan and season with salt and pepper. Cover, bring to the boil and simmer gently for 15 minutes, stirring from time to time. In a cup, blend the cornflour (cornstarch) with a little cold water to make a smooth paste. Stir into the pan and simmer, stirring, for 1–2 minutes.

Meanwhile, cook the spaghetti in boiling salted water until just tender. Drain and divide the spaghetti between four warmed plates and spoon a portion of chicken liver sauce on top of each plate.

Serve the fruit in individual dishes, topped with ice cream to follow.

Chicken and Pineapple Casserole, and Banana Jelly Serves 4 (500 Calories per serving)

Metric/Imperial	American
4 x 225 g/8 oz chicken leg joints, skin removed	4 x 8 oz chicken leg joints, skin removed
1 x 425 g/15 oz can pineapple cubes in natural juice	1 x 15 oz can pineapple cubes in natural juice
1 green pepper, cored, seeded and diced	1 green pepper, seeded and diced
1 medium onion, chopped	1 medium onion, chopped
10 ml/2 teaspoons soy sauce	2 teaspoons soy sauce
1 chicken stock cube	2 chicken bouillon cubes
275 ml/½ pint boiling water	1¼ cups boiling water
salt and pepper	salt and pepper
30 ml/2 level tablespoons cornflour	2 level tablespoons cornstarch
125 g/4 oz long-grain rice	8 tablespoons long-grain rice
450 g/1 lb sliced green beans	2 cups sliced green beans
To follow	To follow
1 packet lemon jelly	1 package lemon-flavored gelatin
1 large banana	1 large banana

First, make up the jelly according to packet instructions and pour into a bowl. When almost set, peel and slice the banana and stir into the jelly. Pour into a wetted mould and leave to set completely.

Place the chicken joints in a casserole with the pineapple and juice. Add the green pepper, onion and soy sauce to the casserole. Dissolve the stock (bouillon) cube in the boiling water and pour into the casserole with salt and pepper. Cover and cook in a preheated moderately hot oven (190°C/375°F/Gas Mark 5) for 45 minutes. In a cup, blend the cornflour (cornstarch) with a little cold water; stir into the casserole and cook for a further 15 minutes. Meanwhile, cook the rice and beans in separate pans of boiling water, then drain and serve with the chicken and pineapple casserole.

Unmould the banana jelly and serve to follow.

Fish and Mushroom Pie, and Apple and Apricot Meringue Serves 4 (500 Calories per serving)

Metric/Imperial	American
4 x 175 g/6 oz white fish steaks	4 x 6 oz white fish steaks
1 x 295 g/10½ oz can condensed cream of mushroom soup	1 x 10½ oz can condensed cream of mushroom soup
15 ml/1 tablespoon skimmed milk	1 tablespoon skimmed milk
75 g/3 oz mature Cheddar cheese, grated	¾ cup grated sharp Cheddar cheese
50 g/2 oz fresh breadcrumbs	1 cup fresh bread crumbs
450 g/1 lb carrots, diced	2⅔ cups diced carrots
450 g/1 lb green beans, sliced	2 cups sliced green beans
Meringue	Meringue
125 g/4 oz dried apricots, soaked in water for several hours	¾ cup dried apricots, soaked in water for several hours
450 g/1 lb cooking apples	1 lb tart apples
15 ml/1 level tablespoon clear honey	1 level tablespoon clear honey
2 egg whites	2 egg whites
50 g/2 oz caster sugar	4 tablespoons caster sugar

Place the fish steaks in a shallow ovenproof dish. Mix together the soup and milk and pour over the fish. Combine the cheese and breadcrumbs and sprinkle over the top. Bake in a preheated moderately hot oven (190°C/375°F/Gas Mark 5) for 20–25 minutes.

Meanwhile, make the apple and apricot meringue: Drain the apricots and reserve 60 ml/4 tablespoons of the soaking liquid. Peel, core and slice the apples and place in a saucepan with the apricots and reserved liquid. Cover and cook until the apples are soft. Stir in the honey and turn the mixture into a shallow ovenproof dish. Whisk the egg whites until stiff. Sprinkle over the sugar and whisk again until stiff. Pile the meringue on top of the fruit and cook alongside the fish for 10–15 minutes. Cook the vegetables in boiling water and serve with the pie. Serve the apple and apricot meringue to follow.

Grilled Lamb Chops with Jacket Potatoes, and Fruit Serves 4 (500 Calories per serving)

Metric/Imperial	American
4 x 175 g/6 oz potatoes	4 x 6 oz potatoes
4 x 150 g/5 oz lamb chops	4 x 5 oz lamb chops
450 g/1 lb frozen mixed vegetables	2 cups frozen mixed vegetables
60 ml/4 tablespoons mint sauce	4 tablespoons mint sauce
To follow	To follow
4 small bananas or 450 g/1 lb grapes or 4 medium oranges	4 small bananas or 4 cups grapes or 4 medium oranges

Bake the potatoes in their jackets in a preheated moderately hot oven (200°C/400°F/Gas Mark 6) for about 50 minutes, until cooked through.

Grill (broil) the chops without added fat under a preheated grill, turning once, until well cooked. Cook the vegetables in boiling salted water, drain and serve with the potatoes, chops and mint sauce.

Serve the fruit to follow.

The Mix and Match Formula

This is a simple, satisfying and very successful way to lose weight. All you have to do is pick one breakfast a day, have a steaming bowl of soup with a wholemeal roll for lunch, then choose a comfortingly hot main meal from the saucy selection starting on page 114. Add two pieces of fresh fruit and 275 ml/½ pint/1¼ cups skimmed milk each day and you have a slimming formula which totals 1,250 Calories and which will help you shed your excess pounds speedily if you have between 1 and 3 stones (6.3–19 kg/14–42 lb) to lose.

All your lunchtime soups are delicious home-made recipes that make 4 servings. Make some up before you begin your diet and freeze them in single-portion containers. Then all you have to do is take one from the freezer when required and reheat it. If you take a packed lunch to work you can carry your soup in a vacuum flask, but remember to take frozen soup from the freezer the night before so that you can quickly heat it up before you dash off in the morning. If you are a bread-lover, though, it may be a good idea to freeze your wholemeal rolls and take one from the freezer just before you leave for work. As the roll will take several hours to thaw, you won't be able to start nibbling away at it before lunchtime!

For your main meal you have a choice of 5 foods to which you add any of 5 sauces. Ring the changes and you'll never get bored. Try serving fish with a curry sauce, or with a creamy mushroom topping. Lamb is delicious in tomato or herby brown sauce, and how about chicken in cider sauce or beefburgers in tomato? If you prefer to eat vegetarian, serve any of the sauces with a helping of red kidney beans plus other vegetables of your choice. There are lots of delicious combinations you can try – make up your own or follow any of the recipes we show you. It is very important to cook the meats as we tell you. Chicken, beefburgers and lamb should be grilled (broiled) before adding to a casserole, otherwise the fatty calories that would have dripped out into the grill (broiler) pan will go straight into your recipe. White fish, however, contains little fat and does not need grilling (broiling) before it is added to a dish.

In our recipes we have selected vegetables for you, but when you do a plain saucy grill you can serve it with any vegetables you wish as long as they don't total more than 175 Calories.

If you normally eat your main meal with family or friends, you can increase servings to include them if you wish.

Check your weight once a week and when you have less than 1 stone (6.3 kg/14 lb) to lose, check the questionnaire on page 14 to see if it is time for you to change to another eating plan.

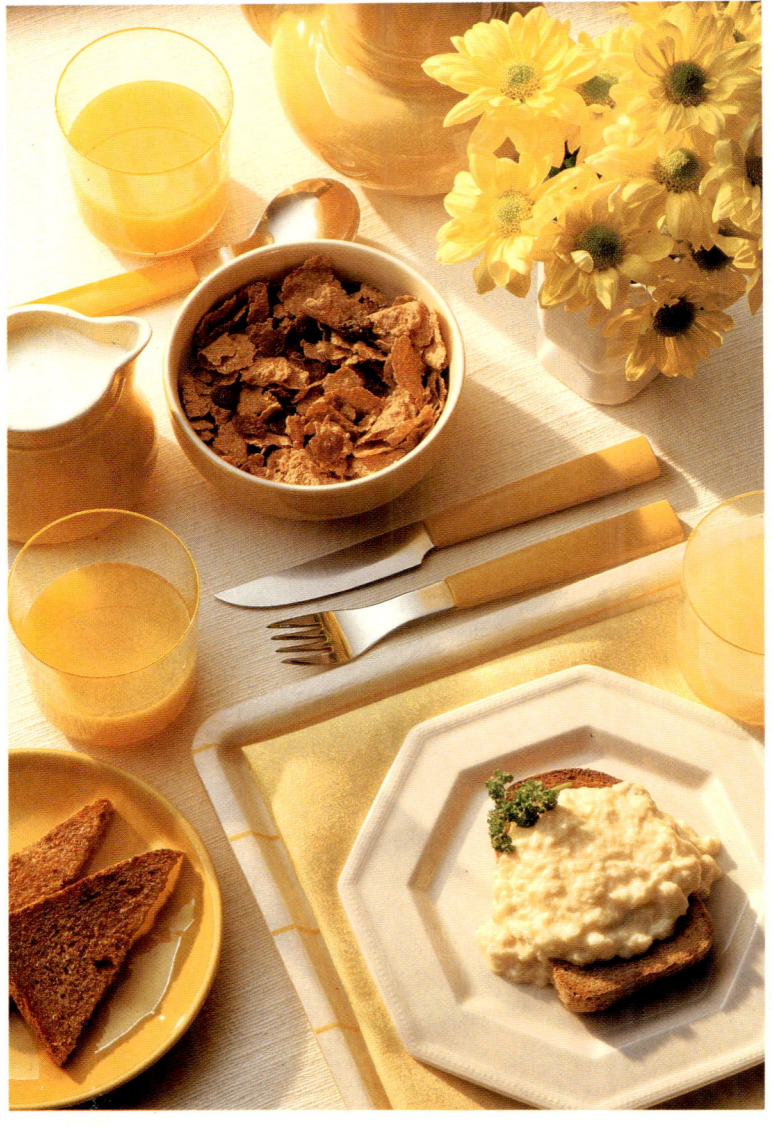

Diet Rules

1 Choose 1 breakfast each day from the selection given below. If you prefer not to eat breakfast, save this meal for later in the day.

2 Choose 1 of the soups on pages 111–114 for lunch and eat it with a wholemeal roll (45 g/1¾ oz). Do not spread any butter or margarine on the roll.

3 For your main meal of the day, choose from the selection on pages 116–119.

4 You are also allowed two pieces of fresh fruit a day. You may eat

250-CALORIE BREAKFASTS: Grapefruit Juice and Scrambled Egg; Orange Juice and Honey Toast; Orange Juice and Fruity Cereal

these as between-meal snacks or as a dessert to follow your main meal or lunch. Pick any two of your favourites, except avocado.

5 Each day you may have 275 ml/ ½ pint/1¼ cups skimmed milk to use in tea or coffee or to drink on its own.

Any milk given in the meals that follow is in addition to this allowance. You may also drink as much water, yeast extract drinks or as many low-calorie squashes or mixers as you wish.

250-Calorie Breakfasts

Choose one of these each day:

GRAPEFRUIT, AND BEANS ON TOAST
Sprinkle $\frac{1}{2}$ a medium grapefruit with 5 ml/1 level teaspoon sugar or artificial sweetener to taste. Heat 1 × 150 g/5 oz can baked beans in tomato sauce in a small saucepan and serve on 1 × 40 g/ $1\frac{1}{2}$ oz slice of wholemeal toast.

GRAPEFRUIT, BOILED EGG AND TOAST
Sprinkle $\frac{1}{2}$ a medium grapefruit with 5 ml/1 level teaspoon sugar or artificial sweetener to taste. Boil 1 size 3 (medium) egg to your liking. Spread 1 × 40 g/$1\frac{1}{2}$ oz slice wholemeal toast with 10 ml/ 2 level teaspoons low-fat spread and serve with the boiled egg.

SUNSHINE BREAKFAST
Serve 150 ml/$\frac{1}{4}$ pint/$\frac{2}{3}$ cup unsweetened orange juice. Mix 1 peeled and sliced small banana with 15 ml/1 level tablespoon raisins or sultanas (golden raisins), 5 ml/1 level teaspoon chopped mixed nuts and 1 × 150 ml/5 oz carton/$\frac{2}{3}$ cup low-fat natural yogurt in an individual serving bowl.

GRAPEFRUIT JUICE, SCRAMBLED EGG ON TOAST
Serve 150 ml/$\frac{1}{4}$ pint/$\frac{2}{3}$ cup unsweetened grapefruit juice. Beat 1 size 3 (medium) egg with 45 ml/3 tablespoons skimmed milk and season with salt and pepper. Melt 5 ml/1 level teaspoon low-fat spread in a small saucepan, add the egg mixture and cook, stirring, over a gentle heat, until just set and creamy. Serve on 1 × 40 g/$1\frac{1}{2}$ oz slice wholemeal toast.

ORANGE JUICE, POACHED EGG ON TOAST
Serve 115 ml/4 fl oz/$\frac{2}{3}$ cup unsweetened orange juice. Poach 1 size 3 (medium) egg. Spread 1 × 40 g/$1\frac{1}{2}$ oz slice wholemeal toast with 10 ml/2 level teaspoons low-fat spread and serve the egg on the toast.

FRUITY STARTER
Combine 1 small peeled and segmented orange, 25 g/1 oz/2 tablespoons muesli (Swiss-style cereal), one 150 ml/5 oz carton/$\frac{2}{3}$ cup low-fat natural yogurt and 15 ml/1 level tablespoon raisins or sultanas (golden raisins) in an individual serving bowl.

TOAST WITH MARMALADE OR JAM
Spread 20 ml/4 level teaspoons low-fat spread and 20 ml/4 level teaspoons marmalade or jam over 2 × 25 g/1 oz slices wholemeal toast.

ORANGE JUICE AND HONEY TOAST
Serve 175 ml/6 fl oz/$\frac{3}{4}$ cup unsweetened orange juice. Spread 1 × 40 g/$1\frac{1}{2}$ oz slice wholemeal toast with 10 ml/ 2 level teaspoons low-fat spread and 15 ml/3 level teaspoons honey.

ORANGE JUICE AND FRUITY CEREAL
Serve 150 ml/$\frac{1}{4}$ pint/$\frac{2}{3}$ cup unsweetened orange juice. Mix 40 g/$1\frac{1}{2}$ oz/3 tablespoons All Bran with 15 ml/1 level tablespoon raisins or sultanas (golden raisins) in an individual serving dish and pour 150 ml/$\frac{1}{4}$ pint/$\frac{2}{3}$ cup skimmed milk over cereal.

Note

Where calorie-reduced crispbreads are mentioned select a brand that provides 20 Calories or less per crispbread.

275-Calorie Lunches

Serve one portion of any of the following soups with a 45 g/$1\frac{3}{4}$ oz wholemeal roll. All soups will freeze, so they can be made in advance, frozen and reheated when you need them. All fruit is extra to your daily snack allowance.

Chicken and Vegetable Chowder Serves 4

Metric/Imperial	*American*
1 medium onion, chopped	1 medium onion, chopped
125 g/4 oz potato (peeled weight), diced	$\frac{2}{3}$ cup diced potato
125 g/4 oz carrot, diced	$\frac{2}{3}$ cup diced carrot
50 g/2 oz swede, diced, peeled weight	$\frac{1}{3}$ cup diced rutabaga, peeled weight
50 g/2 oz leeks, sliced	$\frac{1}{4}$ cup sliced leeks
2 chicken stock cubes	4 chicken bouillon cubes
1 litre/$1\frac{3}{4}$ pints water	4 cups water
150 g/5 oz cooked chicken, diced	$\frac{2}{3}$ cup cooked diced chicken
125 g/4 oz sweetcorn	$\frac{2}{3}$ cup kernel corn

Put the onion, potato, carrot, swede (rutabaga) and leeks into a large saucepan with the water and stock (bouillon) cubes. Bring to the boil, then lower the heat, cover and cook gently for about 20 minutes, until the vegetables are tender.

Purée half the contents of the pan in a food processor or blender, or pass through a sieve.

Return the purée to the pan, add the chicken and corn and heat through, or allow the soup to cool, then divide between 4 freezer containers, label and freeze.

To serve, place a portion of frozen soup in a saucepan and heat through slowly, stirring occasionally, until piping hot.

Kidney and Bacon Soup Serves 4

Metric/Imperial	*American*
10 ml/2 teaspoons oil	2 teaspoons oil
225 g/8 oz ox kidney, diced	1 cup diced ox kidney
2 medium onions, chopped	2 meduim onions, chopped
700 ml/$1\frac{1}{4}$ pints water	3 cups water
1 beef stock cube	2 beef bouillon cubes
4 streaky bacon rashers	4 bacon slices
30 ml/2 level tablespoons cornflour	2 level tablespoons cornstarch
salt and pepper	salt and pepper

Heat the oil in a non-stick saucepan, add the kidney and onion and fry gently for 5 minutes. Add the water and stock (bouillon) cube. Bring to the boil, then lower the heat, cover and simmer for 1 hour.

Grill (broil) the bacon until crisp, then chop. Blend the cornflour (cornstarch) with a little cold water until smooth. Stir into the pan with the bacon, bring to the boil and simmer for 2–3 minutes, stirring, until the soup thickens.

Season with salt and pepper. Allow the soup to cool, then divide between 4 freezer containers, label and freeze.

To serve, place a portion of frozen soup in a saucepan and heat through slowly, stirring occasionally, until piping hot.

Dutch Onion Soup Serves 4

Metric/Imperial	American
450 g/1 lb onions, sliced	4 cups sliced onions
850 ml/1½ pints water	3¾ cups water
2 beef stock cubes	4 beef bouillon cubes
30 ml/2 level tablespoons cornflour	2 level tablespoons cornstarch
salt and pepper	salt and pepper
125 g/4 oz Edam cheese, grated, to garnish	1 cup grated Dutch cheese, to garnish

Put the onions into a saucepan with the water and stock (bouillon) cubes. Bring to the boil, then lower the heat, cover and simmer for 30 minutes.

Blend the cornflour (cornstarch) with a little cold water until smooth. Stir into the soup, then return to the boil and simmer for 2–3 minutes, stirring, until the soup thickens. Season to taste with salt and pepper. Allow the soup to cool, then divide between 4 freezer containers, label and freeze.

To serve, place a portion of frozen soup in a saucepan and heat through slowly, stirring occasionally, until piping hot. Serve each portion sprinkled with 25 g/1 oz/¼ cup grated cheese.

Chinese Leaves and Green Pepper Soup, and Banana Serves 4

Metric/Imperial	American
1 large green pepper, seeded and diced	1 large green pepper, seeded and diced
2 medium onions, chopped	2 medium onions, chopped
½ head Chinese leaves, shredded	½ head Chinese leaves, shredded
575 ml/1 pint water	2½ cups water
1 chicken stock cube	2 chicken bouillon cubes
salt and pepper	salt and pepper
30 ml/2 level tablespoons cornflour	2 level tablespoons cornstarch
To follow	To follow
1 medium banana per serving	1 medium banana per serving

Put the green pepper, onions and Chinese leaves into a saucepan with the water, stock (bouillon) cube, salt and pepper. Bring to the boil, then lower the heat, cover and simmer for 30 minutes.

Purée in a food processor or blender, or by passing through a sieve. Return to the pan. Blend the cornflour (cornstarch) with a little cold water until smooth. Stir into the soup. Return to the boil and simmer for 2–3 minutes, stirring, until the soup thickens. Allow the soup to cool, then divide between 4 freezer containers, label and freeze.

To serve, place a portion of frozen soup in a saucepan and heat through slowly, stirring occasionally, until piping hot. Follow with a medium banana.

Quick Tomato Soup, and Banana Serves 4

Metric/Imperial	American
575 ml/1 pint tomato juice	2½ cups tomato juice
275 ml/½ pint water	1¼ cups water
1 medium onion, finely chopped	1 medium onion, finely chopped
salt and pepper	salt and pepper
10 ml/2 level teaspoons caster sugar	2 level teaspoons sugar
30 ml/2 level tablespoons cornflour	2 level tablespoons cornstarch
To follow	To follow
1 medium banana per serving	1 medium banana per serving

Put the tomato juice, water, onion, salt and pepper, and sugar into a saucepan and bring to the boil. Lower the heat and simmer for 20 minutes.

Blend the cornflour (cornstarch) with a little cold water until smooth and stir into the soup. Return to the boil, then simmer for 2–3 minutes, stirring, until the soup thickens. Allow the soup to cool, then divide between 4 freezer containers. Label and freeze.

To serve, place a portion of frozen soup in a saucepan and heat through slowly, stirring occasionally, until piping hot. Follow with a medium banana.

Asparagus Soup, and Banana Serves 4

Metric/Imperial	American
1 medium onion, finely chopped	1 medium onion, finely chopped
850 ml/1½ pints water	3¾ cups water
1 chicken stock cube	2 chicken bouillon cubes
2.5 ml/½ level teaspoon celery salt	½ level teaspoon celery salt
1.25 ml/¼ level teaspoon nutmeg	¼ level teaspoon ground nutmeg
1 x 340 g/12 oz can asparagus spears	1 x 12 oz can asparagus spears
25 g/1 oz skimmed milk powder	¼ cup skimmed milk powder
30 ml/2 level tablespoons cornflour	2 level tablespoons cornstarch
salt and pepper	salt and pepper
To follow	To follow
1 medium banana per serving	1 medium banana per serving

Put the onion into a saucepan with the water, stock (bouillon) cube, celery salt and nutmeg. Cover, bring to the boil, then lower the heat and simmer for 15 minutes.

Purée the asparagus with the liquid from the can in a food processor or blender. Stir the asparagus purée into the pan.

Blend the skimmed milk powder and cornflour (cornstarch) with a little cold water until smooth and stir into the soup. Return to the boil, then simmer for 2–3 minutes, stirring, until the soup thickens. Season with salt and pepper. Allow the soup to cool, then divide between 4 freezer containers, label and freeze.

To serve, place a portion of frozen soup in a saucepan and heat through slowly, stirring occasionally. Follow with a medium banana.

Vegetable and Wholewheat Pasta Chowder Serves 4

Metric/Imperial	American
125 g/4 oz carrots, diced	⅔ cup diced carrots
125 g/4 oz courgettes, diced	1 cup diced zucchini
125 g/4 oz celery, chopped	1 cup chopped celery
1 medium onion, chopped	1 medium onion, chopped
1.15 litres/2 pints water	5 cups water
2 chicken stock cubes	4 chicken bouillon cubes
275 ml/½ pint tomato juice	1¼ cups tomato juice
125 g/4 oz wholewheat pasta	1 cup wholewheat pasta
salt and pepper	salt and pepper

Put the carrots, courgettes (zucchini), celery and onion into a large saucepan with the water, stock (bouillon) cubes and tomato juice. Bring to the boil, and cook for 5 minutes.

Add the pasta, cover and simmer for a further 20 minutes, or until the pasta is tender. Purée half the contents of the pan in a food processor or blender or pass through a sieve. Stir the purée back into the pan and season with salt and pepper. Allow the soup to cool, then divide between 4 freezer containers, label and freeze.

To serve, place a portion of frozen soup in a saucepan and heat through slowly, stirring occasionally, until piping hot.

Spring Mushroom Soup, and Apple Serves 4

Metric/Imperial	American
6 spring onions, chopped	6 scallions, chopped
50 g/2 oz watercress, chopped	1 cup chopped watercress
225 g/8 oz mushrooms, sliced	2 cups sliced mushrooms
850 ml/1½ pints water	3¾ cups water
2 chicken stock cubes	4 chicken bouillon cubes
salt and pepper	salt and pepper
25 g/1 oz skimmed milk powder	¼ cup skimmed milk powder
30 ml/2 level tablespoons cornflour	2 level tablespoons cornstarch
To follow	To follow
1 large apple per serving	1 large apple per serving

Put the spring onions (scallions), watercress, mushrooms, water and stock (bouillon) cubes into a saucepan. Bring to the boil, then lower the heat, cover and simmer for 10 minutes. Season to taste with salt and pepper.

Blend the skimmed milk powder and cornflour (cornstarch) with a little cold water until smooth. Stir into the soup. Return to the boil and simmer for 2–3 minutes, stirring. Allow the soup to cool slightly, then divide between 4 freezer containers, label and freeze.

To serve, place a portion of frozen soup in a saucepan and heat through slowly, stirring occasionally, until piping hot. Follow with a large apple.

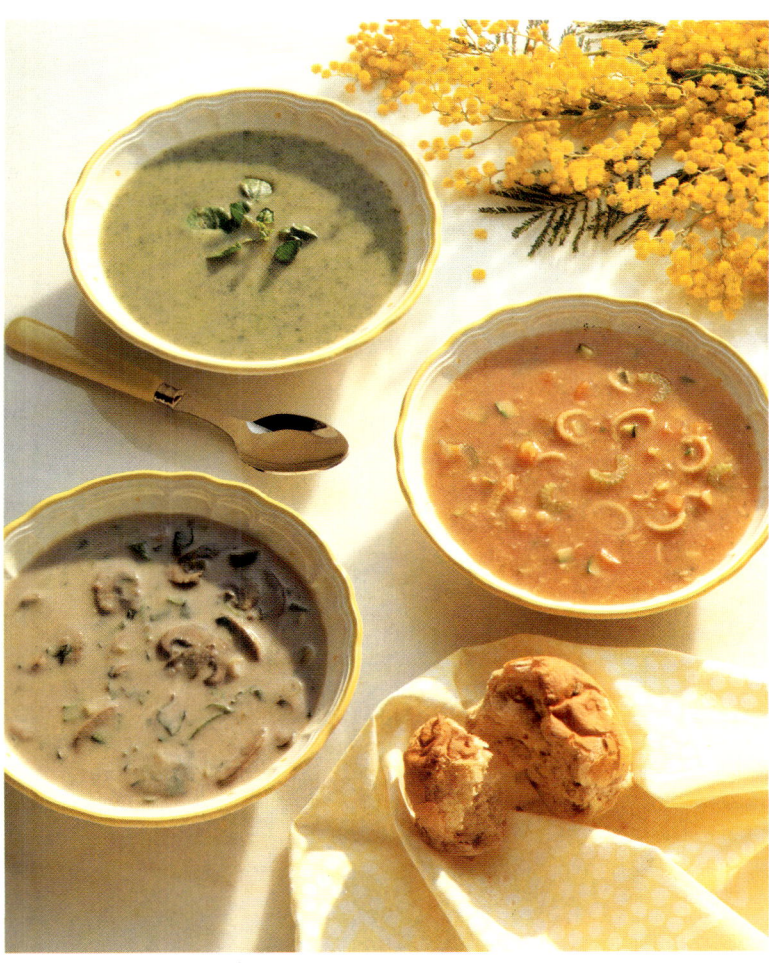

Watercress and Potato Soup Serves 4

Metric/Imperial	American
1 medium onion, chopped	1 medium onion, chopped
2 chicken stock cubes	4 chicken bouillon cubes
850 ml/1½ pints water	3¾ cups water
150 g/5 oz watercress	2 cups watercress
275 g/10 oz potatoes (peeled weight), diced	1⅔ cups peeled diced potato
40 g/1½ oz skimmed milk powder	1½ oz skimmed milk powder
15 ml/1 level tablespoon cornflour	1 level tablespoon cornstarch
salt and pepper	salt and pepper

Put the onion, stock (bouillon) cubes and water into a saucepan. Bring to the boil, then cover and simmer for 10 minutes. Wash watercress and discard yellow leaves and hard stalks.

Add the watercress and potatoes and simmer for a further 10 minutes. Purée the contents of the pan in a food processor or blender, or by passing through a sieve, then return to the pan.

Blend the skimmed milk powder and cornflour (cornstarch) with a little cold water until smooth. Stir into the soup, then return to the boil, lower the heat and simmer for 2–3 minutes, stirring, until the soup thickens. Season with salt and pepper. Allow the soup to cool, then divide between 4 freezer containers, label and freeze.

To serve, place a portion of frozen soup in a saucepan and heat through slowly, stirring occasionally, until piping hot. Serve garnished with a little extra watercress if used.

Creamed Vegetable Soup, and Orange Serves 4

Metric/Imperial	American
225 g/8 oz carrots, diced	1⅓ cups diced carrots
225 g/8 oz leeks, sliced	1 cup sliced leek
1 medium onion, chopped	1 medium onion, chopped
125 g/4 oz celery, chopped	⅔ cup chopped celery
1.15 litres/2 pints water	5 cups water
2 chicken stock cubes	4 chicken bouillon cubes
salt and pepper	salt and pepper
125 g/4 oz cauliflower florets	⅔ cup cauliflower florets
125 g/4 oz mushrooms	1 cup mushrooms
25 g/1 oz skimmed milk powder	25 g/1 oz skimmed milk powder
30 ml/2 level tablespoons cornflour	2 level tablespoons cornstarch
To follow	To follow
1 small orange per serving	1 small orange per serving

Put the carrots, leeks, onion and celery into a large saucepan with the water, stock (bouillon) cubes, salt and pepper. Bring to the boil, then lower the heat, cover and simmer for 10 minutes.

Add the cauliflower and mushrooms to the pan and simmer for a further 10 minutes. Purée the contents of the pan in a food processor or blender.

Return the purée to the pan. Blend the skimmed milk and cornflour (cornstarch) with a little cold water until smooth. Stir into the soup. Return to the boil and simmer for 2–3 minutes, until the soup thickens. Allow the soup to cool slightly, then divide between 4 freezer containers, label and freeze.

To serve, place a portion of frozen soup in a saucepan and heat through slowly, stirring occasionally, until piping hot. Follow with a small orange.

275-CALORIE LUNCHES: Watercress and Potato Soup; Vegetable and Wholewheat Pasta Chowder; Spring Mushroom Soup

Chicken and Mushroom Broth, and Orange Serves 4

Metric/Imperial	American
1 medium onion, chopped	1 medium onion, chopped
1 medium carrot, chopped	1 medium carrot, chopped
2 sticks celery, chopped	2 stalks celery, chopped
1.5 litres/2½ pints water	6¼ cups water
2 chicken stock cubes	4 chicken bouillon cubes
salt and pepper	salt and pepper
175 g/6 oz mushrooms, sliced	1½ cups sliced mushrooms
150 g/5 oz cooked chicken, cut into bite-sized pieces	⅔ cup chopped cooked chicken
30 ml/2 level tablespoons cornflour	2 level tablespoons cornstarch
To follow	*To follow*
1 small orange per serving	1 small orange per serving

Put the onion, carrot and celery into a large saucepan with the water, stock (bouillon) cubes, salt and pepper. Bring to the boil, stirring occasionally, then lower the heat, cover and simmer for 20 minutes.

Add the mushrooms and chicken to the pan and cook for a further 10 minutes. Blend the cornflour (cornstarch) with a little cold water until smooth, then stir into the pan. Return to the boil and simmer for 2–3 minutes, stirring until the soup thickens. Allow the soup to cool, then divide between 4 freezer containers, label and freeze.

To serve, place a portion of frozen soup in a saucepan and heat through slowly, stirring occasionally, until piping hot. Follow with a small orange.

Broad Bean and Leek Soup, and Apple Serves 4

Metric/Imperial	American
125 g/4 oz potato (peeled weight), diced	⅔ cup diced potato
225 g/8 oz leek, sliced	1 cup sliced leek
225 g/8 oz shelled broad beans, fresh or frozen	1½ cups shelled fava beans, fresh or frozen
1.25 ml/¼ level teaspoon dried mixed herbs	¼ level teaspoon dried mixed herbs
850 ml/1½ pints water	3¾ cups water
2 chicken stock cubes	2 chicken bouillon cubes
salt and pepper	salt and pepper
To follow	*To follow*
1 medium apple per serving	1 medium apple per serving

Place all ingredients in a saucepan. Bring to the boil, then lower the heat, cover and simmer for 30 minutes for fresh beans, or 20 minutes for frozen.

Purée the contents of the pan in a food processor or blender, or by passing through a sieve. Return to the pan, reheat and season to taste with salt and pepper. Allow the soup to cool, then divide between 4 freezer containers, label and freeze.

To serve, place a portion of frozen soup in a saucepan and heat through slowly, stirring occasionally, until piping hot. Follow with a medium apple.

Note

Unless otherwise stated, fresh or frozen vegetables can be used.

Cauliflower Cheese Soup Serves 4

Metric/Imperial	American
450 g/1 lb cauliflower	1 lb cauliflower
850 ml/1½ pints water	3¾ cups water
15 ml/1 level tablespoon cornflour	1 level tablespoon cornstarch
25 g/1 oz skimmed milk powder	¼ cup skimmed milk powder
75 g/3 oz mature Cheddar cheese, grated	¾ cup grated sharp Cheddar cheese
salt and pepper	salt and pepper

Separate the cauliflower florets from the stalk. Dice the stalk and cook with the florets in a large saucepan of boiling, salted water for 10–15 minutes until tender.

Reserve half the cauliflower florets, then purée the remainder with the cooking liquid in a food processor or blender or by passing through a sieve. Return the purée to the saucepan.

Blend the cornflour (cornstarch) and skimmed milk powder with a little water until smooth, then stir into the cauliflower purée. Bring to the boil, stirring all the time, until the soup thickens. Stir in the cheese (do not allow the soup to boil again). Season with salt and pepper and add the reserved cauliflower florets. Allow the soup to cool, then divide between 4 freezer containers, label and freeze.

To serve, place a portion of frozen soup in a saucepan and heat through gently, stirring occasionally, until piping hot, but not boiling.

475-Calorie Main Meals

In The Mix and Match Formula we give you the opportunity to create your own main meals by combining a 200-Calorie Main Meal Maker, a 100-Calorie Sauce and a selection of vegetables with a total calorific value of 175 (see page 116). Alternatively opt for the simple life and select one of the 475-Calorie Recipes beginning on page 116.

200-Calorie Main Meal Makers

Choose one from the following options:

150 g/5 oz lamb chop, well grilled (broiled)
2 x 50 g/2 oz beefburgers (hamburgers), well grilled (broiled)
275 g/10 oz chicken leg, grilled (broiled) and skin removed
225 g/8 oz white fish fillet, served grilled (broiled)
225 g/8 oz/1⅓ cups red kidney beans, cooked or canned, drained

100-Calorie Sauces

Serve the meat, fish or beans with one of the following:

Cider Sauce

Metric/Imperial	American
175 ml/6 fl oz dry or sweet cider	¾ cup dry or sweet cider
15 ml/1 level tablespoon cornflour	1 level tablespoon cornstarch

Heat the cider in a saucepan. Blend the cornflour (cornstarch) with a little cold water until smooth. Stir into the cider. Bring to the boil, stirring continuously, and simmer for 2–3 minutes, stirring.

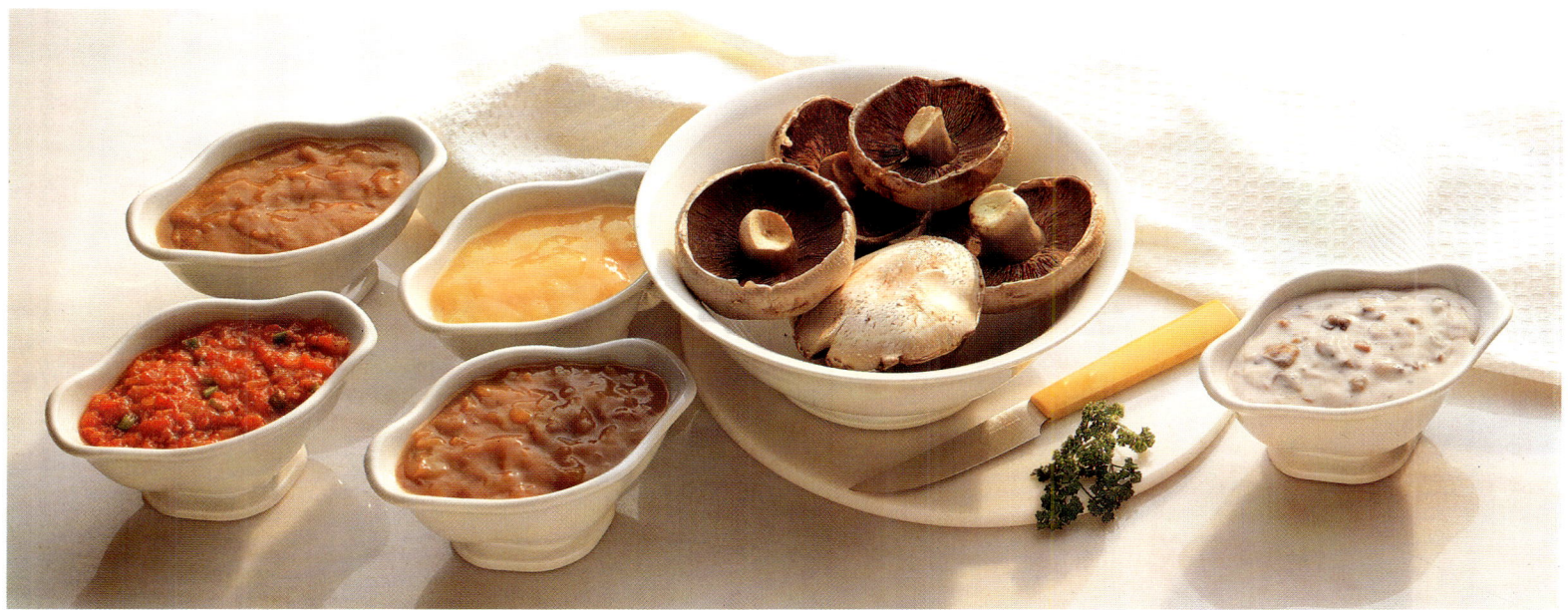

100-CALORIE SAUCES (left to right). Tomato Sauce; Curry Sauce; Herby Brown Sauce; Cider Sauce and Mushroom Sauce

Curry Sauce

Metric/Imperial
5 ml/1 level teaspoon butter
7.5 ml/1½ level teaspoons curry powder
1 small onion, finely chopped
½ chicken stock cube
175 ml/6 fl oz water
5 ml/1 level teaspoon tomato purée
5 ml/1 level teaspoon cornflour

American
1 level teaspoon butter
1½ level teaspoons curry powder
1 small onion, finely chopped
1 chicken bouillon cube
¾ cup water
1 level teaspoon tomato paste
1 level teaspoon cornstarch

Melt the butter in a saucepan, add the curry powder and fry for 1 minute. Add the onion, stock (bouillon) cube, water and tomato purée (paste) and bring to the boil, cover and simmer for 15 minutes.

Blend the cornflour (cornstarch) with a little cold water until smooth. Stir into the sauce. Return to the boil, then simmer for 2–3 minutes, stirring constantly. Add a little extra water if necessary.

Tomato Sauce

Metric/Imperial
1 x 225 g/8 oz can tomatoes
½ onion, finely chopped
¼ green or red pepper, cored, seeded and finely chopped
pinch of dried mixed herbs
10 ml/2 level teaspoons tomato ketchup
2.5 ml/½ teaspoon Worcestershire sauce
5 ml/1 level teaspoon cornflour

American
1 x 8 oz can tomatoes
½ onion, finely chopped
¼ green or red pepper, seeded and finely chopped
pinch of dried mixed herbs
2 level teaspoons tomato ketchup
½ teaspoon Worcestershire sauce
1 level teaspoon cornstarch

Chop the tomatoes and place in a pan with their juice. Add the onion, green pepper, herbs and sauces. Bring to the boil, then lower the heat, cover and simmer for 10 minutes. Uncover and boil for a further 15 minutes, stirring occasionally, to reduce. Blend the cornflour (cornstarch) with a little cold water until smooth. Stir into the sauce. Return to the boil, then simmer for 2–3 minutes, stirring continuously.

Herby Brown Sauce

Metric/Imperial
5 ml/1 level teaspoon margarine
1 small onion, finely chopped
½ garlic clove, crushed (optional)
½ beef stock cube
175 ml/6 fl oz water
10 ml/2 level teaspoons tomato ketchup
pinch of dried mixed herbs
10 ml/2 level teaspoons cornflour

American
1 level teaspoon margarine
1 small onion, finely chopped
½ garlic clove, crushed (optional)
1 beef bouillon cube
¾ cup water
2 level teaspoons tomato ketchup
pinch of dried mixed herbs
2 level teaspoons cornstarch

Melt the margarine in a small saucepan, add the onion and fry for 1 minute. Add the garlic, if using, with the stock (bouillon) cube, water, ketchup and herbs. Bring to the boil, then lower the heat, cover and simmer for 15 minutes. Blend the cornflour (cornstarch) with a little cold water until smooth. Stir into the sauce. Return to the boil, then simmer for 2–3 minutes, stirring constantly. Add a little extra water if necessary to prevent the sauce from sticking.

Mushroom Sauce

Metric/Imperial
15 ml/1 level tablespoon cornflour
175 ml/6 fl oz skimmed milk
50 g/2 oz mushrooms, chopped
pinch of grated nutmeg
salt and pepper

American
1 level tablespoon cornstarch
¾ cup skimmed milk
½ cup finely chopped mushrooms
pinch of grated nutmeg
salt and pepper

Blend the cornflour (cornstarch) with a little of the skimmed milk until smooth. Pour the remaining milk into a saucepan and heat.

Stir the blended cornflour (cornstarch) into the hot milk, beating well to get rid of any lumps. Add the mushrooms and season with the nutmeg and salt and pepper. Return to the boil, then lower the heat and simmer for 2–3 minutes, stirring constantly.

175-Calorie Vegetables

Serve your own choice of vegetables from the following list, adding up to no more than 175 Calories. Do not add oil, butter or fat of any kind to your vegetables during or after cooking.

Vegetables	Calories
Asparagus, per spear	5
Aubergine (eggplant), raw, 25 g/1 oz	4
Aubergine (eggplant), average whole 200 g/7 oz	28
Baked beans in tomato sauce, per 150 g/5 oz can	110
Baked beans in tomato sauce, per 225 g/8 oz can	160
Bean sprouts, raw, 25 g/1 oz	8
Beetroot, boiled, 25 g/1 oz	12
Broad beans (fava beans), boiled, 25 g/1 oz	14
Broccoli, raw, 25 g/1 oz	7
Brussels sprouts, raw, 25 g/1 oz	7
Butter beans, boiled, 25 g/1 oz	27
Cabbage, raw, 25 g/1 oz	6
Carrots, raw, 25 g/1 oz	6
Cauliflower, raw, 25 g/1 oz	4
Celeriac, raw, 25 g/1 oz	8
Celery, per stick (stalk)	5
Chicory (endive), raw, 25 g/1 oz	3
Courgette (zucchini), average whole 65 g/2½ oz	10
Cucumber, 25 g/1 oz	3
French beans (green beans), frozen, 25 g/1 oz	10
Haricot beans, boiled, 25 g/1 oz	26
Leeks, 1 average whole, 75 g/3 oz	25
Lettuce, 25 g/1 oz	3
Marrow (squash), raw, 25 g/1 oz	5
Mixed vegetables, frozen, 25 g/1 oz	15
Mushrooms, raw, 25 g/1 oz	4
Mustard and cress, whole carton	5
Onions, average small onion	15
Onion, pickled, each	5
Onion, spring (scallion), each	3
Parsnips, raw, 25 g/1 oz	14
Peas, frozen, 25 g/1 oz	15
Peppers, average whole, red or green 150 g/5 oz	20
Potatoes, raw, peeled, 25 g/1 oz	25
Potatoes, new, canned, drained 25 g/1 oz	15
Potato, prepared instant mash, per 15 ml/1 level tablespoon	40
Red kidney beans, 1 × 225 g/8 oz can	165
Red kidney beans, boiled or canned, drained, 25 g/1 oz	25
Radishes, each	2
Runner beans, raw, 25 g/1 oz	7
Spinach, raw, 25 g/1 oz	7
Spinach, boiled, 25 g/1 oz	9
Swede (rutabaga), raw, 25 g/1 oz	6
Sweetcorn (whole kernel corn), frozen 25 g/1 oz	25
Sweetcorn (whole kernel corn), canned, 1 × 200 g/7 oz can	155
Sweet potato, raw, 25 g/1 oz	26
Tomatoes, average whole, raw, 50 g/2 oz	8
Tomatoes, 1 × 225 g/8 oz can	25
Turnip, raw, 25 g/1 oz	6
Watercress, 25 g/1 oz	4

475-Calorie Recipes

Try one of the following using the meat, fish, beans and sauces:

Chicken Curry

Metric/Imperial	*American*
1 small apple	1 small apple
15 ml/1 level tablespoon sultanas	1 level tablespoon golden raisins
Curry Sauce (see page 115)	Curry Sauce (see page 115)
1 x 275 g/10 oz chicken leg	1 x 10 oz chicken leg
25 g/1 oz brown rice	1 oz brown rice
lemon wedges to garnish	lemon wedges to garnish

Peel and chop the apple and add with the sultanas (golden raisins) to the Curry Sauce in a saucepan. Cover and simmer gently for 15 minutes.

Meanwhile, grill (broil) the chicken until cooked through and remove and discard the skin. Cook the rice in a small saucepan of boiling, salted water for about 25 minutes or until tender, then drain.

Pour the hot Curry Sauce over the chicken, garnish with lemon and serve with the rice.

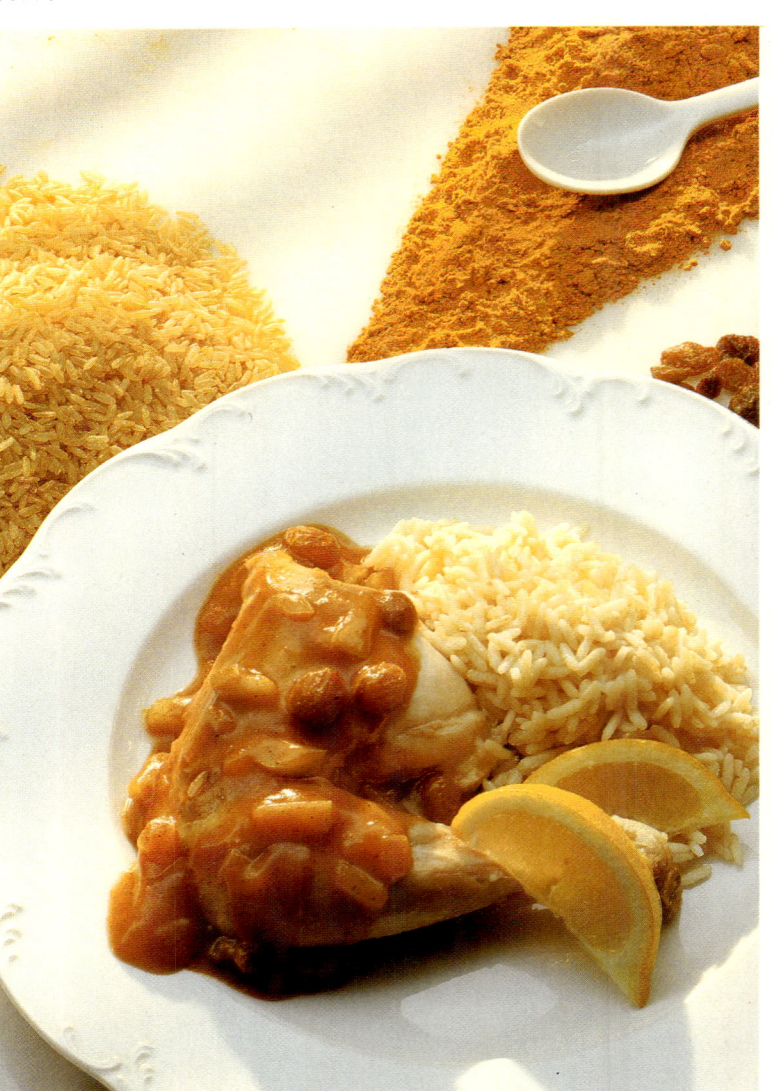

475-CALORIE RECIPE: Chicken Curry

Chicken Casserole

Metric/Imperial	American
125 g/4 oz carrots, diced	$\frac{2}{3}$ cup chopped carrot
75 g/3 oz turnip, diced	$\frac{1}{2}$ cup chopped turnip
1 small onion, chopped	1 small chopped onion
75 g/3 oz parsnips, chopped	$\frac{1}{2}$ cup chopped parsnips
275 g/10 oz chicken leg	10 oz chicken leg
75 g/3 oz canned red kidney beans, drained	$\frac{1}{2}$ cup drained canned red kidney beans
Tomato Sauce (see page 114)	Tomato Sauce (see page 114)

Cook the carrots, turnip, onion and parsnips in a saucepan of boiling salted water for 10 minutes, then drain.

Meanwhile, lightly grill (broil) the chicken and remove and discard the skin.

Put the chicken in a small casserole with the boiled vegetables, kidney beans and the Tomato Sauce. Cover and cook in a preheated moderately hot oven (190°C/375°F/Gas Mark 5) for 25–30 minutes.

Cidered Chicken

Metric/Imperial	American
1 x 275 g/10 oz chicken leg	1 x 10 oz chicken leg
1 medium tomato, thinly sliced	1 medium tomato, thinly sliced
1 small onion, thinly sliced	1 small onion, thinly sliced
25 g/1 oz mushrooms, sliced	$\frac{1}{4}$ cup thinly sliced mushrooms
1 celery stick, sliced	1 stalk celery, sliced
Cider Sauce (see page 115)	Cider Sauce (see page 115)
125 g/4 oz potatoes, (peeled weight), diced	$\frac{2}{3}$ cup diced potatoes
150 g/5 oz French beans, sliced	$\frac{2}{3}$ cup sliced green beans

Lightly grill (broil) the chicken and remove and discard the skin. Add the tomato, onion, mushroom and celery to the Cider Sauce and mix well. Pour over the chicken place in a small casserole and cover and cook in a preheated moderately hot oven (200°C/400°F/Gas Mark 6) for 30 minutes. Meanwhile, cook the potatoes and French (green) beans in separate saucepans of boiling salted water. Drain and serve with the hot Cidered Chicken.

Spicy Chicken and Pasta

Metric/Imperial	American
$\frac{1}{4}$ green pepper, cored, seeded and diced	$\frac{1}{4}$ green pepper, seeded and chopped
1 celery stick, chopped	1 stalk celery, chopped
Tomato Sauce (see page 114)	Tomato Sauce (see page 114)
1.25 ml/$\frac{1}{4}$ level teaspoon chilli powder	$\frac{1}{4}$ level teaspoon chili powder
5 ml/1 teaspoon Worcestershire sauce	1 teaspoon Worcestershire sauce
$\frac{1}{2}$ garlic clove, crushed	$\frac{1}{2}$ garlic clove, crushed
275 g/10 oz chicken leg	10 oz chicken leg
25 g/1 oz wholewheat pasta	$\frac{1}{4}$ cup wholewheat pasta
125 g/4 oz frozen peas	$\frac{3}{4}$ cup frozen peas

Add the green pepper and celery to the Tomato Sauce in a saucepan and stir in the chilli powder, Worcestershire sauce and garlic. Cook over a gentle heat for 15 minutes.

Meanwhile, grill (broil) the chicken until cooked through and remove and discard the skin. Cook the pasta and peas in separate pans of boiling water.

Pour the spicy sauce over the chicken and serve with the well drained pasta and peas.

Lamb Courgette Bake

Metric/Imperial	American
1 x 125 g/4 oz potato	1 x 4 oz potato
1 x 150 g/5 oz lamb chop	1 x 5 oz lamb chop
150 g/5 oz courgettes, sliced	1 cup zucchini, sliced
pinch of dried rosemary	pinch of dried rosemary
Tomato Sauce (see page 114)	Tomato Sauce (see page 114)
150 g/5 oz Brussels sprouts	$\frac{2}{3}$ cup Brussels sprouts

Bake the potato in its jacket in a preheated moderately hot oven (200°C/400°F/Gas Mark 6) for 45 minutes or until cooked through.

Meanwhile, grill (broil) the lamb chop and place with the courgettes (zucchini) and rosemary in a small casserole. Add the hot Tomato Sauce, cover and cook in the oven below the potato for 30 minutes.

Cook the Brussels sprouts in boiling salted water. Drain well and serve with the Lamb Courgette (Zucchini) Bake and the baked potato.

Country Cider Lamb

Metric/Imperial	American
1 x 175 g/6 oz lamb chop	1 x 6 oz lamb chop
1 small onion, sliced	1 small onion, sliced
25 g/1 oz carrot, sliced	$\frac{1}{6}$ cup sliced carrot
50 g/2 oz turnip, diced	$\frac{1}{3}$ cup chopped turnip
1 small apple, peeled, cored and sliced	1 small apple, peeled, cored and sliced
Cider Sauce (see page 115)	Cider Sauce (see page 115)
175 g/6 oz cauliflower florets	1 cup cauliflower florets
150 g/5 oz frozen peas	Scant cup frozen peas

Grill (broil) the lamb chop until well done.

Meanwhile, put the onion carrot, turnip and apple in a saucepan with the Cider Sauce. Cover and simmer for 20 minutes.

Cook the cauliflower and peas in separate saucepans of boiling salted water, then drain. Pour the hot sauce over the chop and serve accompanied by the vegetables.

Herby Lamb Chop and Baked Potato

Metric/Imperial	American
1 x 200 g/7 oz potato	1 x 7 oz potato
1 x 150 g/5 oz lamb chop	1 x 5 oz lamb chop
Herby Brown Sauce (see page 115)	Herby Brown Sauce (see page 115)

Bake the potato in its jacket in a preheated moderately hot oven (200°C/400°F/Gas Mark 6) for 45 minutes or until cooked through.

Grill (broil) the lamb chop until well done. Pour the hot Herby Brown Sauce over the chop and serve with the baked potato.

Lamb Chop and Saucy Vegetables

Metric/Imperial	American
150 g/5 oz cauliflower florets	1 cup cauliflower florets
150 g/5 oz mixed vegetables	1 cup mixed vegetables
75 g/3 oz broad beans (shelled weight)	$\frac{1}{2}$ cup shelled fava beans
1 x 150 g/5 oz lamb chop	1 x 5 oz lamb chop
Mushroom Sauce (see page 115)	Mushroom Sauce (see page 115)

Cook the cauliflower, mixed vegetables and broad (fava) beans in separate saucepans of boiling water, then drain.

Meanwhile, grill (broil) the lamb chop until well done. Pour the hot Mushroom Sauce over the vegetables and serve with the chop.

Herby Lamb Stew

Metric/Imperial
1 x 150 g/5 oz lamb loin chop
1 carrot, sliced
25 g/1 oz leek, sliced
50 g/2 oz turnip, diced
Herby Brown Sauce (see page 115)
pinch of dried rosemary
1 x 175 g/6 oz or 2 x 75 g/3 oz potatoes
50 g/2 oz peas (shelled weight)

American
1 x 5 oz lamb loin chop
1 carrot, sliced
1 oz leek, sliced
⅓ cup chopped turnip
Herby Brown Sauce (see page 115)
pinch of dried rosemary
1 x 6 oz or 2 x 3 oz potatoes
⅓ cup shelled peas

Lightly grill (broil) the lamb chop and place in a casserole. Mix the carrot, leek and turnip with the Herby Brown Sauce and add the rosemary. Pour the mixture over the lamb chop and cook in a moderate oven (180°C/350°F/Gas Mark 4) for 45 minutes.

Bake the potato alongside the stew for 30 minutes (small) or 1 hour (medium). Stir the peas into the stew and cook for a further 5 minutes. Serve with the potatoes.

Fish Parcel and Tomato Sauce

Metric/Imperial
25 g/1 oz mushrooms, finely chopped
1 celery stick, finely chopped
15 ml/1 level tablespoon breadcrumbs
15 ml/1 level tablespoon tomato ketchup
225 g/8 oz plaice or lemon sole fish fillets, skinned
Tomato Sauce (see page 115)
125 g/4 oz broccoli
125 g/4 oz carrots, diced
125 g/4 oz potato (peeled weight), diced

American
¼ cup finely chopped mushrooms
1 stalk celery, finely chopped
1 tablespoon bread crumbs
1 tablespoon tomato ketchup
8 oz plaice or lemon sole fish fillets, skinned
Tomato Sauce (see page 115)
⅔ cup broccoli
⅔ cup chopped carrots
⅔ cup chopped potato

Mix the mushrooms and celery with the breadcrumbs and tomato ketchup. Spoon the stuffing mixture on to the centre of the fish fillet, fold over the edges to form a parcel and secure with wooden cocktail sticks.

Place the stuffed fish in a casserole, cover with Tomato Sauce and cook in a preheated moderately hot oven (200°C/400°F/Gas Mark 6) for 20 minutes.

Meanwhile, cook the broccoli, carrots and potato in separate pans of boiling salted water, then drain. Serve with the Fish Parcel and Tomato Sauce (cocktail sticks removed).

Fish and Mushroom Sauce with Vegetables

Metric/Imperial
225 g/8 oz white fish fillets, skinned
Mushroom Sauce (see page 115)
150 g/5 oz sweetcorn
125 g/4 oz broad beans

American
8 oz white fish fillets, skinned
Mushroom Sauce (see page 115)
1 cup kernel corn
¾ cup fava beans

Put the fish in a small casserole and cover with the Mushroom Sauce. Cover and cook in a preheated moderately hot oven (190°C/375°F/Gas Mark 5) for 25–30 minutes.

Meanwhile, cook the sweetcorn and broad (fava) beans in boiling salted water, then drain. Serve with the Fish in Mushroom Sauce.

Fish Curry and Vegetable Rice

Metric/Imperial
25 g/1 oz long-grain brown rice
275 ml/½ pint cold water
1 onion, chopped
75 g/3 oz frozen peas
75 g/3 oz mushrooms, sliced
225 g/8 oz white fish fillets, skinned
Curry Sauce (see page 115)

American
2 level tablespoons long-grain brown rice
1¼ cups cold water
1 onion, chopped
½ cup frozen peas
¾ cup sliced mushrooms
8 oz white fish fillets, skinned
Curry Sauce (see page 115)

Put the rice in a small saucepan with the water. Cover, bring to the boil and simmer for 20 minutes. Add the onion, peas and mushrooms to the pan. Return to the boil and cook for a further 5 minutes, then drain.

Meanwhile, grill (broil) the fish until cooked through. Pour the hot Curry Sauce over the fish and serve with the rice and vegetables.

Curried Fish Kebabs

Metric/Imperial
40 g/1½ oz brown rice
225 g/8 oz white fish fillet, skinned and cut into bite-sized cubes
½ green pepper, seeded and cut into small squares
8 button mushrooms
1 firm tomato, quartered
4 bay leaves
30 ml/2 tablespoons lemon juice
Curry Sauce (see page 115)

American
3 level tablespoons brown rice
8 oz white fish fillet, skinned and cut into bite-sized cubes
½ green pepper, seeded and cut into small squares
8 button mushrooms
1 firm tomato, quartered
4 bay leaves
2 tablespoons lemon juice
Curry Sauce (see page 115)

Cook the rice in boiling salted water until tender. Thread the fish, green pepper, mushrooms, tomato and bay leaves alternately on to 2 kebab skewers. Sprinkle with lemon juice and grill (broil) under a preheated moderate grill (broiler) for 10 minutes, turning frequently and basting with lemon juice.

Drain the rice and serve with the fish kebabs and the Curry Sauce poured over the top.

Beefburger and Vegetable Bake

Metric/Imperial
2 x 50 g/2 oz beefburgers
½ small onion, thinly sliced
25 g/1 oz carrot, diced
50 g/2 oz potato, diced (peeled weight)
Mushroom Sauce (see page 115)
175 g/6 oz cauliflower
150 g/5 oz mixed vegetables

American
2 x 2 oz hamburgers
½ small onion, thinly sliced
¼ cup chopped carrot
⅓ cup chopped potato (peeled weight)
Mushroom Sauce (see page 115)
1 cup cauliflower
¾ cup mixed vegetables

Well grill (broil) the beefburgers (hamburgers). Cook the onion, carrot and potato together in boiling salted water for 5 minutes, then drain.

Put the beefburgers in a small casserole. Arrange the onion, carrots and potato on top. Pour the Mushroom Sauce over the top. Cover and cook in a preheated moderately hot oven (190°C/375°F/Gas Mark 5) for 30 minutes.

Meanwhile, cook the cauliflower and mixed vegetables in separate saucepans of boiling salted water. Drain and serve with the Beefburger and Vegetable Bake.

Beefburger Hotpot

Metric/Imperial	American
125 g/4 oz carrots, diced	⅔ cups chopped carrots
1 x 125 g/4 oz potato	1 x 4 oz potato
125 g/4 oz frozen peas	⅔ cup frozen peas
2 x 50 g/2 oz beefburgers	2 x 2 oz hamburgers
Herby Brown Sauce (see page 115)	Herby Brown Sauce (see page 115)

Cook the carrots and potato in boiling salted water for 5 minutes. Add the peas, return to the boil, then lower the heat and cook for a further 5 minutes. Drain.

Meanwhile, grill (broil) the beefburgers (hamburgers) well, then cut into chunks and place in a small casserole. Add the peas and carrots and cover with Herby Brown Sauce. Slice the potato thinly and arrange on top of the casserole. Cook in a preheated moderately hot oven (200ºC/400ºF/Gas Mark 6) for 30 minutes or until the potato is cooked through and lightly browned.

Beefburger Casserole

Metric/Imperial	American
1 x 150 g/5 oz potato	1 x 5 oz potato
2 x 50 g/2 oz beefburgers	2 x 2 oz hamburgers
Herby Brown Sauce (see page 115)	Herby Brown Sauce (see page 115)
50 g/2 oz carrot, diced	⅓ chopped carrot
½ small onion, sliced	½ small onion, sliced
50 g/2 oz turnip, diced	⅓ cup chopped turnip
50 g/2 oz frozen peas	⅓ cup frozen peas

Bake the potato in its jacket in a preheated moderately hot oven (200ºC/400ºF/Gas Mark 6) for 45 minutes or until cooked through.

Meanwhile, well grill (broil) the beefburgers (hamburgers) and cut into chunks. Place in a small casserole with the Herby Brown Sauce, carrot, onion and turnip. Cover and cook in the oven below the potato for 20 minutes. Add the peas to the casserole and cook for a further 10 minutes. Serve with baked potato.

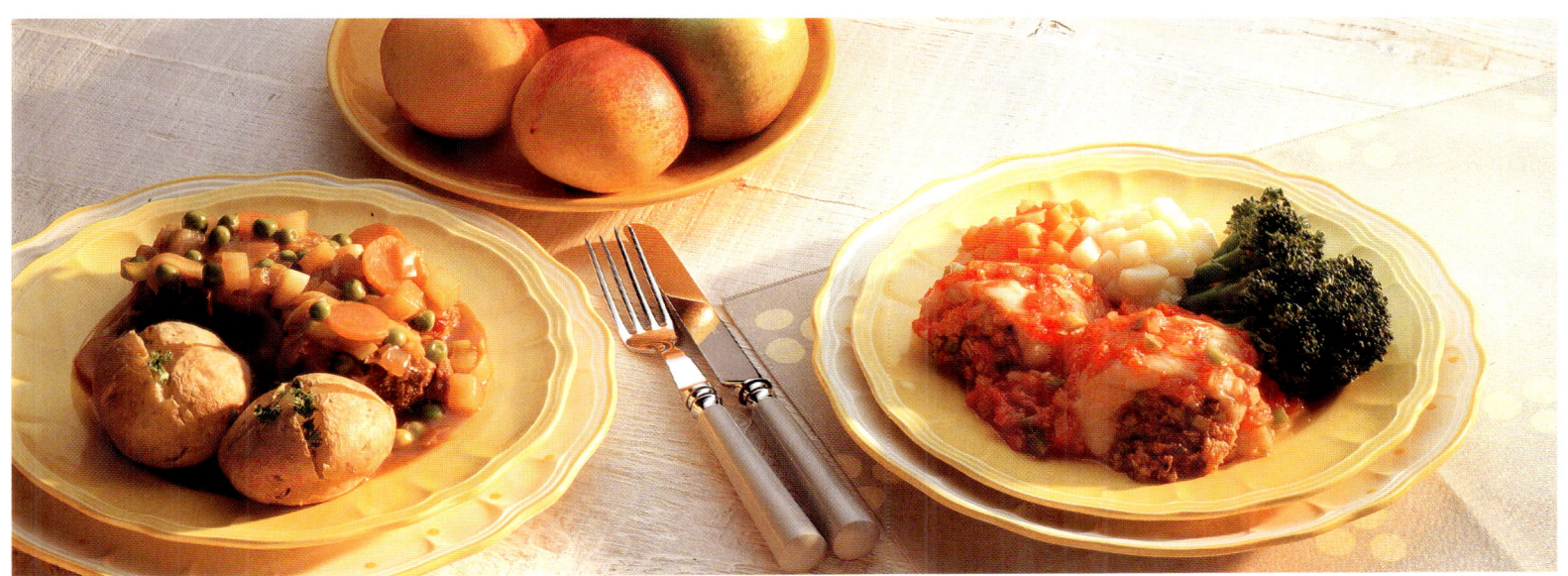

475-CALORIE RECIPES: Herby Lamb Stew; Fish Parcel with Tomato Sauce

Cidered Beans and Pasta

Metric/Imperial	American
225 g/8 oz red kidney beans, cooked or canned and drained	1⅓ cups cooked or canned and drained red kidney beans
Cider Sauce (see page 115)	Cider Sauce (see page 115)
¼ red pepper, cored, seeded diced	¼ red pepper, seeded and chopped
¼ green pepper, cored seeded and diced	¼ green pepper, seeded and chopped
25 g/1 oz mushrooms, sliced	¼ cup sliced mushrooms
50 g/2 oz sweetcorn	⅓ cup kernel corn
25 g/1 oz wholewheat pasta	¼ cup wholewheat pasta
150 g/5 oz cauliflower florets	1 cup cauliflower florets

Mix the kidney beans with the Cider Sauce in a saucepan. Add the red pepper, green pepper, mushrooms and corn. Stir well to mix, bring just to the boil, then lower the heat and cover and simmer for 15 minutes. Meanwhile, cook the pasta and cauliflower florets in separate saucepans of boiling salted water. Drain and serve with the Cidered Beans.

Beany Casserole

Metric/Imperial	American
225 g/8 oz red kidney beans, cooked or canned and drained	1⅓ cups cooked or canned and drained red kidney beans
Herby Brown Sauce (see page 115)	Herby Brown Sauce (see page 115)
50 g/2 oz turnip, diced	⅓ cup chopped turnip
50 g/2 oz frozen peas	⅓ cup frozen peas
1 celery stick, chopped	1 stalk celery, chopped
¼ red pepper, cored, seeded and diced	¼ red pepper, seeded and chopped
1 x 150 g/5 oz potato (peeled weight)	1 x 5 oz potato, peeled

Mix the kidney beans with the Herby Brown Sauce in a casserole. Stir in the turnip, peas, celery and red pepper. Cook in a preheated moderately hot oven (200ºC/400ºF/Gas Mark 6) for 30 minutes. Meanwhile, boil the potato, drain and serve with the Beany Casserole.

The Dine and Diet Plan

This is an ideal diet if you are a businesswoman who has to cope with slap-up business lunches, or if you enjoy eating out or entertaining friends. Over a week, four days are planned to be super-strict, with a breakfast, light meal and main meal. Then for three days during that week you can indulge in a fairly high-calorie restaurant or pub meal or share one of the Dine and Diet menus with family or friends. Your Calories for the week will average out to 1,250 a day – a total at which you will successfully shed weight if you have an excess stone (6.3 kg/14 lb) or more to lose.

It is best to decide before you go into a restaurant what you intend to eat. If you know, for example, that the restaurant you will be visiting serves mainly Italian food, study the Italian menus given on page 125 and decide which of them you would prefer. It helps if you are already familiar with the restaurant's menu because then you can make sure you don't bank on eating something that is unlikely to be obtainable.

All our menus are based on the most popular foods available when you are eating out, but if you find that your well-laid plans are dashed by the whim of a chef who has decided to take your chosen dish off the menu, follow these basic eating out rules: Don't order fried fish, meat or vegetables. Avoid meat and fish that come smothered in a creamy sauce. Be moderate with your portions, except for low-calorie vegetables which you can heap on to your plate in whatever quantity you wish. Make sure salads don't come covered in mayonnaise or an oily dressing. Learn to be impolite and don't have a starter or dessert just to keep someone company. Save all your calories for food which will give you pleasure. Say no to cream in coffee or poured over fruit.

On strict dieting days you must weigh and measure all your food very carefully to ensure that you are consuming just 850 Calories. If you do not usually eat breakfast you can take a packed meal to work to eat mid-morning or save it as a snack to eat in the evening. Some dieters find that they cope far better with strict days if they delay their first meal as long as possible. It doesn't matter if you eat your restaurant or entertaining menu at lunchtime or in the evening, provided that in addition you have only one breakfast meal and a light meal at other times during the day.

All the eating out and entertaining menus allow you an alcoholic drink. You can make wine go much further if you mix it with mineral water (carbonated water tastes nicest) to make a Spritz. Water contains no calories at all, so drink as much of any kind with your meal as you wish. If you like, you can swap a glass of wine for 275 ml/½ pint/1¼ cups lager or cider, or vice versa.

The Dine and Diet Plan is ideal if you have over a stone to lose and want to keep up your social life while you diet; but you will probably have to be a little stricter as you near target weight. Either check the questionnaire on page 14 and choose another diet, cut down your eating out or entertaining meals to two a week or swap your alcoholic drinks for no-calorie water.

Diet Rules

1 For four days of the week you must be super-strict. On the other three days you can indulge in a fairly high-calorie restaurant or pub meal with drinks, or share a Dine and Diet Menu with family or friends.

2 On super-strict days choose one breakfast, one light meal and one main meal. If it's a working day choose a light meal that you can pack and eat at your desk. For weekends we've included some hot light meals.

3 On eating-out or celebration days choose a breakfast, one light meal and one of the restaurant meals listed on page 125 or a Dine and Diet Menu. If you don't feel like eating first thing in the morning pick one of the breakfasts that can be taken to work, or save your breakfast to eat later.

4 In addition to the listed food and drink, each day you are allowed 275 ml/½ pint/1¼ cups skimmed milk to use in drinks. Milk given as part of a recipe or menu is in addition to your daily allowance.

5 You may drink unlimited amounts of tea and coffee, using milk from your allowance and artificial sweetener if you wish. You are also allowed unlimited amounts of water, low-calorie mixers and squashes.

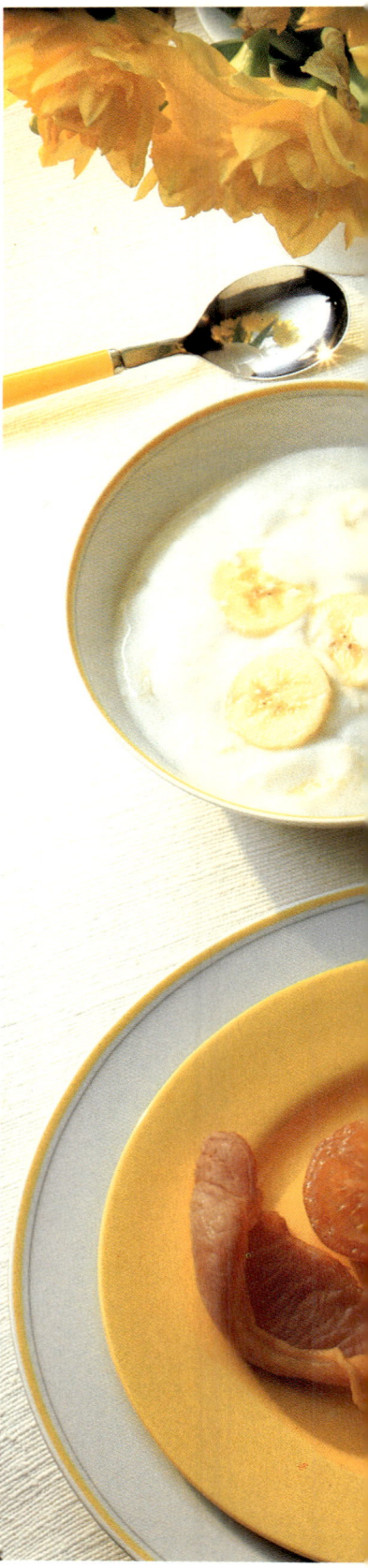

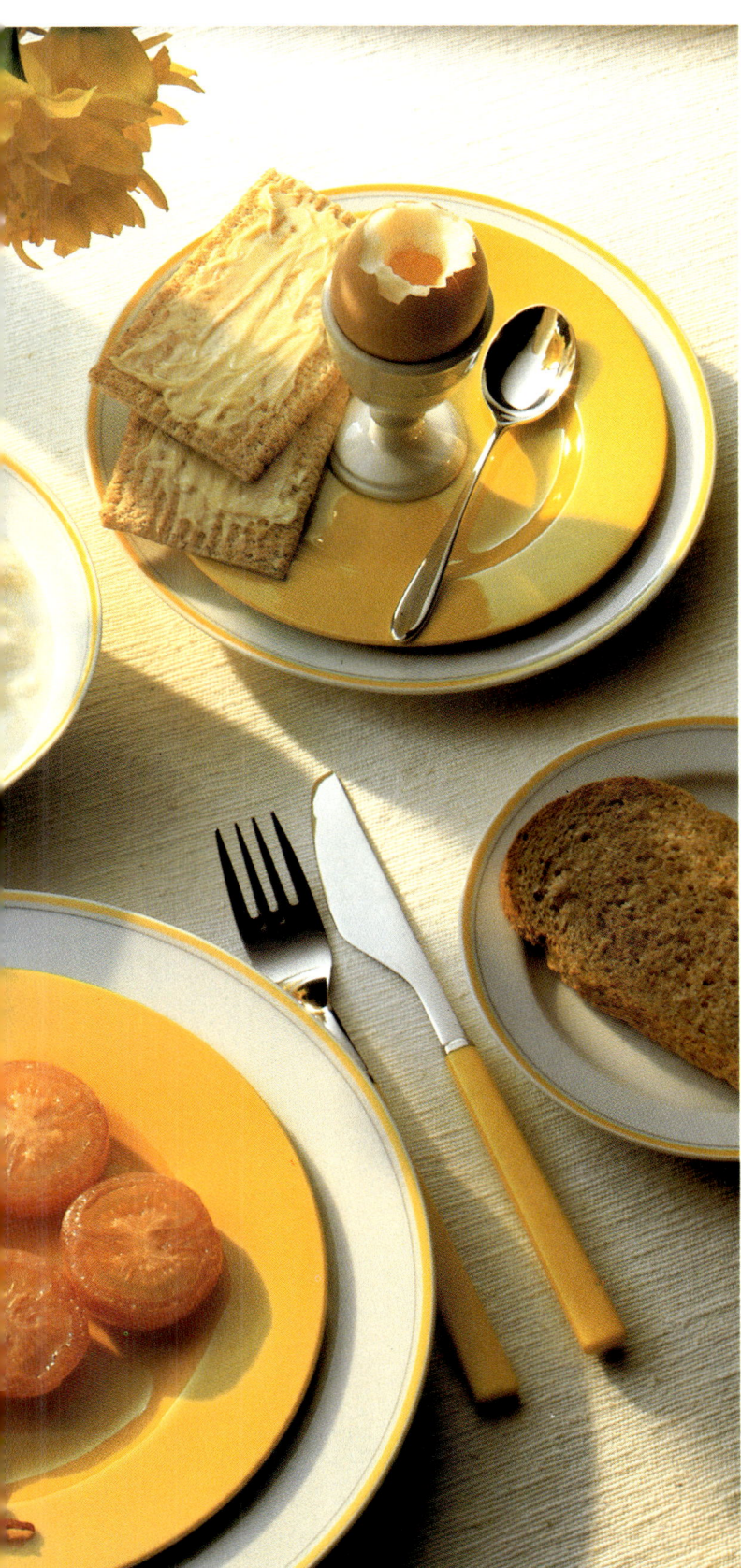

150-Calorie Breakfasts to eat at Home

BOILED EGG AND CRISPBREADS
Boil 1 × size 3 (medium) egg and serve with 2 calorie-reduced crispbreads spread with 10 ml/2 level teaspoons low-fat spread.

BACON AND TOMATOES
Cook 1 rasher (slice) of back bacon and 2 tomatoes under a preheated grill (broiler) until the bacon is crisp. Serve with 1 × 25 g/1 oz slice wholemeal bread.

YOGURT AND BANANA
Pour 1 × 150 g/5 oz carton/⅔ cup low-fat natural yogurt into an individual serving bowl and mix in 1 small peeled and sliced banana.

CEREAL
Put 25 g/1 oz/1 cup Cornflakes or Rice Krispies into an individual serving bowl, sprinkle with 5 ml/1 level teaspoon sugar and pour over 115 ml/4 fl oz/½ cup skimmed milk.

TOAST AND MARMALADE
Spread one 40 g/1½ oz slice wholemeal toast with 10 ml/2 level teaspoons low-fat spread and 10 ml/2 level teaspoons jam, marmalade or honey.

ALL BRAN
Put 40 g/1½ oz/⅓ cup All Bran cereal into an individual serving bowl and pour over 115 ml/4 fl oz/½ cup skimmed milk.

SHREDDED WHEAT AND APRICOTS
Put 1 Shredded Wheat into an individual serving dish, sprinkle with 4 chopped dried apricots and pour over 75 ml/3 fl oz/⅓ cup skimmed milk.

150-Calorie Breakfasts to take to Work

HAM SANDWICH
Spread 1 × 40 g/1½ oz slice wholemeal bread with 5 ml/1 level teaspoon low-fat spread and a little mustard. Cut the slice in half and sandwich together with 25 g/1 oz lean cooked ham, all visible fat removed. Wrap in plastic wrap.

RAISIN AND WHEATGERM YOGURT
Mix 1 × 150 g/5 oz carton/⅔ cup fruit yogurt, 15 ml/1 level tablespoon raisins and 15 ml/1 level tablespoon wheatgerm together and pack in a plastic container.

CHEESE AND CUCUMBER SANDWICH, AND FRUIT
Cut 1 × 35 g/1¼ oz slice wholemeal bread in half and sandwich together with 15 g/½ oz cheese spread and a few slices cucumber. Wrap in plastic wrap. Pack 1 medium peach or pear to follow.

EGG AND CRISPBREADS
Mix 1 size 3 (medium) hard-boiled (hard-cooked) chopped egg with 15 ml/1 level tablespoon low-calorie salad dressing. Pack in a small container. Spread on two crispbreads when ready to eat.

150-CALORIE BREAKFASTS TO EAT AT HOME: Boiled Egg and Crispbreads; Yogurt and Banana; Bacon and Tomatoes

250-Calorie Light Meals

COTTAGE CHEESE WITH CRISPBREADS, AND FRUIT

Spread 4 calorie-reduced crispbreads with 125 g/4 oz/½ cup cottage cheese flavoured with chives or pineapple. Serve 1 medium apple or 1 orange to follow.

COTTAGE CHEESE SALAD, AND FRUIT

Combine 1 quartered tomato, 2 celery sticks (stalks) and ¼ red or green pepper, cored, seeded and diced. Mix with ¼ head shredded lettuce and toss with 15 ml/1 tablespoon oil-free French dressing. Serve with 175 g/6 oz/¾ cup plain or cottage cheese flavoured with chives. Follow with 1 medium peach or pear.

PRAWN AND SWEETCORN SALAD

In an individual salad bowl combine 75 g/3 oz/½ cup peeled prawns (shelled shrimp) with ¼ red or green pepper, cored, seeded and diced. Add 50 g/ 2 oz/½ cup chopped cucumber and 125 g/4 oz/⅔ cup sweetcorn kernels (whole kernel corn). Stir through 15 ml/1 level tablespoon low-calorie seafood sauce and 15 ml/1 level tablespoon low-fat natural yogurt and add salt and pepper to taste.

BAKED BEANS ON TOAST, AND FRUIT

Heat 1 × 225 g/8 oz can baked beans in tomato sauce in a small saucepan and serve on 1 × 25 g/ 1 oz slice wholemeal toast. Follow with 1 kiwifruit or 125 g/ 4 oz/¾ cup raspberries or strawberries, fresh or frozen and thawed.

TUNA SANDWICH, AND FRUIT

Mix 50 g/2 oz/¼ cup drained and flaked tuna in brine with 2 small chopped gherkins and 15 ml/1 level tablespoon low-calorie seafood sauce. Use as a filling between 2 × 25 g/1 oz slices wholemeal bread. Serve 1 medium peach or pear to follow.

SARDINE AND OLIVE SANDWICH

Mash 2 canned sardines in tomato sauce and mix with 2 chopped stuffed olives and 1 teaspoon finely chopped onion. Use as a filling between 2 × 25 g/ 1 oz slices wholemeal bread.

BEEF SANDWICH, AND FRUIT

Make a sandwich using 2 × 25 g/ 1 oz slices wholemeal bread spread with 10 ml/2 level teaspoons low-fat spread and a little mustard, and 1 × 40 g/1½ oz slice lean roast topside (top round) beef, all visible fat removed. Follow with 1 mandarin orange or 75 g/3 oz/¾ cup raspberries or strawberries, fresh or frozen and thawed.

CHEESE AND TOMATO SANDWICH

Mix 40 g/1½ oz/⅓ cup grated Tendale (low calorie Cheddar-like) cheese with 15 ml/1 level tablespoon low-calorie salad dressing. Use with 1 small sliced tomato as a filling between 2 × 25 g/1 oz slices wholemeal bread.

BACON SANDWICH

Grill (broil) 2 rashers (slices) streaky bacon, derinded, until crisp. Make a sandwich using 2 × 25 g/1 oz slices wholemeal bread spread with 15 ml/1 level tablespoon tomato ketchup, and filled with the bacon.

CHEESE AND HAM ROLL

Split 1 crusty brown bread roll and spread with 15 ml/1 level tablespoon processed cheese spread. Fill with 1 × 25 g/1 oz slice lean cooked ham, all visible fat removed, and 15 ml/1 level tablespoon sweet pickle relish.

CHICKEN AND CORN SANDWICH

Make a sandwich using 2 × 25 g/ 1 oz slices wholemeal bread, 30 ml/2 level tablespoons corn relish, 50 g/2 oz/¼ cup chopped cooked chicken (without skin) and a little cress.

PRAWN SALAD, AND FRUIT

Mix 125 g/4 oz/⅔ cup peeled prawns (shelled shrimp) with 30 ml/2 level tablespoons low-calorie seafood sauce and pile the mixture in the centre of a serving platter.

Surround the seafood with 1 quartered tomato, ¼ shredded lettuce, ¼ sliced cucumber, chopped celery sticks (stalks) and ¼ green pepper, cored, seeded and diced. Sprinkle a little mustard and cress over the top and serve. Follow with 1 small banana or 1 medium orange.

PLAICE IN SAUCE WITH VEGETABLES

Cook 175 g/6 oz frozen plaice (flounder) in cream sauce according to the directions on the packet. Serve with 125 g/ 4 oz/⅔ cup boiled peas and 125 g/ 4 oz/½ cup boiled French (green) beans.

RAVIOLI

Heat 1 × 215 g/7½ oz can ravioli in tomato sauce in a small saucepan and transfer to a heatproof dish. Mix 15 g/½ oz grated Edam (Dutch) cheese with 15 ml/1 level tablespoon fresh soft breadcrumbs and sprinkle over the ravioli. Place the dish under a preheated grill (broiler) and cook until the cheese has melted.

FRENCH ONION SOUP WITH CHEESY TOAST

Heat 1 × 425 g/15 oz can French onion soup in a small saucepan. Place 1 × 25 g/1 oz slice wholemeal bread under a preheated grill (broiler) and toast on one side only. Sprinkle the untoasted side with 25 g/1 oz/ ¼ cup grated Edam (Dutch) cheese. Return to the grill (broiler) and cook until cheese melts, then cut into 4 squares. Pour the soup into a warmed soup bowl and float the cheesy toast on top.

SARDINE SANDWICH

Mash 2 sardines canned in tomato sauce with 25 g/1 oz/1 tablespoon plain cottage cheese or cottage cheese with chives. Use as a filling between 2 × 25 g/ 1 oz slices wholemeal bread.

PRAWN AND CURD CHEESE SANDWICH

Mix together 15 g/½ oz chopped cucumber, 50 g/2 oz/¼ cup curd cheese and 25 g/1 oz peeled prawns (shelled shrimp). Season with salt and pepper. Use as a filling between 2 × 25 g/1 oz slices wholemeal bread.

EGG AND YEAST EXTRACT SANDWICH

Hard-boil (hard-cook) 1 size 3 (medium) egg. Chop it and mix with 15 ml/1 level tablespoon low-calorie salad dressing. Spread 1 × 25 g/1 oz slice wholemeal bread with 5 ml/1 level teaspoon yeast extract. Top with the egg mixture and a little cress and make into a sandwich with a second 25 g/1 oz slice of wholemeal bread.

SCRAMBLED EGGS ON TOAST

Place 2 size 3 (medium) eggs in a bowl with 30 ml/2 tablespoons skimmed milk and salt and pepper to taste. Beat lightly. Melt 5 ml/1 level teaspoon low-fat spread in a non-stick saucepan. Pour in the egg mixture and cook over a low heat, stirring until just cooked and creamy. Serve on 1 × 35 g/1¼ oz slice wholemeal toast.

HAM STEAK WITH BUBBLE AND SQUEAK, AND FRUIT

Arrange 1 × 125 g/4 oz ham steak and 2 × 50 g/2 oz patties frozen bubble and squeak (potato cakes) on the rack of a preheated grill (broiler). Cook without added fat, turning once, until done. Serve 1 medium apple or pear to follow.

BACON AND EGG

Poach 1 size 3 (medium) egg. Cook 3 rashers (slices) streaky bacon under a preheated grill (broiler) until crisp. Serve the egg and bacon with 1 calorie-reduced crispbread.

CHEESE CRISPBREADS WITH CELERY, AND FRUIT

Serve 40 g/1½ oz Brie or Camembert cheese with 3 calorie reduced crispbreads and 2 celery sticks (stalks). Follow with 1 medium apple or pear.

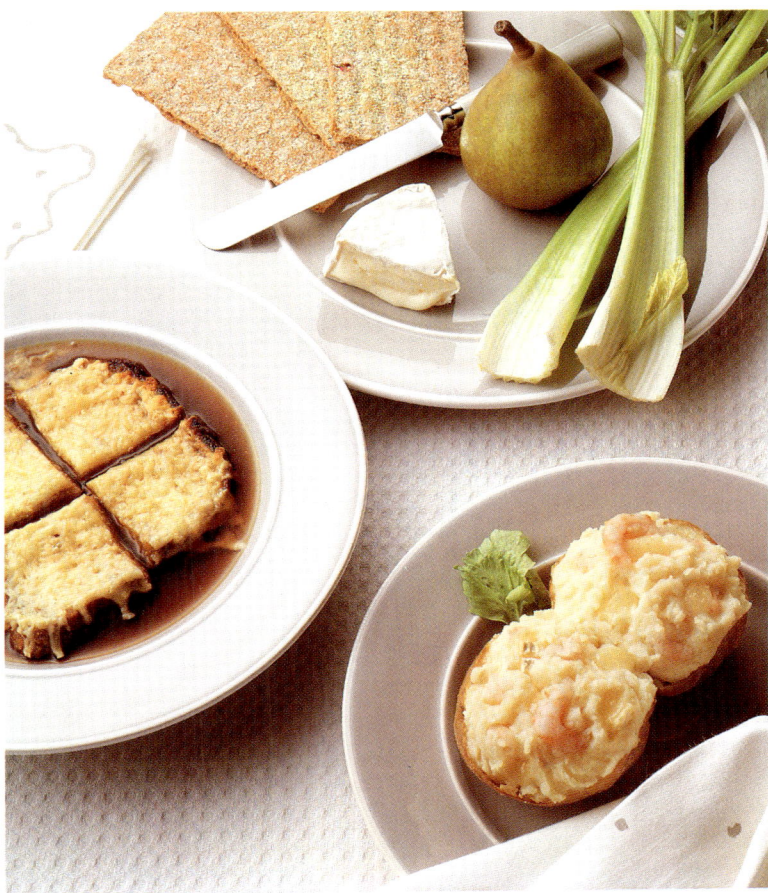

250-CALORIE LIGHT MEALS: Cheese Crispbreads with Celery and Fruit; French Onion Soup with Cheesy Toast. 350-CALORIE MAIN MEAL: Baked Potato with Brie and Prawns

350-Calorie Main Meals for Strict Days

Ham and Egg Salad, and Yogurt

Metric/Imperial	American
1 egg, size 3, hard-boiled	1 medium egg, hard-cooked
50 g/2 oz slices lean cooked ham, all visible fat removed	2 oz lean cooked ham, all visible fat removed
1 tomato, quartered	1 tomato, quartered
¼ small lettuce, shredded	¼ small head lettuce, shredded
¼ small cucumber, sliced	¼ small cucumber, sliced
¼ green or red pepper, cored, seeded and diced	¼ green or red pepper, seeded and diced
15 ml/1 level tablespoon low-calorie salad dressing	1 tablespoon low-calorie salad dressing
To follow	*To follow*
150 g/5 oz carton low-fat natural yogurt	⅔ cup low-fat natural yogurt
10 ml/2 level teaspoons clear honey	2 level teaspoons clear honey

Combine the salad ingredients and serve with the ham, egg and salad dressing. Serve the yogurt mixed with the honey to follow.

Quarterpounder Grill

Metric/Imperial	American
1 x 125 g/4 oz beefburger	1 x 4 oz hamburger
125 g/4 oz frozen peas	⅔ cup frozen peas
125 g/4 oz button mushrooms	1 cup button mushrooms
15 ml/1 level tablespoon tomato ketchup or brown sauce	1 level tablespoon tomato ketchup or brown sauce

Grill (broil) the beefburger under a preheated grill (broiler), turning once, until cooked well. Cook the peas in boiling water. Poach the mushrooms in a little water. Drain the vegetables and serve with the beefburger and tomato ketchup.

Smoked Haddock with Poached Egg and Spinach, and Fruit

Metric/Imperial	American
1 x 175 g/6 oz packet frozen smoked haddock with butter	1 x 6 oz packet frozen finnan haddie with butter
125 g/4 oz chopped spinach, frozen	½ cup frozen chopped spinach
1 egg, size 3	1 medium egg
To follow	*To follow*
1 medium apple or pear	1 medium apple or pear

Cook the fish and spinach according to packet instructions. Drain the spinach well. Poach the egg. Spoon the spinach over the base of an individual serving dish and lay the fish on top. Place the egg on the fish and serve. Follow with fruit.

Prawn and Rice Salad

Metric/Imperial	American
40 g/1½ oz long-grain rice	3 tablespoons long-grain rice
50 g/2 oz frozen peas	⅓ cup frozen peas
¼ red or green pepper, cored, seeded and diced	¼ red or green pepper, seeded and diced
50 g/2 oz cucumber, diced	½ cup diced cucumber
125 g/4 oz peeled prawns	¾ cup shelled shrimp
30 ml/2 tablespoons oil-free French dressing	2 tablespoons oil-free French dressing
salt and pepper	salt and pepper

Cook the rice and peas separately in boiling, salted water. Drain, rinse under cold water and drain again. Combine all the ingredients, season with salt and pepper and stir well to mix.

Baked Potato with Brie and Prawns (Shrimp)

Metric/Imperial	American
1 x 200 g/7 oz potato	1 x 7 oz potato
15 ml/1 tablespoon skimmed milk	1 tablespoon skimmed milk
40 g/1½ oz Brie cheese, diced	⅓ cup diced Brie cheese
25 g/1 oz peeled prawns	⅙ cup peeled shrimp
salt and pepper	salt and pepper

Bake the potato in its jacket in a preheated moderately hot oven (200°C/400°F/Gas Mark 6) for about 1 hour or until cooked. Cut the potato in half lengthways and carefully scoop out the flesh, leaving the cases intact. Mash the potato flesh with the milk. Stir the cheese and prawns (shrimp) into the mashed potato and season with salt and pepper. Pile the mixture back into the potato cases and reheat in the oven for about 10–15 minutes.

Egg and Asparagus in Cheese Sauce

Metric/Imperial
1 egg, size 3, hard-boiled and halved
125 g/4 oz asparagus, canned or cooked
40 g/1¾ oz Brie or Edam cheese, diced
15 ml/1 level tablespoon cornflour
150 ml/¼ pint skimmed milk
salt and pepper
30 ml/2 level tablespoons fresh breadcrumbs

American
1 medium egg, hard-cooked and halved
⅔ cup drained, canned asparagus
½ cup diced Brie or Dutch cheese
1 level tablespoon cornstarch
⅔ cup skimmed milk
salt and pepper
2 level tablespoons fresh breadcrumbs

Put the egg in a heatproof dish with the asparagus. Blend the cornflour (cornstarch) with a little of the milk. Heat the remaining milk and pour on to the cornflour (cornstarch) mixture, stirring. Return to the pan and bring to the boil, stirring continuously. Remove from the heat and stir in the cheese. Pour over the egg and asparagus and sprinkle the breadcrumbs on top. Bake in a preheated moderately hot oven (190°C/375°F/Gas Mark 5) for 15 minutes.

Tomato Omelette with Beans, and Banana

Metric/Imperial
125 g/4 oz frozen broad beans
2 eggs, size 3
pinch of dried mixed herbs
15 ml/1 tablespoon water
salt and pepper
5 ml/1 level teaspoon butter
1 tomato, skinned and chopped
To follow
1 medium banana

American
⅔ cup frozen fava beans
2 medium eggs
pinch of dried mixed herbs
1 tablespoon water
salt and pepper
1 level teaspoon butter
1 tomato, skinned and chopped
To follow
1 medium banana

Cook the beans in boiling water, then drain. Beat the eggs with the water and herbs and season with salt and pepper. Melt the butter in a small non-stick omelette pan and brush over the surface. Pour in the egg mixture and cook until set, tilting the pan and lifting the edges of the omelette so that the uncooked mixture runs underneath. Add the tomato, fold over and serve with the beans. Serve the banana to follow.

Trout with Almonds, and Fruit

Metric/Imperial
1 x 175 g/6 oz trout
15 ml/1 level tablespoon flaked almonds
125 g/4 oz frozen peas
125 g/4 oz French beans
To follow
1 medium nectarine or apple

American
1 x 6 oz trout
1 tablespoon slivered almonds
⅔ cup frozen peas
½ cup green beans
To follow
1 medium nectarine or apple

Grill (broil) the trout without added fat, turning several times until cooked. Place the almonds on a piece of foil and grill carefully until brown. Serve the trout sprinkled with almonds, and with the lightly boiled vegetables. Serve the fruit to follow.

Kidneys, Bacon and Baked Beans

Metric/Imperial
2 lamb's kidneys, trimmed and halved lengthways
2 rashers streaky bacon
1 x 225 g/8 oz can baked beans in tomato sauce

American
2 lamb's kidneys, trimmed and halved lengthways
2 slices bacon
1 x 8 oz can baked beans in tomato sauce

Grill (broil) the kidneys without added fat turning frequently, until cooked. Grill (broil) the bacon until crisp. Heat the beans and serve with the kidneys and bacon.

Eggs Florentine

Metric/Imperial
175 g/6 oz chopped spinach, frozen
pinch of ground nutmeg
salt and pepper
2 eggs, size 3
40 g/1½ oz Edam cheese, grated

American
¾ cup frozen chopped spinach
pinch of ground nutmeg
salt and pepper
2 medium eggs
¼ cup grated Dutch cheese

Cook the spinach according to packet instructions. Drain well and season with nutmeg, salt and pepper. Spoon into a heatproof dish. Poach the eggs and place on the spinach. Sprinkle the cheese on top and grill (broil) until the cheese is melted.

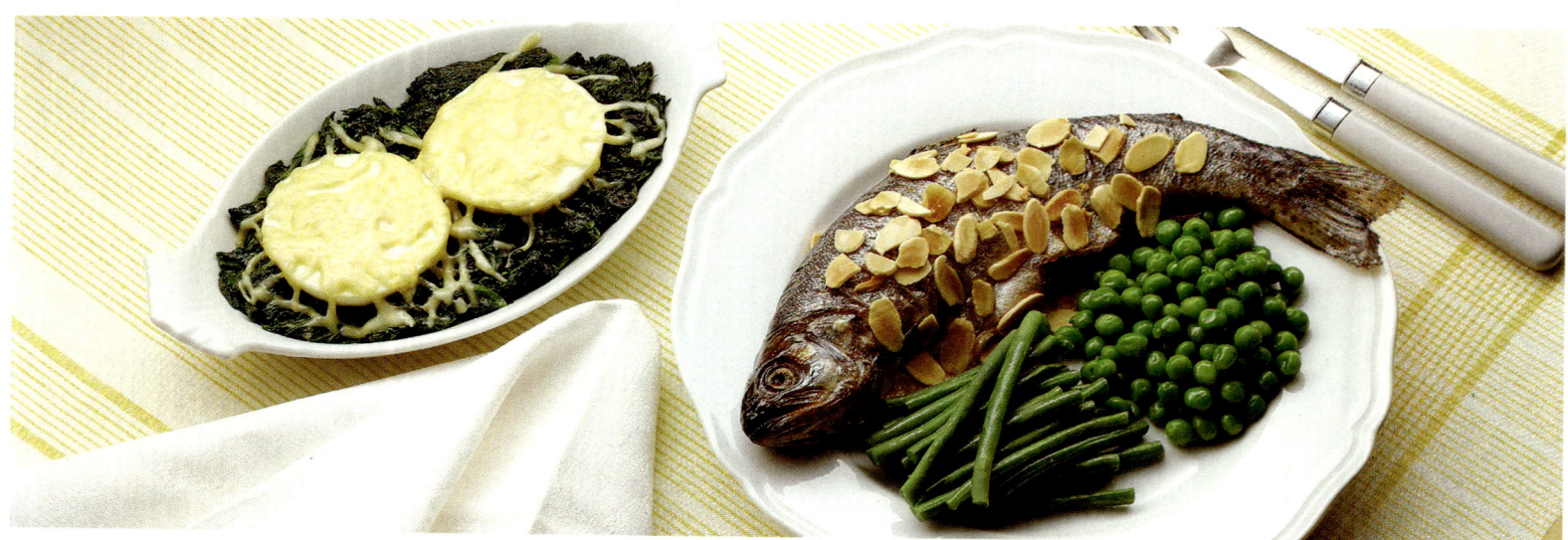

350-CALORIE MAIN MEALS FOR STRICT DAYS: Eggs Florentine; Trout with Almonds

Eating Out

Choose no more than three of these each week as your main meal of the day.

STEAK MEAL
Starter
Smoked salmon (no bread and butter)
or
Consommé
or
Mushrooms à la Grecque

Main course
175 g/6 oz fillet, rump (top round steak) or sirloin steak, all visible fat removed, medium or well-done
Mushrooms, grilled (broiled), poached or fried
Jacket potato (no butter or sour cream)
Side salad (no dressing)

Dessert
Fresh raspberries or strawberries (no cream or ice cream)
or
Sorbet

Drinks
2 glasses wine
Coffee, black or with a little milk

FISH MEAL
Starter
Consommé
or
Melon
or
Grapefruit

Main course
Grilled (broiled) Dover sole (if this is served at the table ask the waiter not to spoon on the buttery juice)
Peas (no butter)
Carrots *or* green beans *or* asparagus *or* broccoli (no butter)

Dessert
Plain ice cream, any flavour
or
Fresh fruit salad (no cream or ice cream)
or
Unsweetened strawberries or raspberries (no cream or ice cream)

ITALIAN MEAL (1)
Starter
Melon and Parma ham, all visible fat removed
1 breadstick

Main course
Calves' liver with sage
Broccoli *or* green beans *or* spinach (no butter)

Dessert
Zabaglione
1 sweet biscuit

Drinks
2 glasses wine
Espresso coffee, black or with a little milk

ITALIAN MEAL (2)
Starter
Melon
or
Consommé or clear soup
2 breadsticks

Main course
Mixed fish salad with dressing
Green salad (no dressing)

Dessert
Cassata
or
Ice cream

Drinks
2 glasses wine
Espresso coffee, black or with a little milk

CHINESE MEAL
While you wait for your meal nibble as many fresh, raw vegetables as you wish and 4 prawn (shrimp) crackers.

Main course
120 ml/4 rounded tablespoons Chicken with Mushrooms
240 ml/8 rounded tablespoons Prawn (Shrimp) Chop Suey
180 ml/6 rounded tablespoons bean sprouts
180 ml/6 rounded tablespoons plain boiled rice
Soy sauce (as much as you like)

Dessert
Lychees

Drinks
2 glasses wine
Unlimited China tea

PUB LUNCH
Ploughman's Lunch
Ploughman's Lunch (made with any cheese of your choice. You may eat all the bread and cheese but do not use any butter.)
Pickled onions, as many as you like
15 ml/1 level tablespoon pickle
Tomato and lettuce garnish

Drinks
2 glasses wine
or
575 ml/1 pint cider
or
575 ml/1 pint/1½ cans lager
or
575 ml/1 pint shandy
or
4 single measures gin, whisky, brandy, vodka or rum (with ice or low-calorie mixers)
or
3 small schooners (175 ml/6 fl oz glasses) sherry
or
2 measures Campari and soda
or
3 measures dry vermouth (with ice or low-calorie mixers)
or
2 measures sweet vermouth or bianco vermouth (with ice or low-calorie mixers)
or
2 measures Dubonnet (neat or with soda or low-calorie mixer)
or
3 dry Babychams
or
2 sweet Babychams

SALAD MEAL
Starter
Prawn cocktail (with one slice of brown bread and butter)

Main course
Prawn *or* crab *or* lobster *or* chicken *or* turkey (no skin) *or* roast beef *or* ham salad (all visible fat removed), without sauce or dressing

Dessert
Lemon mousse
or
Crème caramel

Drinks
2 glasses wine
Coffee, black or with a little milk

CARVERY MEAL
Starter
Melon
or
Tomato juice
or
Fresh grapefruit

Main course
2 slices roast beef, all visible fat removed
1 Yorkshire pudding
1 small roast potato
30 ml/2 tablespoons gravy
Two of the following:
Brussels sprouts, green beans, cabbage, carrots, broccoli

Dessert
Fresh fruit salad (no cream or ice cream)
or
Raspberries or strawberries (no cream or ice cream)
or
Sorbet

Drinks
2 glasses wine
Coffee, black or with a little milk

INDIAN MEAL
Starter
1 poppodum

Main course
Tandoori chicken
Yogurt relish
Tomato and onion sambal
Cucumber raita
1 chapati *or* 120 ml/4 rounded tablespoons plain boiled rice

Drinks
2 glasses wine *or*
575 ml/1 pint/1½ cans lager
Tea or coffee, black or with a little milk

PIZZA EXPRESS MEAL
Main course
1 Pizza Marinara

Drinks
2 glasses wine
Coffee, black or with a little milk

HAMBURGER MEAL
Main course
1 quarter-pound cheeseburger
15 ml/1 level tablespoon relish
Side salad (without dressing)

Dessert/Drinks
Thick milk shake, any flavour

Dine and Diet Menu 1 Serves 6

Mushrooms à la Grecque

Metric/Imperial	*American*
225 ml/8 fl oz dry white wine	1 cup dry white wine
15 ml/1 tablespoon lemon juice	1 tablespoon lemon juice
bouquet garni	bouquet garni
1 clove garlic, peeled	1 clove garlic, peeled
1 small onion, peeled and finely chopped	1 small onion, peeled and finely chopped
salt and pepper	salt and pepper
450 g/1 lb mushrooms	4 cups mushrooms
350 g/12 oz small firm tomatoes, skinned, quartered and seeded	$\frac{3}{4}$ lb small firm tomatoes, peeled, quartered and seeded

Put the wine, lemon juice, bouquet garni, garlic, onion and salt and pepper to taste into a saucepan. Heat to boiling point. Add the mushrooms and tomatoes and simmer gently, uncovered, for 5 minutes. Remove from the heat, turn the mushroom mixture into a bowl and leave to cool completely. Divide between 6 small serving dishes. Remove the bouquet garni and garlic from the mushroom mixture, then spoon into individual dishes and serve.

Beef Bourguignonne with Vegetables

Metric/Imperial	*American*
1 kg/2 lb lean braising steak, all visible fat removed, cubed	2 lb lean braising steak, all visible fat removed, cubed
125 g/4 oz pickling onions or shallots, peeled	1 cup small white onions, peeled
125 g/4 oz button mushrooms	1 cup button mushrooms
bouquet garni	bouquet garni
salt and pepper	salt and pepper
425 ml/$\frac{3}{4}$ pint beef stock	$1\frac{3}{4}$ cups beef stock
15 ml/1 level tablespoon cornflour	1 level tablespoon cornstarch
Marinade	*Marinade*
1 large onion, peeled and sliced	1 large onion, peeled and sliced
1 large carrot, peeled and sliced	1 large carrot, peeled and sliced
1 bay leaf	1 bay leaf
8 whole black peppercorns	8 whole black peppercorns
275 ml/$\frac{1}{2}$ pint red wine	$1\frac{1}{4}$ cups red wine
To serve	*To serve*
cauliflower	cauliflower
green beans	green beans
potatoes	potatoes
chopped parsley to garnish	chopped parsley to garnish

First, combine all the marinade ingredients in a large bowl. Add the meat and mix well. Cover with plastic wrap and leave in a cool place for at least 4 hours, or overnight in the refrigerator.

Put the pickling onions and mushrooms in a casserole. Remove the bay leaf, sliced onion, carrot and peppercorns from the marinade, then add the beef and marinade to the casserole with the bouquet garni and salt and pepper to taste. Pour over the stock and stir well to mix.

Cover and cook in a preheated cool oven (150°C/300°F/Gas Mark 2) for 3 hours. Blend the cornflour (cornstarch) to a smooth paste with a little cold water and stir into the casserole. Remove the bouquet garni. Cover again and return to the oven for 15 minutes. Serve the Beef Bourguignonne straight from the casserole. Accompany with lightly cooked cauliflower, green beans and potatoes sprinkled with parsley.

Apricot Brûlée

Metric/Imperial	*American*
575 g/1$\frac{1}{4}$ lb fresh apricots, halved and stoned, or 125 g/4 oz dried apricots, soaked overnight and drained	1$\frac{1}{4}$ lb fresh apricots, halved and stoned, or $\frac{2}{3}$ cup dried apricots, soaked overnight and drained
artificial sweetener (optional)	artificial sweetener (optional)
3 x 150 g/5 oz cartons low-fat natural yogurt	2 cups low-fat natural yogurt
60 ml/4 level tablespoons soft dark brown sugar	4 level tablespoons soft dark brown sugar

Cook the apricots in a little water until tender. Sweeten them when cooked with a little artificial sweetener if liked.

Arrange the apricots in the bottom of a large shallow heatproof dish or divide between 6 individual ramekin or soufflé dishes.

Pour over the yogurt, then sprinkle evenly with sugar. Chill in the refrigerator until just before serving, then place under a preheated hot grill (broiler) until the sugar melts, watching all the time so that the sugar is not allowed to burn. Serve immediately.

Drinks
2 glasses wine with meal

Dine and Diet Menu 2 Serves 6

Melon and Grapes

Metric/Imperial	*American*
350 g/12 oz large grapes, peeled, halved and pipped	3 cups large green grapes, peeled, halved and seeded
15 ml/1 tablespoon lemon juice	1 tablespoon lemon juice
3 small melons, halved and seeded	3 small melons, halved and seeded

Combine the grapes and stir in the lemon juice. Divide the grapes equally between the melon halves. Cover with plastic wrap and chill before serving.

Chicken Marengo with Vegetables

Metric/Imperial	*American*
1 x 400 g/14 oz can tomatoes, chopped	1 x 14 oz can tomatoes, chopped
1 medium onion, chopped	1 medium onion, chopped
225 g/8 oz carrots, peeled and sliced	1$\frac{1}{3}$ cups sliced carrots
1 x 65 g/2$\frac{1}{4}$ oz can tomato purée	4 tablespoons tomato paste
30 ml/2 level tablespoons cornflour	2 level tablespoons cornstarch
700 ml/1$\frac{1}{4}$ pints chicken stock, made from 2 chicken stock cubes	3 cups chicken stock, made from 4 chicken stock cubes
75 ml/5 tablespoons dry sherry	5 tablespoons dry sherry
salt and pepper	salt and pepper
6 x 225 g/8 oz chicken leg joints, skin removed	6 x 8 oz chicken leg joints, skin removed
175 g/6 oz button mushrooms	1$\frac{1}{2}$ cups button mushrooms
broccoli, to serve	broccoli, to serve

Put the tomatoes into a saucepan with the onion and carrots. Bring to the boil, lower the heat, then cover and simmer gently for about 10 minutes.

Stir in the tomato purée (paste). Blend the cornflour (cornstarch) with a little cold water and stir into the tomato mixture. Add the chicken stock and bring to the boil, stirring continuously, then cover and simmer gently for 10 minutes.

Pass the tomato sauce through a sieve and return the sieved sauce to a large clean pan or flameproof casserole. Add the sherry and season to taste with salt and pepper. Add the chicken joints to the pan and spoon the sauce over to coat completely. Bring to the boil, lower the heat, cover and simmer gently for 40 minutes.

Add the mushrooms to the pan. Simmer for a further 15 minutes or until the chicken is tender. Arrange the chicken on a warmed serving dish and spoon over the sauce. Serve with lightly boiled broccoli and Duchesse potatoes (below).

Duchesse Potatoes

Metric/Imperial	*American*
1 kg/2 lb potatoes, peeled weight	2 lb potatoes, peeled weight
75 ml/5 tablespoons skimmed milk	5 tablespoons skimmed milk
15 ml/1 tablespoon finely chopped fresh parsley	1 tablespoon finely chopped fresh parsley
1 egg, size 3	1 medium egg
1 egg yolk, size 3	1 medium egg yolk
salt and pepper	salt and pepper

Peel and cook the potatoes in boiling, salted water for about 12–15 minutes, until tender. Drain and mash, then beat in the skimmed milk, parsley, egg, egg yolk and salt and pepper to taste. Using a piping (pastry) bag with a large nozzle, pipe the potato into 18 swirls on a non-stick baking tray. Heat through and brown in a hot oven just before serving.

Blackcurrant Sorbet

Metric/Imperial	*American*
275 ml/½ pint water	1¼ cups water
125 g/4 oz caster sugar	½ cup sugar
225 g/8 oz blackcurrants, fresh or frozen	2 cups blackcurrants, fresh or frozen
5 ml/1 teaspoon lemon juice	1 teaspoon lemon juice
2 egg whites	2 egg whites
6 sprigs mint, to garnish	6 sprigs mint, to garnish

Put the water and sugar into a small saucepan. Stir over a low heat until the sugar is dissolved, then bring to boiling point and boil gently for 10 minutes. Set the syrup aside to cool. Put the blackcurrants into a saucepan with 45 ml/3 tablespoons water and cook, covered, over a low heat for 10 minutes. Rub the blackcurrants through a sieve, or purée in a food processor or electric blender, then sieve. Stir the blackcurrant purée into the cooled sugar syrup and make up to 575 ml/ 1 pint/2½ cups with cold water. Leave to cool then stir in the lemon juice.

Pour the mixture into a shallow freezer container. Place in the freezer until nearly firm. Beat the egg whites until stiff peaks form. Turn the partly frozen blackcurrant mixture into a chilled mixing bowl, and beat with a fork until mushy, breaking down the large ice crystals. Fold in the beaten egg whites. Return the mixture to the container and freeze until firm.

30 minutes before serving, place the blackcurrant sorbet in the main part of the refrigerator to soften slightly. Spoon into individual serving dishes and serve decorated with a sprig of fresh mint.

Drinks
2 glasses wine with meal

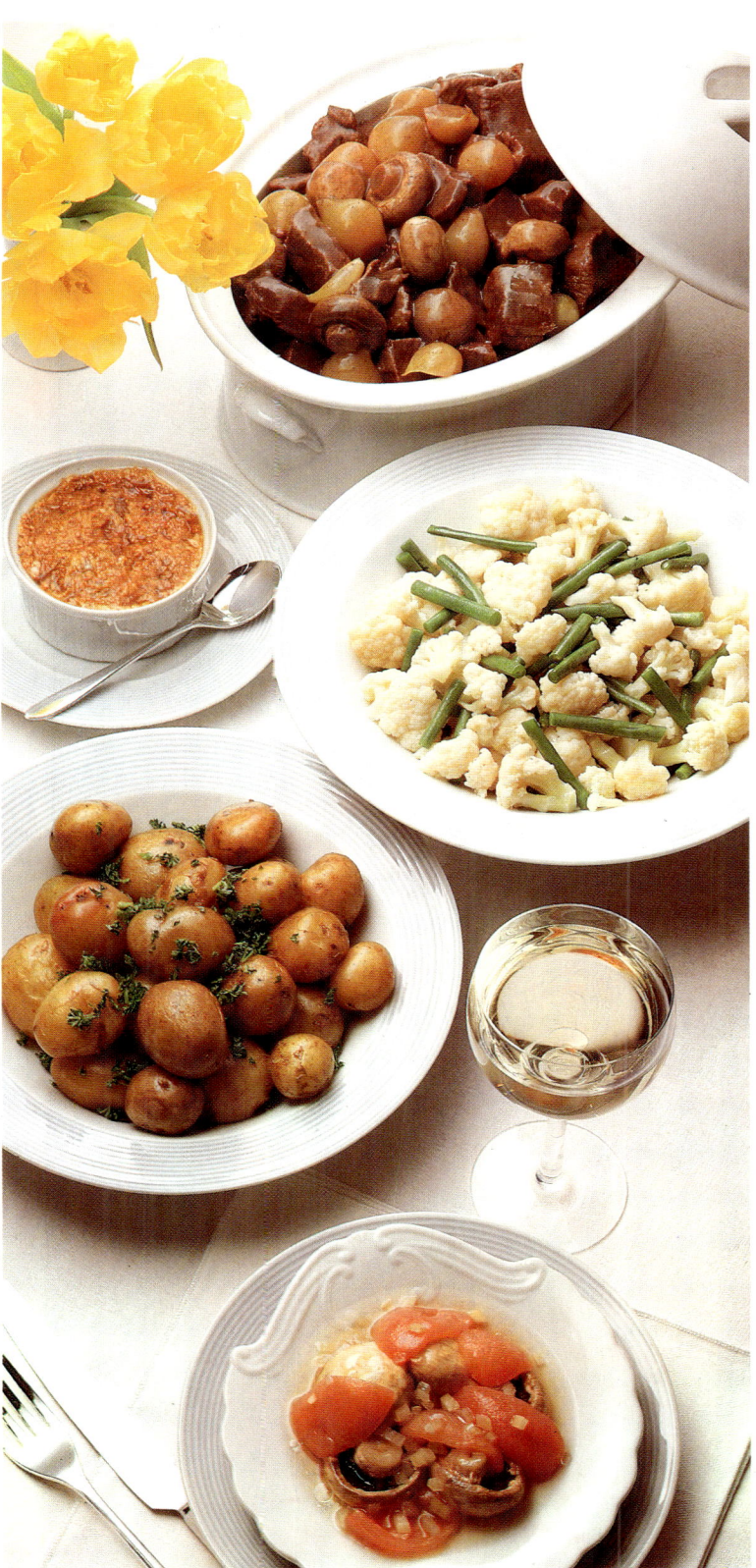

DINE AND DIET MENU 1: *Mushrooms à la Grecque; Beef Bourguignonne with Vegetables; Apricot Brûlée*

Dine and Diet Menu 3 Serves 6

Dressed Artichoke Hearts

Metric/Imperial
2 x 400 g/14 oz cans whole
    artichoke hearts, drained and
    halved lengthways
1 x 150 g/5 oz carton low-fat
    natural yogurt
15 ml/1 tablespoon lemon juice
5 ml/1 level teaspoon grated
    lemon rind
5 ml/1 level teaspoon grated
    onion
dash of Tabasco sauce
salt and pepper

American
2 x 14 oz cans whole artichoke
    hearts, drained and halved
    lengthways
⅔ cup low-fat natural yogurt
1 tablespoon lemon juice
1 level teaspoon grated lemon
    rind
1 level teaspoon grated onion
dash of Tabasco sauce
salt and pepper

Arrange the artichokes in a serving dish, cut side up. Mix the yogurt with remaining ingredients. Spoon the dressing over the artichokes.

Kidneys Marsala with Rice

Metric/Imperial
675 g/1½ lb lambs' kidneys,
    skinned, cored and halved
    lengthways
350 g/12 oz brown rice
350 g/12 oz button mushrooms
1 large onion, chopped
575 ml/1 pint beef stock
175 ml/6 fl oz Marsala or sweet
    sherry
1.25 ml/¼ level teaspoon dried
    mixed herbs
30 ml/2 level tablespoons tomato
    purée
salt and pepper
30 ml/2 level tablespoons
    cornflour
To serve
green salad
60 ml/4 tablespoons oil-free
    French dressing

American
1½ lb lambs' kidneys, skinned,
    cored and halved lengthways
1½ cups brown rice
3 cups button mushrooms
1 large onion, finely chopped
2½ cups beef stock
¾ cup Marsala or sweet sherry
¼ level teaspoon dried mixed
    herbs
2 level tablespoons tomato paste
salt and pepper
2 level tablespoons cornstarch
To serve
green salad
60 ml/4 tablespoons oil-free
    French dressing

Put the kidneys into a bowl and pour in boiling water to cover. Leave for 10 minutes. Cook the rice in boiling water until tender.

Drain the kidneys and put them in a saucepan with the mushrooms and onion. Add the stock, Marsala or sherry, herbs, tomato purée (paste) and salt and pepper to taste. Bring to the boil, lower the heat, cover and simmer very gently for 15 minutes. Blend the cornflour (cornstarch) with a little cold water. Stir into the saucepan, bring to the boil and simmer gently for 2–3 minutes, stirring constantly. Serve the kidneys in a ring of rice, with a green salad tossed in dressing.

Orange Sorbet Cups

Metric/Imperial
6 medium oranges
40 g/1½ oz sugar
175 ml/6 fl oz water
30 ml/2 tablespoons lemon juice
2 egg whites

American
6 medium oranges
3 level tablespoons sugar
¾ cup water
2 tablespoons lemon juice
2 egg whites

Wash and dry the oranges. Cut a slice off the top of each, squeeze out the juice and reserve with the orange 'shells' and tops for lids.

Put the sugar and water in a small saucepan and heat until the sugar is dissolved, then leave until cool. Stir the orange and lemon juices into the sugar syrup. Pour into a shallow freezer container and freeze for about 1 hour until nearly firm.

Beat the egg whites until stiff. Turn the partly frozen orange mixture into a chilled bowl and beat with a fork to break down large ice crystals. Fold in the egg whites until evenly blended. Return to the container and freeze until firm.

Remove the membranes from the orange shells and place them in the freezer with their lids until required. Place the orange sorbet in the main part of the refrigerator for 30 minutes before serving to soften slightly. Spoon the orange sorbet into the frozen orange shells, cover with the lids and serve.

Drinks
2 glasses wine with meal.

Dine and Diet Menu 4 Serves 6
(Suitable for a barbecue)

Smoked Trout Mousse

Metric/Imperial
2 smoked trout, filleted and
    skinned
125 g/4 oz natural cottage cheese
1 x 150 g/5 oz carton low-fat
    natural yogurt
15 ml/1 tablespoon lemon juice
pinch of cayenne pepper
freshly ground black pepper
lime or lemon twists, to garnish

American
2 smoked trout, filleted and
    skinned
½ cup natural cottage cheese
⅔ cup low-fat natural yogurt
1 tablespoon lemon juice
pinch of cayenne
freshly ground black pepper
lime or lemon twists, to garnish

Flake the smoked trout and put into a food processor or blender and add the cottage cheese, yogurt, lemon juice and cayenne pepper. Blend until smooth and season to taste with black pepper. Cover and chill for at least 1 hour. Garnish with twists of lime or lemon. Serve with unbuttered crispbreads or melba toast.

Spicy Lamb Kebabs

Metric/Imperial
675 g/1½ lb boned leg of lamb, all
    visible fat discarded and cut
    into 2.5 cm/1 inch cubes
2 green peppers, cored, seeded,
    and cut into squares
6 small firm tomatoes, halved
1 x 225 g/8 oz can pineapple
    cubes in natural juice, drained
6 small pickling onions
6 bay leaves, halved
Marinade
150 g/5 oz carton low-fat natural
    yogurt
45 ml/3 tablespoons lemon juice
5 ml/1 level teaspoon salt
2.5 ml/½ teaspoon freshly ground
    black pepper
5 ml/1 level teaspoon curry
    powder

American
1½ lb boneless lamb for stew, all
    visible fat discarded and cut
    into 1 inch cubes
2 green peppers, seeded, and
    cut into squares
6 small firm tomatoes, halved
1 x 8 oz can pineapple cubes in
    natural juice, drained
6 small white onions
6 bay leaves, halved
Marinade
⅔ cup low-fat natural yogurt
3 tablespoons lemon juice
1 level teaspoon salt
½ teaspoon freshly ground black
    pepper
1 level teaspoon curry powder

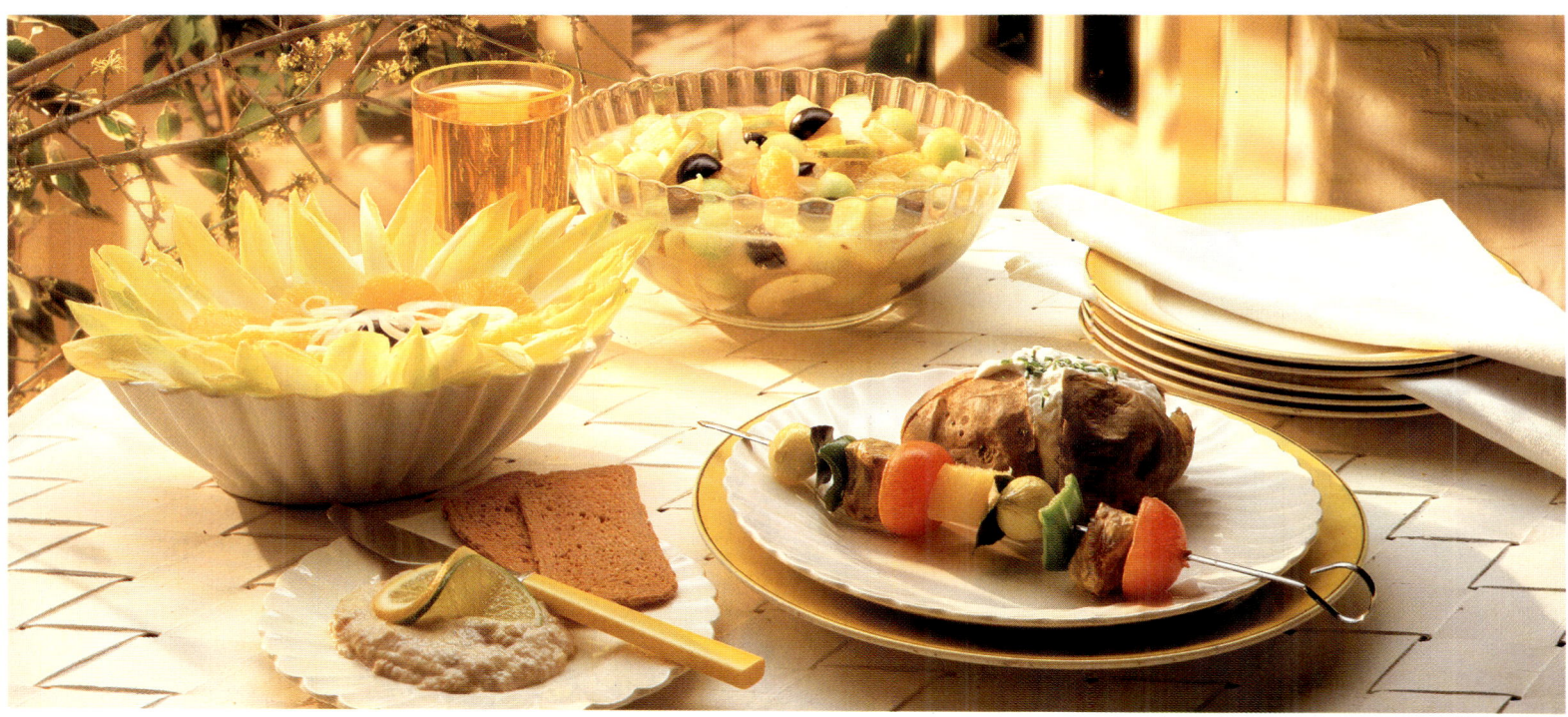

First, combine all the marinade ingredients together in a large bowl. Add the cubed lamb and stir well to coat. Cover with plastic wrap and leave in a cool place overnight.

Lift the lamb from the marinade and thread on to 6 large skewers, alternating with green pepper, tomato, pineapple, onions and 2 bay leaf halves on each.

Cook the kebabs under a preheated hot grill (broiler) or on a barbecue for 10–15 minutes, turning frequently and brushing with the marinade to prevent drying out. Serve with chicory, orange and onion salad and baked potatoes with soured cream.

Chicory, Orange and Onion Salad

Metric/Imperial	American
2–3 heads chicory, leaves separated	2–3 heads endive, leaves separated
2 large oranges, peeled and thinly sliced	2 large oranges, peeled and thinly sliced
1 medium onion, peeled and sliced into thin rings	1 medium onion, peeled and sliced into thin rings
30 ml/2 tablespoons lemon juice	2 tablespoons lemon juice
2 tablespoons oil-free French dressing	2 tablespoons oil-free French dressing
6 black olives	6 ripe olives

Arrange the chicory, orange and onion rings in a salad bowl. Toss the salad in the French dressing combined with the lemon juice. Garnish with the olives

Baked Jacket Potatoes with Soured Cream

Metric/Imperial	American
6 medium potatoes	6 medium potatoes
salt and pepper	salt and pepper
150 ml/5 fl oz soured cream	⅔ cup sour cream
snipped fresh chives	snipped fresh chives

DINE AND DIET MENU 4: Smoked Trout Mousse; Spicy Lamb Kebabs; Chicory, Orange and Onion Salad; Baked Potatoes with Soured Cream; Gingered Fresh Fruit Salad

Bake the potatoes in a preheated moderately hot oven (200°C/400°F/ Gas Mark 6) for about 50 minutes or until cooked, or wrap in foil and bake over a barbecue. Cut a cross in the top of each potato, open up and season with salt and pepper. Add a portion of soured cream to each potato and sprinkle with snipped chives.

Gingered Fresh Fruit Salad

Metric/Imperial	American
2 red-skinned apples	2 red-skinned apples
1 pear	1 pear
30 ml/2 tablespoons lemon juice	2 tablespoons lemon juice
2 medium oranges, peeled and segmented	2 medium oranges, peeled and segmented
250 g/8 oz melon, cubed	½ lb melon, cubed
½ fresh pineapple, chopped	½ fresh pineapple, chopped
125 g/4 oz black grapes, halved and pipped	1 cup purple grapes, halved and seeded
10 ml/2 level teaspoons granulated sweetener	2 level teaspoons granulated sweetener
1 piece stem ginger, chopped	1 piece stem ginger, chopped
425 ml/¾ pint low-calorie ginger ale	1¾ cups low-calorie ginger ale

Core and slice the apples and pear and place in a large bowl. Toss the apples and pear in the lemon juice until well coated.

Add the oranges, melon, pineapple and grapes and stir well. Stir the sweetener and ginger into the low-calorie ginger ale and pour over the prepared fruit. Stir well to mix, cover and chill before serving.

Drinks
1 glass wine or 275 ml/½ pint lager or cider with meal.

The Eat-all-day Diet

If nagging, gnawing hunger is what until now has always stoppd you sticking to a slimming diet, here is your long-awaited answer to those surplus pounds: an irresistible plan that keeps you eating. Do precisely what we say and we can pretty well guarantee that your surplus weight will shift speedily, because this is a diet that never says no to nibbling. In fact, we insist on it.

You must eat 225 g/8 oz raw vegetables every day. Clean and trim any of the raw vegetables given in the list opposite and fill a plastic box or bag with them. You needn't include any vegetables you dislike, but you must select enough to make up the weight. You can chop the vegetables into bite-sized chunks; or cut them into sticks for easy nibbling. Eat some of these raw vegetables with meals if you wish, and the remainder between meals throughout the day. If your taste for raw vegetables isn't highly developed, try accompanying them with one of the delicious dips we list, and count it as one daily meal. Keep the dip in a lidded plastic tub, which can be popped into your vegetable pack. If you go out to work you may find it convenient to make up the vegetable packs in advance, two or three at a time; these will stay fresh in the refrigerator for several days.

You must eat 225 g/8 oz potatoes each day, either boiled or jacket-backed. Serve the potatoes with any of the meals you are allowed, or if you save a little of your raw vegetable dip you could use it to top a baked potato for a between-meal snack.

You must eat 1 medium apple a day. This is in addition to any fruit included in the meals you select. Eat the apple as a dessert to follow a meal or save it for a snack at any time.

You must also eat each day 3 of the meals from the selection that follows – they all contain 200 Calories. These may be eaten at any time of day that you wish. Variety is the key to good nutrition, so ring the changes on your meal choices. As offal (variety meats) is a good source of iron and other nutrients, try to include at least 1 liver or kidney meal a week.

In addition you are allowed 275 ml/½ pint/1¼ cups skimmed milk a day. You can use this in tea and coffee throughout the day or save it for a bedtime drink. Black tea and coffee can be drunk freely, as can water, yeast extract drinks and soft drinks with a low-calorie label. Do not add sugar to drinks, but you may use artificial sweetener if you wish.

That's all there is to the Eat-All-Day Diet – it's simplicity itself. Stick to all our rules and you will be consuming a fast-losing 1,000 Calories a day.

DIPS: Cottage Cheese and Pineapple Dip, Spicy Tomato Dip and Fruity Sauce Dip with a selection of raw vegetables

Raw Vegetables

Choose from the following:
Mushrooms
Cucumber
Spring onions (scallions)
Carrots
White cabbage
Red cabbage
Celery
Peppers, green, red, yellow
Cauliflower
Radishes
Chicory (endive)
Celeriac
Chinese leaves

Dips

You may use one of these to eat with raw vegetables from your daily allowance, but each dip must be counted as one meal.

SPICY TOMATO DIP
Process 70 g/2½ oz/⅓ cup curd (small curd cottage) cheese, 30 ml/2 level tablespoons tomato ketchup, 15 ml/1 level tablespoon tomato purée (paste), 5 ml/1 teaspoon Worcestershire sauce and 30 ml/2 tablespoons skimmed milk in a blender or food processor until smooth. Keep in a covered container in the refrigerator.

FRUITY SAUCE DIP
Process 150 g/5 oz/⅔ cup low-fat natural yogurt, 20 ml/4 level teaspoons low-calorie mayonnaise and 60 ml/4 level tablespoons fruity sauce or brown sauce in a blender until smooth. Keep in a covered container in the refrigerator. Serve garnished with a little finely sliced spring onion (scallion).

COTTAGE CHEESE AND PINEAPPLE DIP
Combine 2 drained and finely chopped rings canned pineapple in natural juice, with 125 g/4 oz/½ cup natural cottage cheese and 20 ml/4 level teaspoons soured cream in a bowl. Season to taste with salt and pepper. Garnish with 1 tablespoon finely diced green or red pepper, cover and keep in the refrigerator.

Cereal Meals

ALL BRAN AND SULTANAS
Mix 30 ml/2 level tablespoons raisins or sultanas (golden raisins) with 40 g/1½ oz All Bran in an individual serving bowl and pour over 150 ml/¼ pint/⅔ cup skimmed milk to serve.

CEREAL AND BANANA
Put 1 Weetabix (wheat breakfast biscuit) in an individual serving bowl, top with 1 medium banana, peeled and sliced, and pour over 150 ml/¼ pint/⅔ cup hot or cold skimmed milk to serve.

MUESLI AND APRICOTS
Mix 5 chopped dried apricots with 25 g/1 oz muesli (Swiss-style cereal) in an individual serving bowl. Pour over 150 ml/¼ pint/⅔ cup skimmed milk

MUESLI YOGURT
Combine 25 g/1 oz muesli (Swiss-style cereal) with 150 g/5 oz/⅔ cup low-fat natural yogurt in an individual serving bowl.

FRUIT JUICE AND CORNFLAKES
Drink 115 ml/4 fl oz unsweetened orange or grapefruit juice. Serve 25 g/1 oz/1 cup Cornflakes with 5 ml/1 level teaspoon sugar and 115 ml/4 fl oz/½ cup skimmed milk in an individual serving bowl

SHREDDED WHEAT AND MILK
Serve 2 Shredded Wheat with 115 ml/4 fl oz/½ cup skimmed milk in an individual serving bowl.

BRAN FLAKES WITH BANANA
Mix 1 small banana, peeled and sliced, with 25 g/1 oz/1 cup Bran Flakes in an individual serving bowl and pour over 150 ml/¼ pint/⅔ cup skimmed milk to serve.

CALIFORNIAN CRUNCH
Halve and pip 50 g/2 oz/½ cup grapes. Add to 25 g/1 oz Bran Buds in an individual serving bowl, with 125 g/4 oz/¾ cup fresh or frozen and thawed raspberries. Pour over 90 ml/6 level tablespoons low-fat natural yogurt to serve.

BRAN AND RAISINS, AND BOILED EGG
Mix 25 g/1 oz All Bran with 15 ml/1 level tablespoon raisins in an individual serving bowl. Pour over 75 ml/3 fl oz/⅓ cup skimmed milk to serve. Boil 1 size 3 (medium) egg to your liking and eat after the cereal.

BREAKFAST SUNSHINE
Mix 30 ml/2 level tablespoons rolled oats with 15 ml/1 level tablespoon sultanas (golden raisins) and 5 ml/1 level teaspoon clear honey in an individual serving bowl. Stir in 1 small orange, peeled and segmented and 3 chopped hazelnuts. Pour over 150 ml/¼ pint/⅔ cup skimmed milk to serve.

SWISS APPLE MUESLI
Soak 30 ml/2 level tablespoons rolled oats in a little water overnight, then drain. Core and chop 1 medium dessert apple and mix with the oats, 90 ml/6 tablespoons skimmed milk, 5 ml/1 level teaspoon clear honey, 1 tablespoon sultanas (golden raisins) and 5 ml/1 level teaspoon mixed nuts in an individual serving bowl.

Toast Meals

SARDINES ON TOAST
Mash 50 g/2 oz sardines, canned in tomato sauce, and spread on 1 × 40 g/1½ oz slice wholemeal toast. Top with cucumber slices.

BAKED BEANS AND CHEESE TOASTED SANDWICH
Mix 15 g/½ oz/¼ cup finely grated Edam (Dutch) cheese with 40 g/1½ oz/¼ cup baked beans in tomato sauce. Spread the mixture on 1 × 25 g/1 oz slice wholemeal bread and sandwich together with another 25 g/1 oz slice. Toast the sandwich on both sides under a grill (broiler).

GARLIC SAUSAGE AND TOMATO PIZZA TOASTIE
Split 1 wholemeal bread roll and spread each cut half with 5 ml/1 level teaspoon low-fat spread. Top each with ½ medium sliced tomato and 15 g/½ oz garlic sausage and grill (broil).

HAM AND PEPPER PIZZA TOASTIE
Split 1 wholemeal bread roll and spread with 5 ml/1 level teaspoon low-fat spread. Discard all visible fat from 25 g/1 oz ham and divide between roll halves. Top with a little green pepper and grill (broil).

BAKED BEANS ON TOAST
Heat 1 × 150 g/5 oz canned baked beans in tomato sauce in a saucepan. Top 1 × 40 g/1½ oz slice wholemeal toast with beans.

PÂTÉ AND TOAST
Spread 1 × 40 g/1½ oz slice wholemeal toast with 40 g/1½ oz ham and tongue pâté and top with 1 medium sliced tomato and a few cucumber slices.

CHEESE AND TOMATO ON TOAST
Toast 1 × 40 g/1½ oz slice wholemeal bread on one side. Top the untoasted side with 25 g/1 oz/¼ cup finely grated Edam (Dutch) cheese and 1 sliced tomato. Grill (broil) until the cheese is melted and bubbling.

PEANUT BUTTER TOASTED SANDWICH
Spread 10 ml/2 level teaspoons peanut butter on 1 × 25 g/1 oz slice wholemeal bread and sandwich together with another 25 g/1 oz slice. Toast on both sides.

HERRING ROES ON TOAST
Melt 5 ml/1 level teaspoon low-fat spread in a non-stick frying pan (skillet), add 125 g/4 oz/½ cup herring roes and fry over a gentle heat, turning from time to time, for 4–5 minutes. Top 1 × 40 g/1½ oz slice wholemeal toast with the roes.

EGG WITH TOAST
Boil or poach 1 size 3 (medium) egg. Spread 1 × 40 g/1½ oz slice wholemeal toast with 10 ml/2 level teaspoons low-fat spread and serve the egg with the toast.

COTTAGE CHEESE TOASTIE
Spread 1 × 40 g/1½ oz slice wholemeal toast with 5 ml/1 level teaspoons yeast extract. Top with 125 g/4 oz/½ cup cottage cheese.

Packed Lunches

FISH SPREAD CRISPBREADS, AND GRAPES

Spread 4 calorie-reduced crispbreads with 1 × 53 g/1⅞ oz pot fish spread (any flavour), and top each with a few cucumber slices. Serve 125 g/4 oz/½ cup grapes to follow.

CHICKEN SANDWICH

Spread 2 × 25 g/1 oz slices wholemeal bread each with 5 ml/1 level teaspoon low-fat spread. Place 25 g/1 oz roast chicken without skin on one slice of bread and sandwich together with the remaining slice.

PRAWN SANDWICH

Mix 50 g/2 oz/⅓ cup peeled prawns (shrimp) with 15 ml/1 level tablespoon low-calorie seafood sauce. Spread on 1 × 25 g/1 oz slice wholemeal bread. Sandwich together with another 25 g/1 oz bread slice.

EGG AND CRISPBREADS, AND SATSUMA ORANGE

Hard-boil (hard-cook) 1 size 3 (medium) egg, shell, chop and mix with 15 ml/1 level tablespoon low-calorie salad dressing. Divide between 4 calorie-reduced crispbreads and top each with 2 cucumber slices. Serve 1 satsuma to follow.

TUNA SANDWICH

Mix 50 g/2 oz/¼ cup tuna in brine, drained and flaked, with 15 ml/1 level tablespoon low-calorie seafood sauce. Spread the mixture on 1 × 25 g/1 oz slice wholemeal bread, top with a few cucumber slices and sandwich together with another 25 g/1 oz slice wholemeal bread.

PINEAPPLE CRISPBREADS

Mix 2 drained and chopped pineapple rings canned in natural juice with 75 g/3 oz/⅓ cup cottage cheese. Spread over 4 calorie-reduced crispbreads.

Meat Meals

Chicken with Coleslaw

Metric/Imperial	American
125 g/4 oz white cabbage, finely shredded	1½ cups finely shredded white cabbage
1 medium carrot, scraped and grated	1 medium carrot, scraped and grated
½ small onion, peeled and finely chopped	½ small onion, peeled and finely chopped
15 ml/1 level tablespoon low-calorie salad dressing	1 level tablespoon low-calorie salad dressing
15 ml/1 level tablespoon low-fat natural yogurt	1 level tablespoon low-fat natural yogurt
2 chicken drumsticks	2 chicken drumsticks

Combine the cabbage, carrot, onion, salad dressing and yogurt in a bowl and stir well to mix. Chill in the refrigerator for at least 1 hour. Grill (broil) the chicken drumsticks, turning from time to time, until cooked. Remove and discard the skin. Serve the chicken with the coleslaw.

Chicken Liver with Vegetables

Metric/Imperial	American
125 g/4 oz chicken livers, trimmed	½ cup chicken livers, trimmed
1.25 ml/¼ teaspoon oil	¼ teaspoon oil
2 tomatoes, halved	2 tomatoes, halved
125 g/4 oz Brussels sprouts	⅔ cup Brussels sprouts

Brush chicken livers with oil and grill (broil) with the tomatoes until cooked. Meanwhile, cook the sprouts in a saucepan of boiling water, then drain. Serve the chicken livers with the sprouts and tomatoes.

Steak and Kidney Stew

Metric/Imperial	American
75 g/3 oz lean stewing steak, all fat discarded, cubed	3 oz lean stewing steak, all fat discarded, cubed
50 g/2 oz kidney, cored and chopped	¼ cup chopped kidney
50 g/2 oz mushrooms, sliced	½ cup sliced mushrooms
150 ml/¼ pint water	⅔ cup water
½ beef stock cube, crumbled	1 beef bouillon cube, crumbled
pinch of dried mixed herbs	pinch of dried mixed herbs
10 ml/2 level teaspoons cornflour	salt and pepper
	2 level teaspoons cornstarch

Place all the ingredients, except the cornflour (cornstarch), in a casserole. Cover and cook at 150°C/300°F/Gas Mark 2 for 2½ hours. Blend the cornflour to a smooth paste with a little cold water, and stir into the the casserole. Return to the oven for 15 minutes.

Kidneys in Sherry Sauce

Metric/Imperial	American
5 ml/1 level teaspoon butter	1 level teaspoon butter
2 lamb's kidneys, skinned, cored and quartered	2 lamb's kidneys, skinned, cored and quartered
25 g/1 oz chopped onion	2 level tablespoons chopped onion
25 g/1 oz mushrooms, chopped	¼ cup chopped mushrooms
50 ml/2 fl oz beef stock	¼ cup beef bouillon
15 ml/1 tablespoon sherry	1 tablespoon dry sherry
15 ml/1 level tablespoon tomato purée	1 level tablespoon tomato paste
salt and pepper	salt and pepper
5 ml/1 level teaspoon cornflour	1 level teaspoon cornstarch
175 g/6 oz cauliflower florets	1 cup cauliflower florets

Heat the butter in a small non-stick frying pan (skillet), add the kidneys and onion and fry over a gentle heat for 2–3 minutes. Turn into a saucepan. Add the mushrooms, stock, sherry, tomato purée (paste) and salt and pepper. Stir well, cover and simmer for 10 minutes. Blend the cornflour (cornstarch) to a smooth paste with a little cold water and stir into the saucepan. Simmer for 2–3 minutes, stirring all the time, until thickened. Meanwhile, lightly boil the cauliflower and serve with the kidneys.

Minced Beef with Vegetables

Metric/Imperial	American
75 g/3 oz very lean minced beef	¼ cup very lean ground beef
50 g/2 oz button mushrooms, sliced	½ cup sliced button mushrooms
½ small onion, peeled and finely chopped	½ small onion, peeled and finely chopped
1 x 225 g/8 oz can tomatoes, chopped	1 x 8 oz can chopped tomatoes
½ beef stock cube, crumbled	1 beef bouillon cube, crumbled
pinch of dried mixed herbs	pinch of dried mixed herbs
salt and pepper	salt and pepper
175 g/6 oz cauliflower	1 cup cauliflower

Fry the beef in a non-stick frying pan (skillet) until brown, then drain off the fat. Put the beef in a saucepan with the mushrooms, onion, tomatoes with their juice, stock (bouillon) cube, herbs and salt and pepper to taste. Cover and simmer for 20 minutes. Meanwhile, cook the cauliflower in boiling water, serve with the beef.

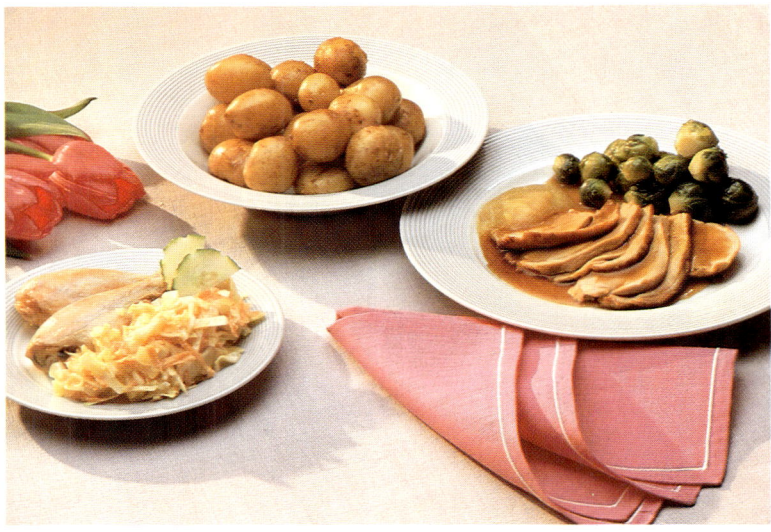

MEAT MEALS: Chicken with Coleslaw; Roast Pork, Apple Sauce and Sprouts.

Beefburger Kebab with Tomato Sauce

Metric/Imperial	American
1 x 50 g/2 oz beefburger, quartered	1 x 2 oz hamburger, quartered
1 tomato, quartered	1 tomato, quartered
½ small green pepper, cored, seeded and cut into 4 pieces	½ small green pepper, seeded and cut into 4 pieces
8 button mushrooms	8 button mushrooms
4 pickled onions	4 pickled onions
10 ml/2 level teaspoons cornflour	2 level teaspoons cornstarch
115 ml/4 fl oz tomato juice	½ cup tomato juice
2.5 ml/½ teaspoon Worcestershire sauce	½ teaspoon Worcestershire sauce

Thread the beefburger, tomato, pepper, mushrooms and pickled onions alternately on to a kebab skewer. Cook under a moderate grill (broiler) for 10 minutes, turning occasionally. Meanwhile, prepare the tomato sauce: blend the cornflour (cornstarch) with a little of the tomato juice to a smooth paste and pour into a saucepan with the remaining tomato juice and Worcestershire sauce. Bring to the boil, then simmer for 2–3 minutes, stirring. Serve the kebab with the tomato sauce.

Lamb's Liver Casserole

Metric/Imperial	American
50 g/2 oz lamb's liver, sliced	2 oz lamb's liver, sliced
1 small onion, finely chopped	1 small onion, finely chopped
50 g/2 oz mushrooms, sliced	½ cup sliced mushrooms
1 x 225 g/8 oz can tomatoes	1 x 8 oz can tomatoes
1 bay leaf	1 bay leaf
½ beef stock cube, crumbled	1 beef bouillon cube, crumbled
salt and pepper	salt and pepper
150 g/5 oz carrots, sliced	¾ cup sliced carrots

Place the liver in a casserole and cover with the onion, mushrooms, tomatoes with their juice, bay leaf and stock (bouillon) cube. Season with salt and pepper. Cover and cook in a preheated moderate oven at (170°C/325°F/Gas Mark 3), for 45 minutes. Meanwhile, cook the carrots in a saucepan of boiling water, then drain. Serve with the carrots.

Roast Lamb, Redcurrant Jelly and Cauliflower

Metric/Imperial	American
75 g/3 oz lean roast leg of lamb, sliced	3 oz lean roast leg of lamb, sliced
125 g/4 oz cauliflower	¾ cup cauliflower
30 ml/2 tablespoons thin, fat-free gravy	2 tablespoons thin gravy made without fat
5 ml/1 level teaspoon redcurrant jelly	1 level teaspoon red currant jelly

Remove all visible fat from the lamb. Lightly boil the cauliflower and serve with the lamb, hot gravy and redcurrant jelly.

Roast Pork, Apple Sauce and Sprouts

Metric/Imperial	American
75 g/3 oz lean roast leg of pork, sliced	3 oz lean roast leg of pork, sliced
150 g/5 oz Brussels sprouts	scant cup Brussels sprouts
30 ml/2 tablespoons thin fat-free gravy	2 tablespoons thin gravy made without fat
15 ml/1 level tablespoon unsweetened apple sauce	1 level tablespoon unsweetened applesauce

Remove all visible fat from the pork. Cook the sprouts in boiling water. Drain and serve with pork, gravy and apple sauce.

Roast Chicken with Vegetables

Metric/Imperial	American
75 g/3 oz roast chicken, sliced	3 oz roast chicken, sliced
125 g/4 oz broccoli spears	⅔ cup broccoli spears
75 g/3 oz frozen peas	½ cup frozen peas
30 ml/2 tablespoons thin, fat-free gravy	2 tablespoons thin, fat-free gravy

Remove all the skin from the roast chicken. Cook the broccoli in a little boiling, salted water, heat through the corn and serve with the chicken and gravy.

Grilled Chicken with Tomatoes and Mushrooms

Metric/Imperial	American
1 x 225 g/8 oz chicken leg joint	1 x 8 oz chicken leg joint
2 tomatoes, halved	2 tomatoes, halved
50 g/2 oz button mushrooms	½ cup button mushrooms
15 ml/1 level tablespoon tomato ketchup	1 level tablespoon tomato ketchup

Grill (broil) the chicken joint, tomatoes and mushrooms until cooked through. Discard the chicken skin and serve the chicken with the grilled (broiled) tomatoes and mushrooms and the tomato ketchup.

Garlic Sausage and Tomato Crispbreads

Metric/Imperial	American
4 calorie-reduced crispbreads	4 calorie-reduced crispbreads
30 ml/2 level tablespoons low-calorie salad dressing	2 level tablespoons low-calorie salad dressing
25 g/1 oz slices garlic sausage	1 oz garlic sausage
1 tomato, sliced	1 tomato, sliced

Spread the crispbreads with the salad dressing. Top with sliced garlic sausage and tomato.

Fish Meals

Salmon Salad

Metric/Imperial
1 tomato, sliced
mixed green salad, e.g. lettuce, cucumber, cress, celery
1 x 100 g/3½ oz can pink or red salmon, drained and flaked
15 ml/1 tablespoon low-calorie seafood sauce

American
1 tomato, sliced
mixed green salad, e.g. lettuce, cucumber, cress, celery
1 x 3½ oz can salmon, drained and flaked
1 tablespoon low-calorie seafood sauce

Arrange the tomato with as much green salad as you wish on a plate. Top with the salmon and pour over the dressing.

Smoked Haddock with rice; Pasta and Prawn Salad; Cod Provençal

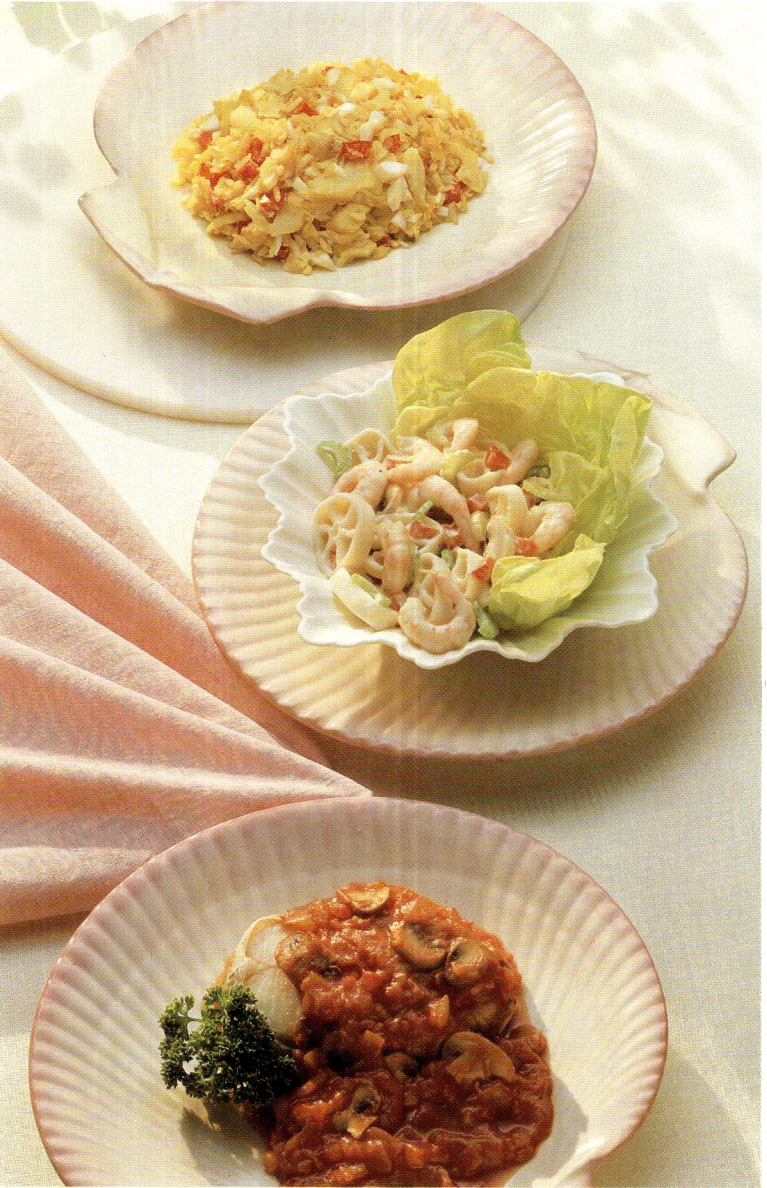

Seafood Salad

Metric/Imperial
175 g/6 oz white fish fillet, cut into 2.5 cm/1 inch cubes
10 ml/2 teaspoons lemon juice
salt and pepper
5 ml/1 level teaspoon gherkin, diced
1 tomato, chopped
50 g/2 oz cucumber
5 ml/1 level teaspoon chopped onion
5 ml/1 level teaspoon capers
15 ml/1 level tablespoon low-calorie seafood sauce
15 ml/1 level tablespoon natural yogurt
lettuce leaves
15 g/½ oz unpeeled prawns

American
6 oz white fish fillet, cut into 1 inch cubes
2 teaspoons lemon juice
salt and pepper
1 level teaspoon chopped gherkin
1 tomato, chopped
⅓ cup cucumber
1 level teaspoon chopped onion
1 level teaspoon capers
1 level tablespoon low-calorie seafood sauce
1 tablespoon natural yogurt
lettuce leaves
4 shrimp

Put the fish into a saucepan with the lemon juice, a little water and salt and pepper and simmer gently for 10–15 minutes, until cooked through. Mix the gherkin, tomato, cucumber, onion and capers together in a bowl. Blend the seafood sauce with the yogurt and stir into the chopped vegetables. Drain the fish, allow to cool and coat with the sauce. Pile into a serving dish lined with lettuce and garnish with prawns (shrimp).

Pasta and Prawn Salad

Metric/Imperial
25 g/1 oz pasta rings or shells
50 g/2 oz peeled prawns
50 g/2 oz mushrooms, sliced
½ small red pepper, cored, seeded and diced
1 celery stick, chopped
30 ml/2 tablespoons natural yogurt
pinch of curry powder
salt and pepper
lettuce leaves

American
¼ cup pasta rings or shells
⅓ cup shelled shrimp
½ cup sliced mushrooms
½ small red pepper, seeded and diced
1 stalk celery, chopped
2 level tablespoons plain yogurt
pinch of curry powder
salt and pepper
lettuce leaves

Cook the pasta in boiling water until just tender, then drain, rinse under cold water and drain again. Combine the pasta with the prawns (shrimp), mushrooms, red pepper and celery. Blend the yogurt with the curry powder and season to taste. Mix with the pasta and prawns (shrimp) until well blended. Serve on a bed of lettuce leaves.

Fish Kebabs

Metric/Imperial
200 g/7 oz cod fillet, skinned and cut into 2.5 cm/1 inch cubes
½ green pepper, cut into 2.5 cm/1 inch pieces
2 tomatoes, quartered
6 button mushrooms
2 bay leaves
30 ml/2 tablespoons lemon juice

American
7 oz cod fillet, skinned and cut into 1 inch cubes
½ green pepper, cut into 1 inch pieces
2 tomatoes, quartered
6 button mushrooms
2 bay leaves
2 tablespoons lemon juice

Thread all the ingredients on to 2 kebab skewers. Brush with lemon juice. Cook under a moderate grill (broiler) until fish is cooked, turning regularly and brushing with more lemon juice.

Smoked Haddock with Rice

Metric/Imperial	American
75 g/3 oz smoked haddock fillet	3 oz smoked haddock fillet
1 egg, size 3	1 medium egg
15 g/½ oz long-grain brown rice	1 tablespoon long-grain brown rice
¼ red pepper, cored, seeded and diced	¼ red pepper, seeded and chopped

Boil rice until tender, then drain. Put the haddock into a saucepan with enough water to just cover and simmer gently for 12–15 minutes until the fish is cooked through. Drain and flake the fish into small pieces. While the fish is cooking, hard-boil (hard-cook) the egg, then chop. Mix the fish, egg, rice and pepper together, reheat gently and serve.

Sole Veronica with Broccoli

Metric/Imperial	American
1 x 150 g/5 oz sole fillet	1 x 5 oz sole fillet
50 ml/2 fl oz white grape juice	4 tablespoons green grape juice
salt and pepper	salt and pepper
50 g/2 oz white grapes, halved	¾ cup green grapes, halved
125 g/4 oz broccoli	⅔ cup broccoli

Put the sole into a saucepan, pour over the grape juice, season with salt and pepper and simmer for about 15 minutes or until the fish is cooked through. Add the grapes to the pan and cook for a further 5 minutes. Place the fish on a serving dish and pour over the sauce and grapes. Serve with boiled broccoli.

Devilled Fish, Peas and Grilled Tomatoes

Metric/Imperial	American
1 x 150 g/5 oz cod fillet	1 x 5 oz cod fillet
30 ml/2 tablespoons lemon juice	2 tablespoons lemon juice
5 ml/1 teaspoon Worcestershire sauce	1 teaspoon Worcestershire sauce
2.5 ml/½ level teaspoon French mustard	½ level teaspoon Dijon mustard
2.5 ml/½ level teaspoon sugar	½ level teaspoon sugar
1 tomato	1 tomato
125 g/4 oz frozen peas	¾ cup frozen peas

Place the cod in a shallow dish. Combine the lemon juice, Worcestershire sauce, mustard and sugar and pour over the cod. Leave to marinate for 2 hours. Cook under a moderate grill (broiler) for 15–20 minutes, basting with the marinade, until cooked through. Grill (broil) the tomato and boil the peas and serve with the cod.

Haddock au Gratin

Metric/Imperial	American
1 x 125 g/4 oz haddock fillet	1 x 4 oz haddock fillet
125 g/4 oz canned tomatoes	½ cup canned tomatoes
salt and pepper	salt and pepper
pinch of dried thyme	pinch of dried thyme
15 g/½ oz Edam cheese, grated	⅛ cup grated Dutch cheese
75 g/3 oz sweetcorn, frozen	½ cup frozen whole kernel corn

Place the haddock in a small ovenproof casserole, cover with the tomatoes and their juice and season with salt, pepper and thyme. Sprinkle the cheese on top. Bake in a preheated moderate oven (180°C/350°F/Gas Mark 4), for 20 minutes or until the haddock is cooked. Meanwhile, cook the corn in a little boiling water, drain and serve with the fish.

Cod in Seafood Sauce with Mixed Vegetables

Metric/Imperial	American
1 x 170 g/6 oz packet frozen cod steak in seafood sauce	1 x 6 oz package frozen cod steak in seafood sauce
150 g/5 oz frozen mixed vegetables	⅔ cup frozen mixed vegetables

Cook the fish according to pack instructions. Meanwhile, cook the mixed vegetables in boiling water, then drain. Serve with the fish and sauce.

Grilled Plaice with Broccoli

Metric/Imperial	American
1 x 150 g/5 oz plaice fillet	1 x 5 oz flounder fillet
5 ml/1 level teaspoon low-fat spread	1 level teaspoon low-fat spread
1 tomato, halved	1 tomato, halved
150 g/5 oz broccoli spears	1 cup broccoli spears
lemon wedge	1 lemon wedge

Spread the fish fillet with the low-fat spread and grill (broil) with the tomato under a moderate heat until cooked through. Meanwhile, cook the broccoli in boiling water, then drain. Serve with the fish, tomato and lemon.

Grilled Trout, Mushrooms and Tomatoes

Metric/Imperial	American
1 x 175 g/6 oz trout, cleaned	1 x 6 oz trout, cleaned
5 ml/1 level teaspoon low-fat spread	1 level teaspoon low-fat spread
2 tomatoes, halved	2 tomatoes, halved
125 g/4 oz button mushrooms	1 cup button mushrooms

Dot the trout with the low-fat spread and grill (broil) with the tomatoes and mushrooms until cooked through. Serve.

Cod Provençal

Metric/Imperial	American
1 x 125 g/4 oz cod cutlet	1 x 4 oz cod cutlet
7.5 ml/1½ teaspoons oil	1½ teaspoons oil
½ garlic clove, crushed	½ clove garlic, crushed
½ small onion, chopped	½ small onion, chopped
50 g/2 oz mushrooms, sliced	½ cup sliced mushrooms
60 ml/4 tablespoons fish or chicken stock	4 tablespoons fish or chicken stock
30 ml/2 tablespoons cider or water	2 tablespoons cider or water
5 ml/1 level teaspoon tomato purée	1 level teaspoon tomato paste
1 bay leaf	1 bay leaf
salt and pepper	salt and pepper
parsley to garnish	parsley to garnish
125 g/4 oz green beans	1 cup green beans

Cook the fish under a moderate grill (broiler) for 15–20 minutes or until cooked through. Meanwhile, heat the oil in a saucepan, add the garlic and onion and fry for 5 minutes until soft. Add the remaining ingredients (except beans) and simmer, uncovered, for 10–15 minutes. Stir occasionally and add a little extra water if necessary. Discard the bay leaf, taste and adjust the seasoning and spoon the sauce over the fish, top with parsley and serve with the lightly boiled beans.

Egg Meals

Egg and Saucy Beans

Metric/Imperial	American
1 x 150 g/5 oz can baked beans in tomato sauce	1 x 5 oz can baked beans in tomato sauce
5 ml/1 level teaspoon sweet pickle	1 level teaspoon sweet pickle relish
5 ml/1 level teaspoon Worcestershire sauce	1 teaspoon Worcestershire sauce
1 egg, size 3	1 medium egg

Heat the beans with the sweet pickle (relish) and Worcestershire sauce in a saucepan. Poach the egg and serve on the beans.

Scrambled Egg and Cheese with Crispbread

Metric/Imperial	American
1 egg, size 3	1 medium egg
15 ml/1 tablespoon skimmed milk	1 tablespoon skimmed milk
25 g/1 oz Edam cheese, grated	$\frac{1}{4}$ cup grated Dutch cheese
1 calorie-reduced crispbread	1 calorie-reduced crispbread

Beat the egg with the milk. Pour into a non-stick saucepan and stir over a gentle heat until just set but still creamy. Stir in the cheese and serve with the crispbread.

Egg and Bacon

Metric/Imperial	American
1 x 125 g/4 oz bacon or ham steak	1 x 4 oz bacon or ham steak
1 egg, size 3	1 medium egg

Well grill (broil) the bacon (ham) steak. Poach the egg and serve with the meat.

Poached Egg on Toast

Metric/Imperial	American
2 x 25 g/1 oz slices wholemeal bread	2 x 1 oz slices wholemeal bread
1 egg, size 3	1 medium egg

Toast the bread. Poach the egg and serve with the toast.

Egg Florentine

Metric/Imperial	American
25 g/1 oz wholewheat spaghetti	$\frac{1}{4}$ cup wholewheat spaghetti
75 g/3 oz fresh or frozen spinach	3 oz spinach
salt and pepper	salt and pepper
1 egg, size 3	1 medium egg

Cook the spaghetti in boiling salted water for about 10 minutes or until tender. Meanwhile, cook the spinach, and drain well, chop. Season well with salt and pepper. Poach the egg. Arrange the spaghetti on a heated serving dish and top with the spinach and poached egg.

Boiled Eggs and Crispbread

Metric/Imperial	American
2 eggs, size 3	2 medium eggs
2 calorie-reduced crispbreads	2 calorie-reduced crispbreads

Boil the eggs and serve with the crispbreads.

Mushroom Omelette

Metric/Imperial	American
75 g/3 oz mushrooms, sliced	$\frac{3}{4}$ cup sliced mushrooms
5 ml/1 level teaspoon butter	1 level teaspoon butter
2 eggs, size 3	2 medium eggs
15 ml/1 tablespoon water	15 ml/1 tablespoon water
salt and pepper	salt and pepper

Poach the mushrooms for 3–5 minutes in a little boiling water seasoned with salt and pepper. Drain. Meanwhile, melt the butter in a non-stick omelette pan. Beat the eggs and water, pour into the pan and make an omelette. Slide the omelette on to a serving dish, place the mushrooms on one half of the omelette and fold over.

Cheese, Chutney and Egg on Toast

Metric/Imperial	American
1 x 25 g/1 oz slice wholemeal bread	1 x 1 oz slice wholemeal bread
15 g/$\frac{1}{2}$ oz Edam cheese, grated	$\frac{1}{8}$ cup grated Dutch cheese
15 ml/1 level tablespoon tomato and chilli chutney	1 level tablespoon tomato relish
1 egg, size 3	1 medium egg

Toast the bread on one side only. Sprinkle the cheese over the untoasted side and grill (broil) until melted. Spread the chutney on to the cheese. Poach the egg and serve on the toasted cheese.

Buck Rarebit

Metric/Imperial	American
1 x 25 g/1 oz slice wholemeal bread	1 x 1 oz slice wholemeal bread
25 g/1 oz Tendale cheese, grated	$\frac{1}{4}$ cup grated low-calorie Cheddar-type cheese
1 egg, size 3	1 medium egg

Toast the bread on one side only. Sprinkle the cheese over the untoasted side and grill (broil) until melted. Poach the egg and serve on top of the cheese and toast.

Egg Savoury

Metric/Imperial	American
50 g/2 oz mushrooms, sliced	$\frac{1}{2}$ cup sliced mushrooms
15 ml/1 tablespoon skimmed milk	1 tablespoon skimmed milk
1 egg, size 3	1 medium egg
1 medium tomato, sliced	1 medium tomato, sliced
25 g/1 oz Edam cheese, grated	$\frac{1}{4}$ cup grated Dutch cheese

Put the mushrooms in a saucepan with the milk. Bring to the boil, then remove from the heat. Remove the mushrooms with a slotted spoon and place in a small heatproof dish. Beat the egg with the mushroom milk and stir over a gentle heat until just set but still creamy. Spoon the scrambled egg over the mushrooms. Top with slices of tomato. Sprinkle with the cheese and brown under a hot grill (broiler).

Cheese Meals

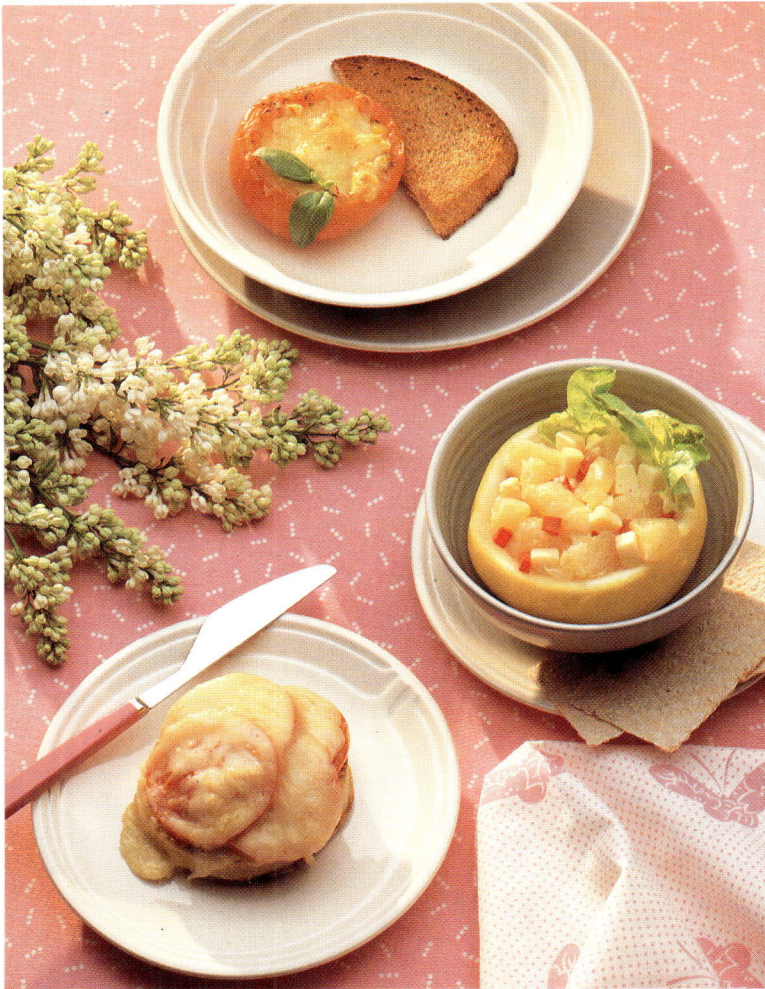

CHEESE MEALS: Cheesy Tomato; Cheese and Grapefruit Cup with Crispbreads; Quick Cheesy Crumpet

Cottage Cheese Crispbreads with Salad

Metric/Imperial	American
4 calorie-reduced crispbreads	4 calorie-reduced crispbreads
125 g/4 oz natural cottage cheese	½ cup natural cottage cheese
1 tomato, sliced	1 tomato, sliced
25 g/1 oz cucumber, sliced	¼ cup sliced cucumber

Spread the crispbreads with the cottage cheese. Top with sliced tomato and cucumber.

Cheese and Pickle on Toast

Metric/Imperial	American
1 x 40 g/1½ oz slice wholemeal bread	1 x 1½ oz slice wholewheat bread
25 g/1 oz Edam cheese, grated	¼ cup grated Dutch cheese
15 ml/1 level tablespoon pickle	1 level tablespoon relish

Toast the bread on one side. Sprinkle the cheese over the untoasted side. Grill (broil) until the cheese is melted. Top with pickle.

Cheesy Tomato

Metric/Imperial	American
1 large tomato	1 large tomato
30 ml/2 level tablespoons sweetcorn	2 level tablespoons whole kernel corn
pinch of dried mixed herbs	pinch of dried mixed herbs
25 g/1 oz Tendale cheese, grated	¼ cup grated sharp low-calorie Cheddar-type cheese
1 x 40 g/1½ oz slice wholemeal toast	1 x 1½ oz slice wholemeal toast
fresh basil or chopped parsley to garnish	fresh basil or chopped parsley to garnish

Cut the tomato in half and scoop out and discard the seeds. Spoon 15 ml/1 level tablespoon corn into each tomato half and sprinkle with the mixed herbs.

Cover with the grated cheese and place under a hot grill (broiler) until the cheese melts and is lightly browned. Top with the basil or parsley and serve with the toast.

Quick Cheesy Crumpet

Metric/Imperial	American
1 x 40 g/1½ oz crumpet	1 x 1½ oz muffin
1 tomato, sliced	1 tomato, sliced
salt and pepper	salt and pepper
25 g/1 oz Cheshire cheese, grated	¼ cup grated Cheshire cheese

Toast the crumpet (muffin) on both sides. Cover with sliced tomato. Season with salt and pepper, then cover with grated cheese. Place under a hot grill (broiler) until the cheese is melted.

Cheese and Grapefruit Cup with Crispbreads

Metric/Imperial	American
½ medium grapefruit	½ medium grapefruit
25 g/1 oz Cheddar cheese, diced	¼ cup chopped sharp Cheddar cheese
¼ red pepper, cored, seeded and diced	¼ red pepper, seeded and chopped
1 large lettuce leaf	1 large lettuce leaf
2 calorie-reduced crispbreads	2 calorie-reduced crispbreads
5 ml/1 level teaspoon low-fat spread	1 level teaspoon low-fat spread

Carefully remove the segments from the grapefruit half and place in a bowl. Discard the pips and cut away the membranes.

Mix the diced cheese and chopped red pepper with the grapefruit segments. Line the grapefruit shell with the lettuce leaf and pile the grapefruit mixture back into the shell. Spread the crispbreads with the low-fat spread and serve with the cheese and grapefruit cup.

Fruity Cheese Open Sandwich

Metric/Imperial	American
1 x 25 g/1 oz slice wholemeal bread	1 x 1 oz slice wholemeal bread
50 g/2 oz natural cottage cheese	¼ cup cottage cheese
1 small banana, peeled and sliced	1 small banana, peeled and sliced
15 ml/1 level tablespoon sultanas	1 level tablespoon golden raisins

Spread the bread with the cottage cheese and top with the sliced banana and sultanas (golden raisins).

Garlic Sausage and Cheese Open Sandwich

Metric/Imperial	American
1 x 25 g/1 oz slice wholemeal bread	1 x 1 oz slice wholemeal bread
25 g/1 oz garlic sausage, sliced	1 oz garlic sausage, sliced
50 g/2 oz natural cottage cheese	¼ cup natural cottage cheese
1 tomato, quartered	1 tomato, quartered

Top the bread with garlic sausage. Spoon over the cottage cheese and arrange the tomato quarters on top.

Slimmer's Ploughman's Lunch

Metric/Imperial	American
25 g/1 oz Tendale cheese	1 oz low-calorie cheese
1 x 40 g/1½ oz slice French bread	1 x 1½ oz slice French bread
1 pickled onion	1 pickled onion
1 medium tomato	1 medium tomato

Serve the cheese, bread, pickled onion and tomato together.

Hot Cheese Cup

Metric/Imperial	American
1 egg, size 3	1 medium egg
30 ml/2 tablespoons skimmed milk	2 tablespoons skimmed milk
25 g/1 oz Cheshire cheese, grated	¼ cup grated Cheshire cheese

Beat the egg with the skimmed milk and three-quarters of the cheese. Season. Pour into an individual heatproof dish. Sprinkle with the remaining cheese. Bake in the centre of a preheated, moderately hot oven (200°C/400°F/Gas Mark 6), for 20 minutes. Serve immediately.

Cheese with Crispbreads and Yeast Extract

Metric/Imperial	American
3 calorie-reduced crispbreads	3 calorie-reduced crispbreads
15 ml/1 level tablespoon yeast extract	1 level tablespoon yeast extract
125 g/4 oz cottage cheese	½ cup cottage cheese

Spread the crispbreads with the yeast extract and the cottage cheese.

Cheese and Pickle Crispbreads

Metric/Imperial	American
25 g/1 oz mature Cheddar cheese, grated	¼ cup grated sharp Cheddar cheese
2 calorie-reduced crispbreads	2 calorie-reduced crispbreads
25 g/1 oz sweet pickle	1 tablespoon sweet pickle relish

Divide the cheese between the crispbreads. Top with the pickle.

Cheese and Crackers

Metric/Imperial	American
3 cream crackers	3 crackers
25 g/1oz Edam cheese, grated	¼ cup grated Dutch cheese
1 celery stick, chopped	1 stalk celery, chopped

Top the crackers with the cheese and celery.

Sweet Meals

Peach and Pear Iced Yogurt

Metric/Imperial	American
1 medium peach	1 medium peach
1 medium pear	1 medium pear
25 g/1 oz vanilla ice cream	1 scoop vanilla ice cream
150 g/5 oz low-fat natural yogurt	⅔ cup low-fat natural yogurt

Skin, halve and stone the peach. Chop the flesh. Core and chop the pear. Beat the ice cream with the yogurt and stir in the fruits.

Grape and Apricot Yogurt

Metric/Imperial	American
175 g/6 oz fresh apricots, stoned and finely chopped	1 cup finely chopped fresh apricots
1 x 150 g/5 oz low-fat natural yogurt	⅔ cup low-fat natural yogurt
1 egg white	1 egg white
75 g/3 oz black grapes, halved	¾ cup grapes, halved

Stir the apricots into the yogurt. Whisk the egg white until stiff and fold into the yogurt mixture. Layer the yogurt mixture and the grapes in an individual glass serving dish, finishing with a layer of grapes.

Yogurt with Banana and Raisins

Metric/Imperial	American
1 medium banana, peeled and sliced	1 medium banana, peeled and sliced
1 x 150 g/5 oz low-fat natural yogurt	⅔ cup low-fat natural yogurt
15 ml/1 tablespoon unsweetened orange juice	1 tablespoon unsweetened orange juice
15 ml/1 level tablespoon raisins	1 level tablespoon raisins

Mix the banana with the yogurt, orange juice and raisins. Serve immediately.

Yogurt with Apricots and Almonds

Metric/Imperial	American
30 ml/2 level tablespoons flaked almonds	2 level tablespoons flaked almonds
4 dried apricots, chopped	4 chopped dried apricots
1 x 150 g/5 oz carton low-fat natural yogurt	⅔ cup low-fat natural yogurt

Toast the almonds until golden brown. (Watch them carefully in case they burn). Allow to cool. Mix the chopped apricots with the yogurt and the toasted almonds.

Jewel Fruit Salad

Metric/Imperial	American
1 kiwifruit, peeled and sliced	1 kiwifruit, peeled and sliced
75 g/3 oz black grapes, halved and pipped	¾ cup black grapes, halved and seeded
125 g/4 oz raspberries	¾ cup raspberries
150 g/5 oz canned lychees	5 oz canned lychees

Mix all the fruit together in an individual serving dish.

Winter Fruit Salad

Metric/Imperial	American
150 g/5 oz canned pineapple rings in natural juice (reserve juice)	5 oz canned pineapple rings in natural juice (reserve juice)
3 dried apricots, chopped	3 dried apricots, chopped
2 prunes, chopped	2 prunes, chopped
1 small orange, peeled and segmented	1 small orange, peeled and segmented
15 ml/1 tablespoon rum	1 tablespoon rum

Cut pineapple rings in quarters and place in a saucepan with juice. Add other ingredients, cover and simmer for 15 minutes. Serve hot.

Raspberry Tilt

Metric/Imperial	American
$\frac{1}{4}$ packet raspberry jelly	$\frac{1}{4}$ package raspberry gelatin
115 ml/4 fl oz boiling water	$\frac{1}{2}$ cup boiling water
1 x 150 g/5 oz low-fat natural yogurt	$\frac{2}{3}$ cup low-fat natural yogurt
25 g/1 oz raspberries	$\frac{1}{4}$ cup raspberries

Dissolve the jelly (gelatin) in the water then allow to cool slightly. Pour into a glass, and tilt the glass to one side so that the jelly sets at an angle. When the jelly has set fill the remaining half of the glass with the yogurt. Chill and serve topped with raspberries.

Slimmer's Knickerbocker Glory

Metric/Imperial	American
$\frac{1}{4}$ packet strawberry jelly	$\frac{1}{4}$ package strawberry gelatin
115 ml/4 fl oz boiling water	$\frac{1}{2}$ cup boiling water
25 g/1 oz vanilla ice cream	1 scoop vanilla ice cream
25 g/1 oz grapes, halved	$\frac{1}{4}$ cup grapes, halved
50 g/2 oz strawberries, sliced	$\frac{1}{3}$ cup sliced strawberries

Dissolve the jelly (gelatin) in the water. Pour into a shallow dish and leave to set. Cut the jelly (gelatin) and ice cream into cubes. Arrange alternate layers of grapes, jelly, strawberries and ice cream in a tall narrow glass. Serve immediately.

Honey Banana Split

Metric/Imperial	American
1 medium banana, peeled and halved lengthways	1 medium banana, peeled and halved lengthways
50 g/2 oz vanilla ice cream	2 scoops vanilla ice cream
7.5 ml/1$\frac{1}{2}$ level teaspoons clear honey	1$\frac{1}{2}$ level teaspoons clear honey

Place the banana in a serving dish. Top with the ice cream and drizzle over the honey. Serve immediately.

Orange Rice Pudding

Metric/Imperial	American
1 x 170 g/6 oz can creamed rice	1 x 6 oz can creamed rice
1 small orange	1 small orange

Heat the creamed rice in a saucepan. Peel and segment the orange. Stir the orange segments into the rice and serve immediately.

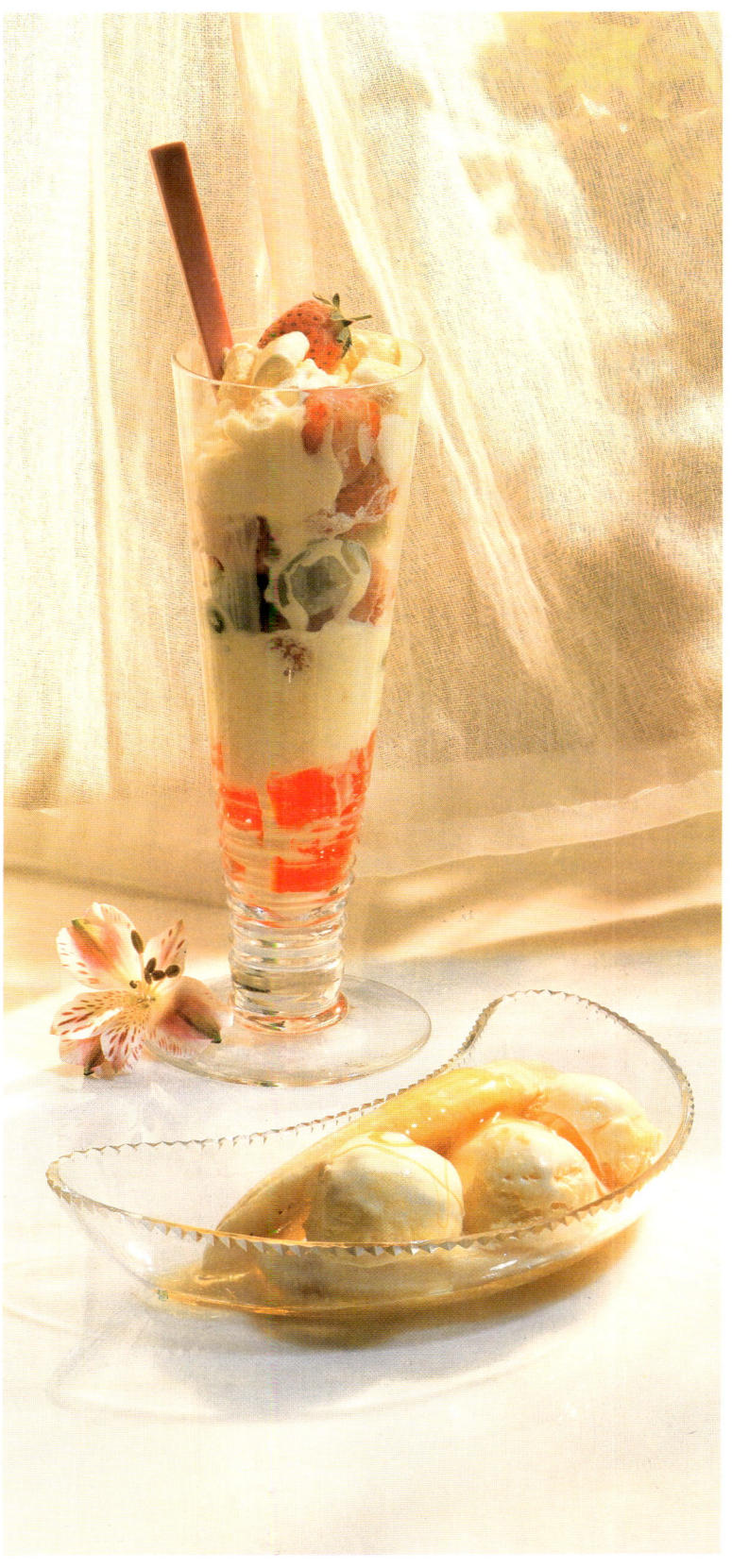

SWEET MEALS: Slimmer's Knickerbocker Glory; Honey Banana Split

The Bully-off Plan

So you have just under a stone (6.3 kg/14 lb) to lose and you want to get down to your target weight at a speedy rate. If you are prepared to do *exactly* what we tell you, you will lose those excess pounds.

DON'T think you are special

Do not give up if you have dieted successfully until now but are finding it difficult to shift the last few pounds. Many slimmers experience this feeling when they have only a little more weight to lose so don't get despondent, simply be extra strict with yourself as you approach your target weight. The problem is that you are just not carrying as much weight as you used to and your body uses fewer calories to move.

DON'T let your problem grow

If you have recently gained weight, do something about it. The Bully-off Plan will get you back to your ideal weight in no time.

DO follow this diet carefully

For the Bully-off Plan to succeed you must be prepared to stick to set menus each day. At the beginning of the week choose any seven menus from the following selection. Write them down in a notebook and make out a shopping list. There are vegetarian days you can select if you wish, and meal quantities can be increased if you have company.

DO vary your choice of foods

Good nutrition depends on you eating a varied selection of foods, so although you may repeat a favourite menu if you wish, make your choice of foods for the week as wide as possible. Most women will benefit nutritionally from having at least one high-iron liver or kidney meal each week.

DON'T swap meals

Each day's menu has been carefully devised to give you 1,000 Calories, but the calories for each meal may vary from day to day. So you must keep to each day's complete menu; though the order in which you eat the meals doesn't matter.

DON'T add ingredients

That means no knobs of butter added during cooking unless stated in the recipe. Any added fat absorbed by the foods you are cooking will greatly increase their calorie content. Weigh all the fats that you use very carefully for they are the highest-calorie foods of all.

DO shop only when necessary

Make a list and shop only when you have to. A supermarket can be a very dangerous place for a slimmer. It's surprising how many extra items mysteriously find their way into shopping trolleys en route to the checkout. Always shop with your diet list and try not to deviate from it.

DO weigh and measure

Guessing the weights and measures of foods is one way of ensuring a diet *does not* work. If the Bully-off Plan is going to be successful we insist you weigh and measure every item on your menu.

DO be realistic

If you live a rather erratic life this is not your best plan and you should choose another diet. If you are prepared to follow this diet to the letter you will find that you lose weight quickly – that's a promise.

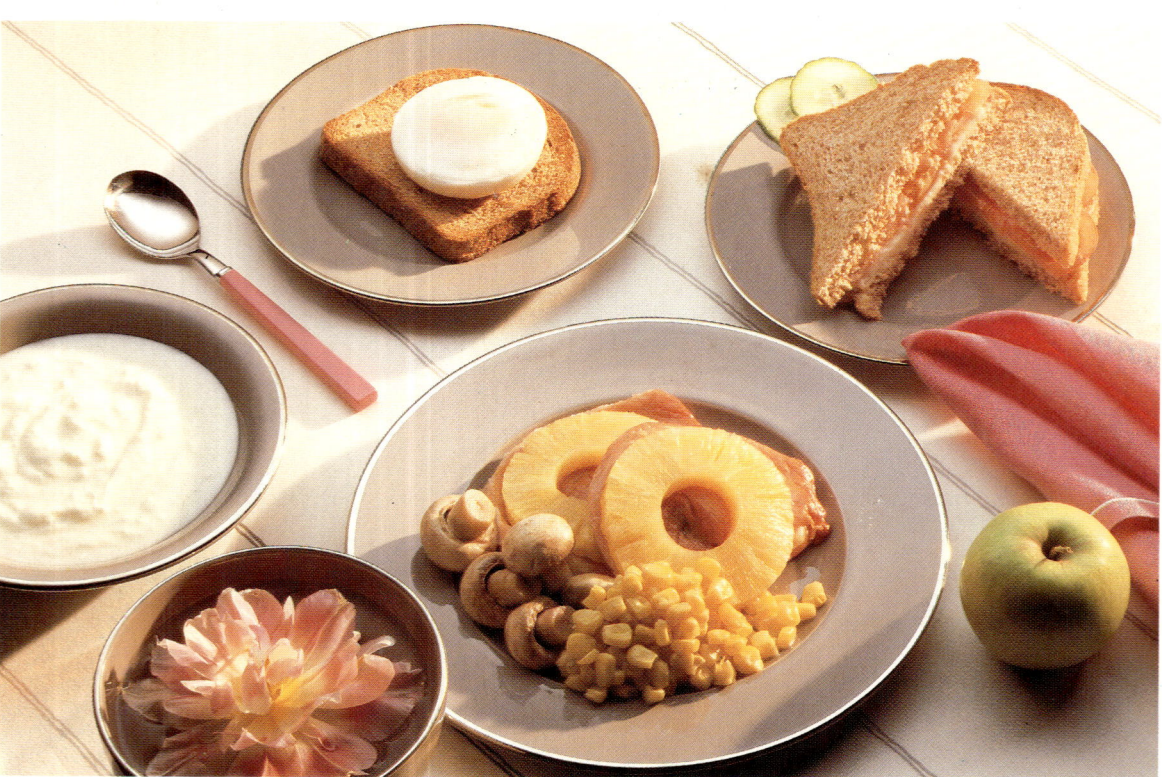

Diet Rules

1 Follow each day's menu plan precisely. You may eat the meals at any time you like. If you do not wish to eat breakfast you may save that meal to eat as an evening snack. Each menu gives you 1,000 Calories a day.

2 You may have 275 ml/$\frac{1}{2}$ pint/1$\frac{1}{4}$ cups skimmed milk or 190 ml/$\frac{1}{3}$ pint/$\frac{7}{8}$ cup semi-skimmed milk each day in addition to any milk given in the menus.

3 You can drink as much tea and coffee as you wish, using milk from the above allowance and using artificial sweetener only. You can also drink unlimited amounts of yeast extract dissolved in water and low-calorie mixers or squashes.

DAY 2: Poached Egg on Toast; Cheese and Tomato Sandwich, and Apple; Ham with Pineapple, and Yogurt

Breakfast

CEREAL
Serve 25 g/1 oz/1 cup Bran Flakes, Cornflakes, Puffed Wheat or Rice Krispies with 115 ml/ 4 fl oz/½ cup skimmed milk.

Light Meal

CHEESE AND CUCUMBER SANDWICH
Make a sandwich with 2 × 40 g/ 1½ oz slices wholemeal bread, 50 g/2 oz/¼ cup curd cheese, 5 ml/1 level teaspoon yeast extract and a few cucumber slices.

Main Meal

Chicken, Broccoli and Baked Potato, and Fruit Yogurt

Metric/Imperial
1 x 175 g/6 oz potato
1 x 175 g/6 oz chicken breast
125 g/4 oz broccoli spears
15 ml/1 level tablespoon corn or barbecue relish
150 g/5 oz carton low-fat natural yogurt
To follow
1 small orange, peeled and segmented
15 ml/1 level tablespoon raisins

American
1 x 6 oz potato
1 x 6 oz chicken breast
¾ cup broccoli spears
1 level tablespoon corn or barbecue relish
⅔ cup low-fat natural yogurt
To follow
1 small orange, peeled and segmented
1 level tablespoon raisins

Bake the potato in its jacket in a preheated moderately hot oven (200°C/ 400°F/Gas Mark 6), for about 50 minutes, until soft when pinched. Bake the chicken breast alongside potato for 25 minutes until cooked and discard the skin. Top the potato with 15 ml/1 level tablespoon yogurt and serve with the chicken, lightly boiled broccoli and relish. Mix the orange with the remaining yogurt and the raisins and serve to follow.

Breakfast

POACHED EGG ON TOAST
Poach 1 size 3 (medium) egg. Spread 10 ml/2 level teaspoons low-fat spread on 1 × 35 g/1¼ oz slice wholemeal toast. Top with the poached egg.

Light Meal

CHEESE AND TOMATO SANDWICH, AND APPLE
Make a sandwich using 2 × 35 g/ 1¼ oz slices wholemeal bread, 15 ml/1 level tablespoon cheese spread and 1 sliced tomato. Serve 1 medium apple to follow.

Main Meal

Ham with Pineapple, and Yogurt

Metric/Imperial
2 x 100 g/3½ oz bacon or ham steaks
2 rings pineapple, canned in natural juice, drained
125 g/4 oz sweetcorn kernels
50 g/2 oz button mushrooms
To follow
1 x 150 g/5 oz carton low-fat natural yogurt

American
2 x 3½ oz ham steaks
2 rings pineapple, canned in natural juice, drained
¾ cup whole kernel corn
½ cup button mushrooms
To follow
⅔ cup low-fat natural yogurt

Grill (broil) the steaks. Heat the pineapple under the grill (broiler). Lightly boil the corn (heat through if canned) and poach the mushrooms in a little water. Serve with the bacon or ham steaks topped with pineapple. Serve the yogurt to follow.

Breakfast

GRAPEFRUIT WITH CEREAL
Start with the segments of ½ grapefruit with artificial sweetener, if liked. Follow with 25 g/1 oz/1 cup Bran Flakes, Cornflakes, Puffed Wheat or Rice Krispies and 115 ml/4 fl oz/½ cup skimmed milk.

Light Meal

BAKED BEANS ON TOAST
Heat 1 × 225 g/8 oz can beans in tomato sauce in a saucepan. Serve on 1 × 40 g/1½ oz slice wholemeal toast.

Main Meal

Grilled Lamb Chop with Vegetables, and Choc Ice

Metric/Imperial
1 x 150 g/5 oz lamb loin chop
125 g/4 oz frozen mixed vegetables
45 ml/3 level tablespoons dried potato powder
15 ml/1 tablespoon mint sauce
To follow
1 small choc ice

American
1 x 5 oz lamb loin chop
1 cup frozen mixed vegetables
3 level tablespoons dried potato powder
1 tablespoon mint sauce
To follow
1 small choc ice

Grill (broil) the chop well. Cook the vegetables in boiling, water and make up the potato according to packet instructions. Serve the vegetables with the chop and mint sauce. Serve the choc ice to follow.

Day 4

Breakfast

BOILED EGG WITH CRISPBREADS
Boil 1 size 3 (medium) egg to your liking and serve with 2 calorie-reduced crispbreads, each spread with 5 ml/1 level teaspoon low-fat spread.

Light Meal

CHEESE, HAM AND TOMATO SANDWICH, AND FRUIT
Spread 1 × 40 g/1½ oz slice wholemeal bread with 15 ml/1 level tablespoon cheese spread. Make into a sandwich with 25 g/1 oz lean cooked ham and a sliced tomato and another 40 g/1½ oz slice bread. Follow with a medium peach or pear.

Main Meal

Cod in Sauce with Vegetables, and Ice Cream

Metric/Imperial	*American*
1 x 175 g/6 oz packet cod in sauce, any flavour	1 x 6 oz package cod in sauce, any flavor
125 g/4 oz frozen peas and baby carrots	¾ cup frozen peas and baby carrots
125 g/4 oz sweetcorn, canned or frozen	¾ cup kernel corn, canned or frozen
To follow	*To follow*
50 g/2 oz vanilla ice cream	2 scoops vanilla ice cream

Cook the fish and vegetables according to packet instructions. Serve the ice cream to follow.

Day 5

Breakfast

BACON AND TOMATOES
Grill (broil) 3 rashers (slices) streaky bacon until crisp, with 2 halved tomatoes. Serve with 1 × 40 g/1½ oz slice unbuttered wholemeal bread.

Light Meal

RAVIOLI AU GRATIN
Mix 1 chopped tomato with 215 g/7½ oz can ravioli in tomato sauce and heat in a small saucepan. Turn into a heatproof dish. Grate 15 g/½ oz/⅛ cup Cheddar cheese, mix with 30 ml/2 level tablespoons/¼ cup fresh breadcrumbs and sprinkle on top of the ravioli. Grill (broil) until the cheese is melted and the crumbs are browned.

Main Meal

Pork Chop with Vegetables, and Pear

Metric/Imperial	*American*
1 x 185 g/6½ oz pork chop	1 x 6½ oz pork chop
125 g/4 oz Brussels sprouts	1 cup Brussels sprouts
125 g/4 oz carrots	⅔ cup carrots
50 ml/2 fl oz fat-free gravy made from gravy powder or granules	¼ cup fat-free gravy, made from gravy powder or granules
To follow	*To follow*
1 medium pear	1 medium pear

Grill (broil) the chop well. Meanwhile, cook the sprouts and carrots in separate saucepans of boiling, salted water, then drain. Serve the vegetables with the chop and gravy. Serve the pear to follow.

Day 6

Breakfast

SWISS APPLE MUESLI
Leave 30 ml/2 level tablespoons rolled oats to soak in a little water overnight. In the morning drain. Core and chop 1 small apple. Mix the oats and apple with 15 ml/1 level tablespoon All Bran, 115 ml/4 fl oz/½ cup skimmed milk, 5 ml/1 level teaspoon clear honey, 15 ml/1 level tablespoon sultanas (golden raisins) and 5 ml/1 level teaspoon mixed nuts in a serving dish.

Light Meal

SOUP AND CHEESE CRISPBREADS, AND APPLE
Heat 1 × 275 g/10 oz can low-calorie vegetable soup in a saucepan. Spread 1 triangle cheese spread and 15 ml/1 level tablespoon sweet pickle (relish) over 2 calorie-reduced crispbreads and serve with the soup. Serve 1 medium apple to follow.

Main Meal

Mexican Bean Pot with Baked Potato, and Pear

Metric/Imperial	*American*
1 x 225 g/8 oz potato	1 x 8 oz potato
175 g/6 oz canned red kidney beans, drained	1 cup canned red kidney beans, drained
½ small onion, thinly sliced	½ small onion, thinly sliced
50 g/2 oz carrots, sliced	⅓ cup sliced carrots
1 small green pepper, cored, seeded and diced	1 small green pepper, seeded and chopped
225 g/8 oz canned tomatoes	1 cup canned tomatoes
½ garlic clove	½ garlic clove
pinch of chilli powder	pinch of chili powder
2.5 ml/½ teaspoon Worcestershire sauce	½ teaspoon Worcestershire sauce
5 ml/1 level teaspoon yeast extract	1 level teaspoon yeast extract
To follow	*To follow*
1 medium pear	1 medium pear

Bake the potato in its jacket in a preheated moderately hot oven (200°C/400°F/Gas Mark 6), for about 1 hour, until soft when pinched. Place all the remaining ingredients into a saucepan, bring to the boil, then lower the heat, cover and simmer for 20 minutes. Serve with the baked potato. Serve the pear to follow.

Breakfast

BOILED EGG AND TOAST
Boil 1 size 3 (medium) egg to your liking. Spread 1 × 40 g/1½ oz slice wholemeal toast with 5 ml/1 level teaspoon yeast extract. Serve with the egg.

Light Meal

WALDORF SALAD
Core and dice 2 medium apples and dip in lemon juice if not using immediately. Chop 4 celery sticks (stalks) and 25 g/ 1 oz/¼ cup walnuts. Mix all the ingredients with 30 ml/2 level tablespoons low-calorie salad dressing.

Main Meal

Roast Lamb with Vegetables

Metric/Imperial	American
125 g/4 oz lean roast leg of lamb	¼ lb lean roast leg of lamb
125 g/4 oz cabbage	1 cup cabbage
125 g/4 oz carrots	⅔ cup carrots
150 g/5 oz potatoes	1 cup potatoes
30 ml/2 tablespoons fat-free gravy	2 tablespoons fat-free gravy
15 ml/1 tablespoon mint sauce	1 tablespoon mint sauce

Trim all visible fat from the lamb. Lightly boil the vegetables then drain. Serve with the lamb, hot gravy and mint sauce.

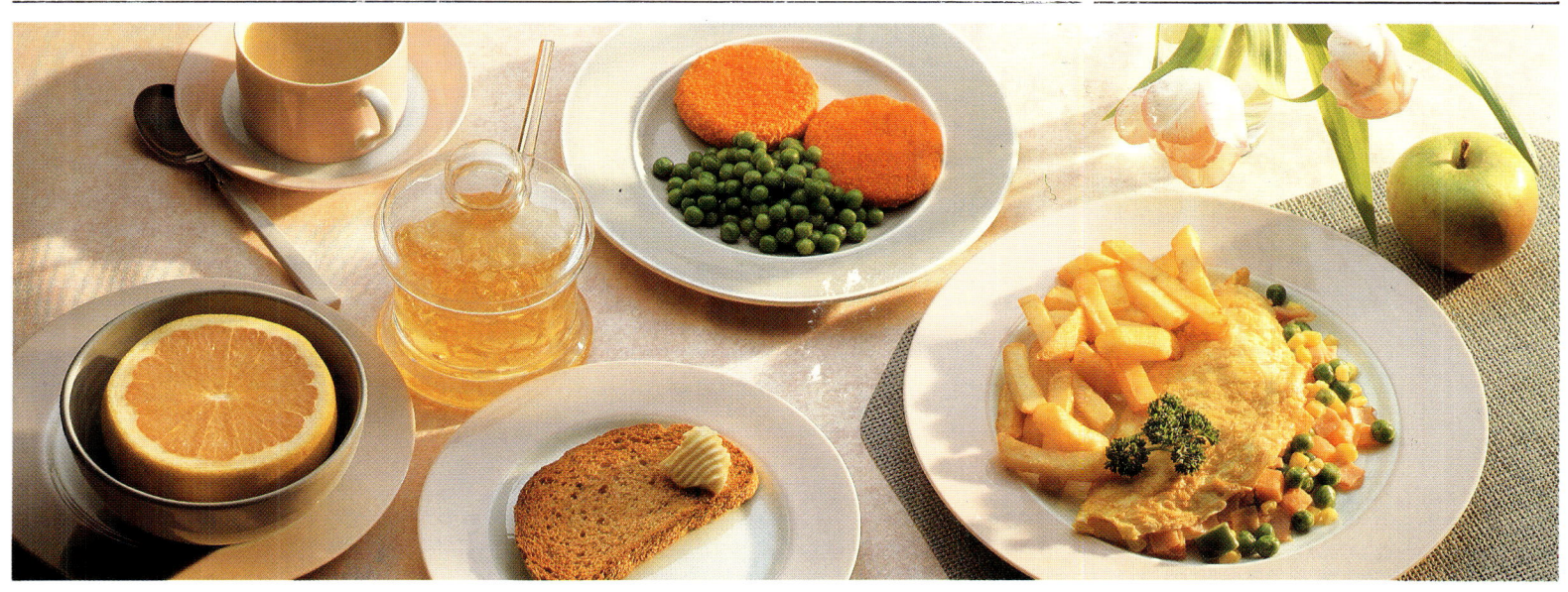

Breakfast

GRAPEFRUIT AND TOAST WITH MARMALADE
Serve ½ grapefruit, adding artificial sweetener if liked, followed by 1 × 40 g/1½ oz slice wholemeal toast spread with 10 ml/2 level teaspoons low-fat spread and 10 ml/2 level teaspoons marmalade or jam.

Light Meal

FISH CAKES WITH PEAS
Grill (broil) 2 frozen fish cakes, without added fat. Cook 125 g/ 4 oz/¾ cup frozen peas according to packet instructions, then drain and serve with the fish cakes and 15 ml/1 level tablespoon tomato ketchup.

Main Meal

Ham Omelette with Chips, and Apple

Metric/Imperial	American
125 g/4 oz frozen mixed vegetables	1 cup frozen mixed vegetables
125 g/4 oz oven or grill chips	1 cup oven French fries
2 eggs, size 3	2 medium eggs
15 ml/1 tablespoon water	15 ml/1 tablespoon water
salt and pepper	salt and pepper
5 ml/1 level teaspoon butter	1 level teaspoon butter
25 g/1 oz lean cooked ham, visible fat discarded, chopped	25 g/1 oz slice lean cooked ham, visible fat discarded, chopped
1 sprig parsley	1 sprig parsley
To follow	*To follow*
1 medium apple	1 medium apple

DAY 8: Grapefruit and Toast with Marmalade; Fish Cakes with Peas; Ham Omelette with Chips, and Apple

Cook the mixed vegetables and chips according to packet instructions. Lightly beat the eggs with the water and season with salt and pepper. Melt the butter in a small non-stick omelette pan and pour in the eggs. Cook until lightly set. Place the ham in the centre of the omelette, fold over, top with parsley and serve with the mixed vegetables and chips. Serve the apple to follow.

Day 9

Breakfast

CEREAL
Serve 25 g/1 oz/1 cup Bran Flakes, Cornflakes, Puffed Wheat or Rice Krispies with 115 ml/4 fl oz/½ cup skimmed milk

Light Meal

EGG SANDWICH
Hard-boil (hard-cook), shell and chop 1 size 3 (medium) egg. Mix with 15 ml/1 level tablespoon low-calorie salad dressing. Make into a sandwich with 2 × 40 g/1½ oz slices wholemeal bread, adding a little mustard and cress, if wished.

Main Meal

Chicken Drumsticks with Vegetables, and Yogurt

Metric/Imperial	American
2 chicken drumsticks	2 chicken drumsticks
125 g/4 oz frozen peas	¾ cup frozen peas
125 g/4 oz sweetcorn, frozen or canned	¾ cup whole kernel corn, frozen or canned
15 ml/1 level tablespoon corn or tomato relish	1 level tablespoon corn or tomato relish
To follow	*To follow*
1 x 150 g/5 oz carton low-fat yogurt, any flavour	⅔ cup low-fat yogurt, any flavour

Grill (broil) the drumsticks until cooked through and discard skin. Meanwhile, cook the peas and corn according to packet instructions, or drain and heat the corn if canned. Serve the vegetables with the drumsticks and relish. Serve the yogurt to follow.

Day 10

Breakfast

MUESLI YOGURT
Chop 1 dried apricot and stir into 1 × 150 g/5 oz carton/⅔ cup low-fat natural yogurt with 15 g/½ oz/4 tablespoons All Bran and 10 ml/2 level teaspoons raisins.

Light Meal

CHEESY SANDWICH, AND ORANGE
Grate 25 g/1 oz/¼ cup Edam (Dutch) cheese and chop 25 g/1 oz/¼ cup cucumber. Mix with 15 ml/1 level tablespoon low-calorie salad dressing. Spread the mixture over 1 × 40 g/1½ oz slice wholemeal bread, top with shredded lettuce and sandwich together with another 40 g/1½ oz slice wholemeal bread. Serve 1 medium orange to follow.

Main Meal

Pork Chop with Vegetables, and Fruit Salad

Metric/Imperial	American
1 x 185 g/6½ oz pork chop, weighed raw	1 x 6½ oz pork chop, weighed raw
125 g/4 oz broccoli spears	¾ cup broccoli spears
125 g/4 oz frozen mixed vegetables	1 cup frozen mixed vegetables
15 ml/1 level tablespoon unsweetened apple sauce	1 level tablespoon unsweetened apple sauce
To follow	*To follow*
1 x 225 g/8 oz can fruit cocktail in low-calorie syrup	1 cup canned fruit cocktail in low-calorie syrup

Grill (broil) the pork chop well. Meanwhile, cook the broccoli and mixed vegetables in separate saucepans of boiling, salted water, then drain and serve with the chop and apple sauce. Serve the fruit cocktail to follow.

Day 11

Breakfast

POACHED EGG ON TOAST
Poach 1 size 3 (medium) egg. Top 1 × 40 g/1½ oz slice wholemeal toast with the poached egg.

Light Meal

SMOKED HADDOCK WITH BREAD, AND PEAR
Cook 1 × 175 g/6 oz packet frozen smoked haddock with butter, according to packet instructions and serve with 1 × 40 g/1½ oz slice wholemeal bread spread with 10 ml/2 level teaspoons low-fat spread. Serve 1 medium pear to follow.

Main Meal

Grilled Kidneys and Sausages, and Fruit

Metric/Imperial	American
1 x 150 g/5 oz potato	1 x 5 oz potato
2 lamb's kidneys, skinned, cored and halved	2 lamb's kidneys, skinned, cored and halved
2 beef chipolata sausages	2 small beef sausages
2 tomatoes, halved	2 tomatoes, halved
125 g/4 oz button mushrooms	1 cup button mushrooms
To follow	*To follow*
1 small orange or 2 tangerines	1 small orange or 2 tangerines

Bake the potato in its jacket in a preheated moderately hot oven (200°C/400°F/Gas Mark 6), for about 50 minutes, until soft when pinched. Grill (broil) the kidneys, sausages and tomatoes without added fat. Poach the mushrooms in a little boiling, salted water, then drain and serve with the kidneys, sausages, tomatoes and the potato. Follow with the orange or tangerines.

Breakfast

GRAPEFRUIT AND CEREAL
Serve ½ medium grapefruit, adding artificial sweetener if liked, followed by 25 g/1 oz/1 cup Bran Flakes, Cornflakes or Puffed Wheat with 115 ml/4 fl oz/½ cup skimmed milk.

Light Meal

CHICKEN SANDWICH, AND FRUIT
Mix 50 g/2 oz/¼ cup cooked chicken, no skin, with ⅛ diced green pepper and 15 ml/1 level tablespoon low-calorie salad dressing. Use as a sandwich filling between 2 × 35 g/1¼ oz slices wholemeal bread. Serve 1 medium pear and 50 g/2 oz/½ cup black grapes to follow.

Main Meal

Toad-in-the-Hole with Vegetables

Metric/Imperial	American
2 pork chipolata sausages	2 small pork sausages
15 ml/1 teaspoon oil	1 teaspoon oil
25 g/1 oz plain flour	2 level tablespoons all-purpose flour
pinch of salt	pinch of salt
45 ml/3 tablespoons water	3 tablespoons water
1 egg, size 3	1 medium egg
125 g/4 oz carrots	⅔ cup carrots
50 g/2 oz frozen peas	⅓ cup frozen peas

Grill (broil) the sausages well. Brush a small baking dish with the oil and heat in a preheated hot oven (220°C/425°F/Gas Mark 7). Mix the flour and salt to a smooth paste with 30 ml/2 tablespoons of the water. Gradually beat in the egg and the remaining water to make a smooth batter. Place the sausages in the hot fat, pour over the batter and cook in the oven for 20–25 minutes until well risen and golden. Meanwhile, boil the vegetables, drain. Serve with the toad-in-the-hole.

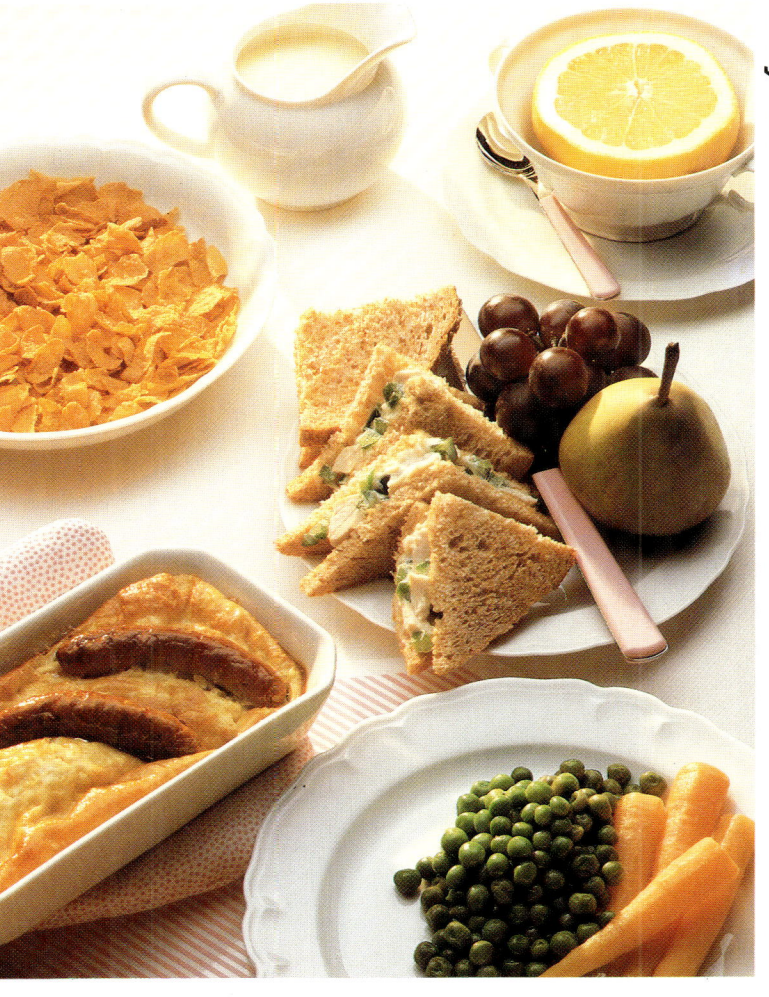

DAY 12: Grapefruit and Cereal; Chicken Sandwich, and Fruit; Toad-in-the-Hole

Breakfast

BREAD AND MARMALADE
Spread 15 ml/1 level tablespoon low-fat spread and 15 ml/1 level tablespoon marmalade over 2 × 25 g/1 oz slices wholemeal bread.

Light Meal

MEXICAN SALAD, AND APPLE
Drain 200 g/7 oz/1¼ cups can sweetcorn (whole kernel corn) with peppers. Chop 3 celery sticks (stalks), 1 spring onion (scallion) and 50 g/2 oz/½ cup cucumber, add to the corn with 50 g/2 oz/⅓ cup peeled prawns (shelled shrimp) and 30 ml/2 tablespoons oil-free French dressing; stir well to mix. Serve a medium apple to follow.

Main Meal

Italian Liver Risotto

Metric/Imperial	American
125 g/4 oz lamb's liver, cut into thin strips	4 oz lamb's liver, cut into thin strips
¼ red pepper, cored, seeded and diced	¼ red pepper, seeded and chopped
125 g/4 oz frozen rice, peas and mushrooms	1 cup frozen rice, peas and mushrooms
½ chicken stock cube	1 chicken bouillon cube
150 ml/¼ pint water	⅔ cup water
5 ml/1 level teaspoon grated Parmesan cheese	1 level teaspoon grated Parmesan cheese

Put the liver and pepper into a small saucepan with the rice and vegetables, the stock (bouillon) cube and the water. Bring to the boil, then lower the heat, cover and simmer gently for 10 minutes or until the liver is cooked and the liquid is absorbed. Add a little more water if necessary to prevent the mixture from sticking. Sprinkle with the Parmesan cheese before serving.

Day 14

Breakfast

BOILED EGG AND CRISPBREAD
Boil 1 size 3 (medium) egg to your liking. Spread 1 calorie-reduced crispbread with 5 ml/1 level teaspoon low-fat spread and serve with the egg.

Light Meal

BACON SANDWICH
Grill (broil) 3 rashers streaky bacon until crisp. Make into a sandwich using 2 × 40 g/1½ oz slices wholemeal bread with 15 ml/1 level tablespoon tomato ketchup.

Main Meal

Grilled Liver with Vegetables, and Apple

Metric/Imperial	American
1 x 175 g/6 oz potato	1 x 6 oz potato
125 g/4 oz lamb's liver	4 oz lamb's liver
2.5 ml/½ teaspoon oil	½ teaspoon oil
2 tomatoes	2 tomatoes
50 g/2 oz mushrooms	½ cup mushrooms
To follow	*To follow*
1 medium apple	1 medium apple

Bake the potato in a preheated moderately hot oven, (200°C/400°F/Gas Mark 6) for about 50 minutes, until soft when pinched. Brush the liver with the oil and grill (broil) with the tomatoes until done. Poach the mushrooms in a little boiling water. Serve the apple to follow.

Day 15

Breakfast

BANANA AND YOGURT
Mix 1 medium peeled and sliced banana with 1 × 150 g/5 oz carton/⅔ cup low-fat natural yogurt.

Light Meal

SOUP AND CHEESY CRISPBREADS
Heat 1 × 275 g/10 oz can low-calorie soup, any flavour, in a saucepan. Spread 2 calorie-reduced crispbreads with 10 ml/2 level teaspoons cheese spread each and top each with 5 ml/1 level teaspoon sweet pickle.

Main Meal

Sausages with Baked Beans and Potato, and Fruit

Metric/Imperial	American
2 large pork sausages	2 large pork sausages
1 x 225 g/8 oz can baked beans in tomato sauce	1 x 8 oz can baked beans in tomato sauce
30 ml/2 level tablespoons dried potato powder	2 level tablespoons dried potato powder
To follow	*To follow*
2 tangerines or 1 small orange	2 tangerines or 1 small orange

Grill (broil) the sausages well. Heat the baked beans. Make up the potato according to packet instructions. Serve the fruit to follow.

Day 16

Breakfast

BAKED BEANS ON TOAST
Heat 1 × 225 g/8 oz can baked beans in tomato sauce and serve on 1 × 40 g/1½ oz slice wholemeal toast.

Light Meal

NUTTY FRUIT SANDWICH
Peel and mash 1 small banana and mix with 15 ml/1 level tablespoon raisins and 15 ml/1 level tablespoon chopped walnuts. Make into a sandwich with 2 × 40 g/1½ oz slices wholemeal bread.

Main Meal

Tomato Macaroni Cheese, and Yogurt

Metric/Imperial	American
40 g/1½ oz wholewheat macaroni	½ cup wholewheat macaroni
1 x 275 g/10 oz can low-calorie tomato soup	1 x 10 oz can low-calorie tomato soup
15 ml/1 level tablespoon cornflour	1 level tablespoon cornstarch
2 tomatoes, sliced	2 tomatoes, sliced
25 g/1 oz mature Cheddar cheese, grated	¼ cup grated sharp Cheddar cheese
1 x 150 g/5 oz carton low-fat natural yogurt	⅔ cup low-fat natural yogurt

Cook the macaroni in a saucepan of boiling, salted water for 10–15 minutes or until tender, then drain. Pour half the soup into a small saucepan. Mix 25 ml/1 fl oz of the remaining soup with the cornflour (cornstarch) to make a smooth paste. Stir into the saucepan. Bring to the boil, stirring continuously, then lower the heat and simmer for 2–3 minutes until thickened. Mix with the macaroni and place in an ovenproof dish. Arrange the sliced tomatoes on top and sprinkle with the cheese. Grill (broil) until the cheese is golden. Remaining soup can be saved for a snack later. Serve the yogurt to follow.

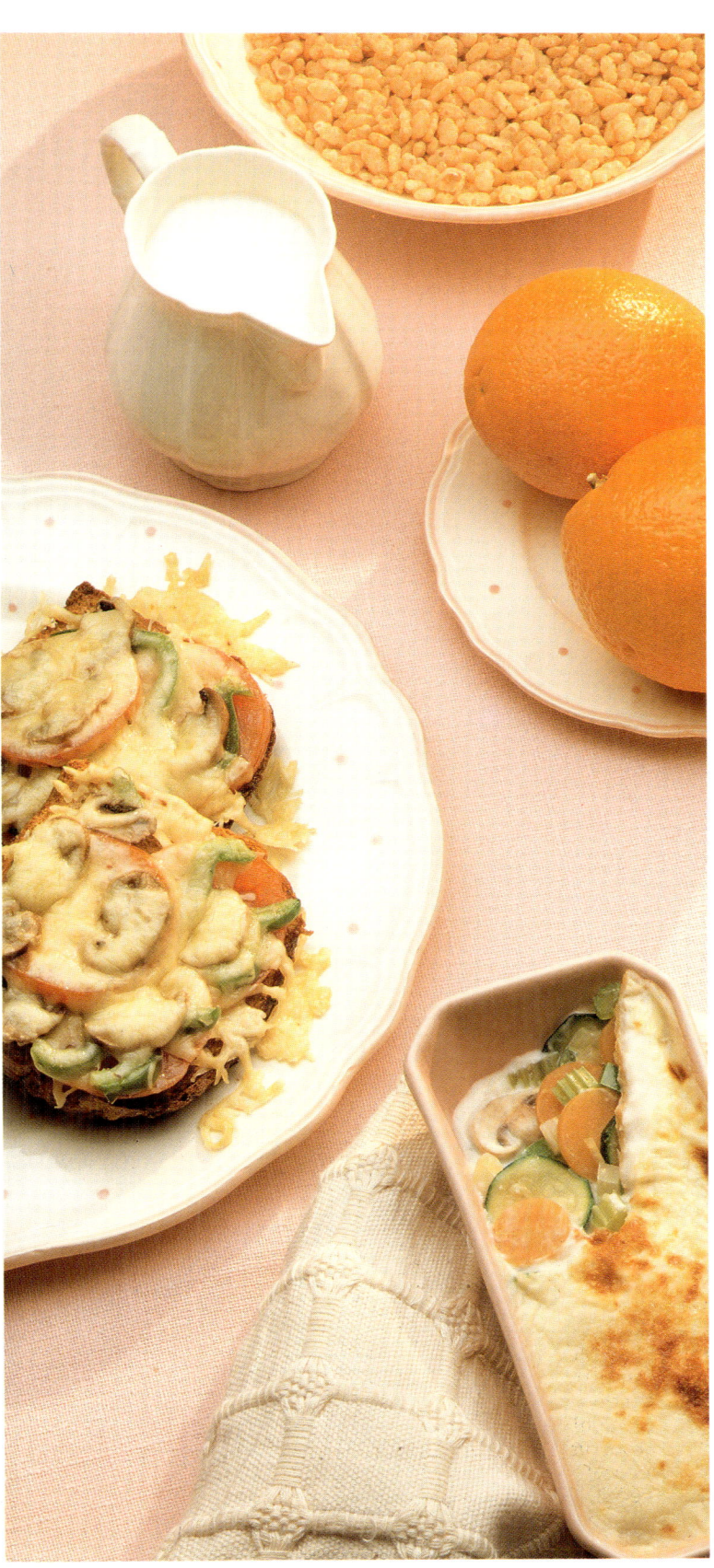

Breakfast

CEREAL

Serve 25 g/1 oz/1 cup Bran Flakes, Cornflakes, Puffed Wheat or Rice Krispies with 115 ml/ 4 fl oz/½ cup skimmed milk.

Light Meal

SAVOURY TOAST, AND ORANGE

Arrange ¼ of a sliced pepper, 1 sliced tomato and 25 g/1 oz/¼ cup sliced mushrooms on 2 × 25 g/ 1 oz slices wholemeal bread. Sprinkle with 25 g/1 oz/ /¼ cup grated Edam (Dutch) cheese and toast under a low grill (broiler) until the cheese is melted and browned. Serve 1 medium orange to follow.

Main Meal

Vegetable Lasagne, and Orange

Metric/Imperial	American
25 g/1 oz wholewheat lasagne	⅓ cup wholewheat lasagne, raw
75 g/3 oz carrots, thinly sliced	½ cup thinly sliced carrots
75 g/3 oz courgettes, sliced	¾ cup sliced zucchini
¼ onion, diced	¼ onion, chopped
½ green pepper, cored seeded and diced	½ green pepper, seeded and chopped
50 g/2 oz celery, diced	⅓ cup chopped celery
50 g/2 oz mushrooms, sliced	½ cup sliced mushrooms
115 ml/4 fl oz boiling water	½ cup boiling water
2.5 ml/½ level teaspoon yeast extract	½ level teaspoon yeast extract
15 ml/1 level tablespoon low-fat spread	1 level tablespoon low-fat spread
15 g/½ oz plain flour	2 level tablespoons all-purpose flour
150 ml/¼ pint skimmed milk	⅔ cup skimmed milk
15 g/½ oz mature Cheddar cheese	2 level tablespoons grated sharp Cheddar cheese
5 ml/1 level teaspoon grated Parmesan cheese	1 level teaspoon grated Parmesan cheese
To follow	To follow
1 medium orange	1 medium orange

Cook the lasagne in a large saucepan of boiling, salted water for 10–15 minutes, or until tender. Put all the vegetables into a saucepan with the water and yeast extract. Bring to the boil, then lower the heat, cover and simmer for 10 minutes. Put the low-fat spread, flour and skimmed milk into a small saucepan and bring to the boil, whisking all the time. Drain the vegetables and stir 45 ml/3 tablespoons of the cooking liquid into the sauce. Add the Cheddar cheese and stir until melted. Make alternate layers of vegetables, lasagne and cheese sauce in a small shallow ovenproof dish. Top with sauce and sprinkle with the Parmesan cheese. Bake in a preheated moderately hot oven (190°C/375°F/ Gas Mark 5), for 20 minutes. Serve the orange to follow.

DAY 17: Cereal; Savoury Toast, and Orange; Vegetable Lasagne, and Orange

Day 18

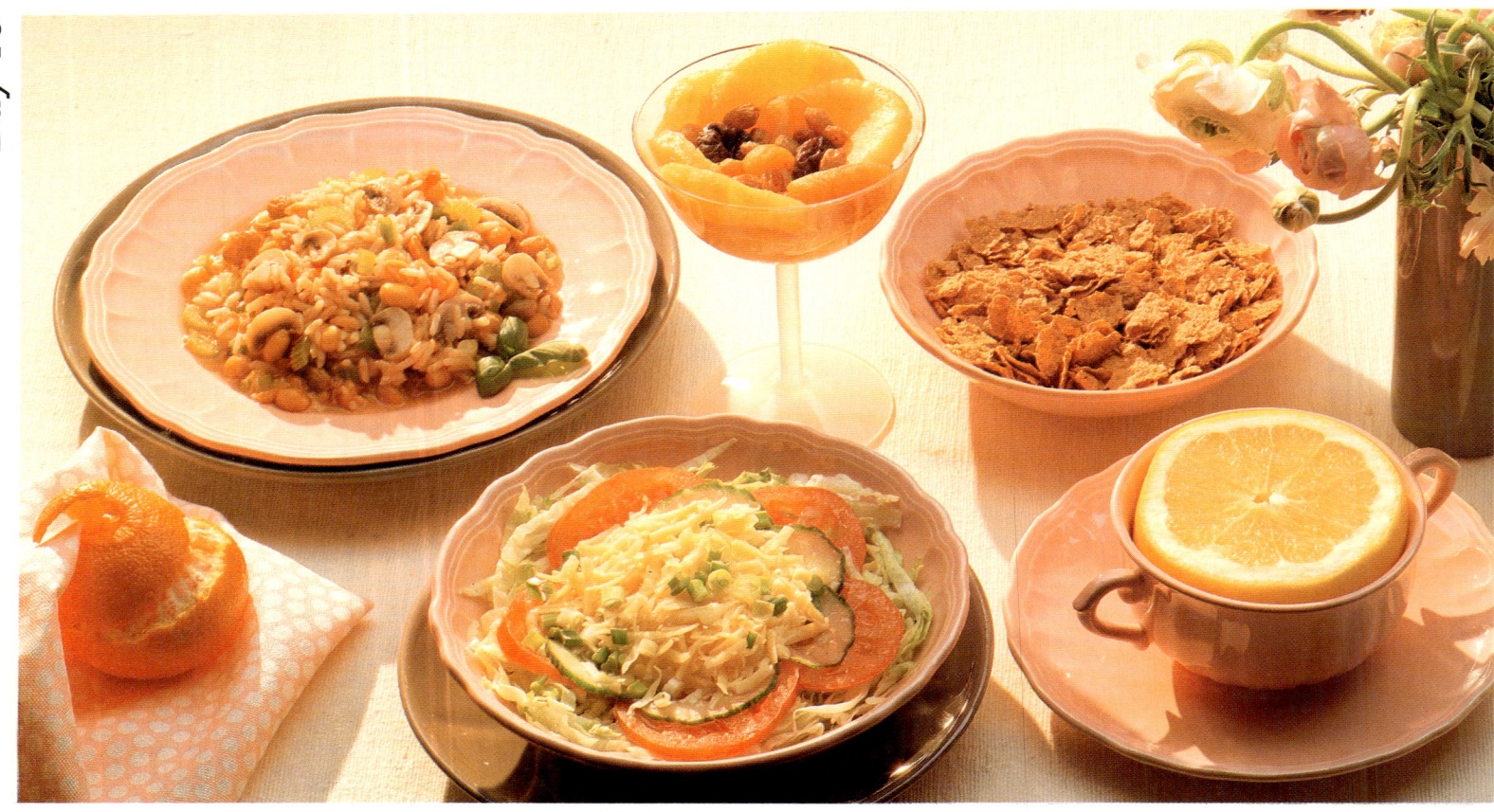

Breakfast

GRAPEFRUIT AND CEREAL

Serve ½ grapefruit, adding 5 ml/1 level teaspoon sugar if liked, followed by 25 g/1 oz/1 cup Bran Flakes, Cornflakes, Puffed Wheat or Rice Krispies and 115 ml/4 fl oz/½ cup skimmed milk.

Light Meal

CHEESE SALAD

Grate 50 g/2 oz/½ cup Edam (Dutch) cheese. Arrange the cheese on a plate with shredded lettuce, 1 sliced tomato, 2 chopped spring onions (scallions) and a few cucumber slices. Spoon over 15 ml/1 level tablespoon low-calorie salad dressing. Follow with a medium peach or small orange.

Main Meal

Savoury Rice, and Hot Fruit Salad

Metric/Imperial
50 g/2 oz brown rice
1 small green pepper, cored, seeded and diced
50 g/2 oz mushrooms, sliced
1 celery stick, chopped
2 spring onions, chopped
115 ml/4 fl oz boiling water
15 ml/1 level tablespoon sultanas
2 tomatoes, skinned and chopped
15 ml/1 level tablespoon salted peanuts
To follow
1 x 255 g/8 oz can pineapple in low-calorie syrup
3 dried apricots
5 ml/1 level teaspoon sultanas
2 prunes

American
4 tablespoons brown rice
1 small green pepper, seeded and chopped
½ cup sliced mushrooms
1 stalk celery, chopped
2 scallions, chopped
½ cup boiling water
1 level tablespoon golden raisins
2 tomatoes, peeled and chopped
1 level tablespoon salted peanuts
To follow
1 x 8 oz can pineapple in low-calorie syrup
3 dried apricots
1 level teaspoon golden raisins
2 prunes

Cook the rice in boiling, salted water for 20–25 minutes or until tender. Drain and rinse with boiling water, then drain again. Meanwhile, put all the vegetables, except the tomatoes, into a saucepan with the boiling water and sultanas (golden raisins). Bring to the boil, then lower the heat, cover and simmer for 5–7 minutes until the vegetables are tender. Drain and mix with the rice, tomatoes and peanuts. For the fruit salad, simmer all the ingredients for 15 minutes. Serve hot.

DAY 18: Grapefruit and Cereal; Cheese Salad; Savoury Rice, and Hot Fruit Salad

Breakfast

YOGURT MUESLI
Combine 15 ml/1 level tablespoon raisins, 150 g/5 oz/ ⅔ cup low-fat natural yogurt and 45 ml/3 level tablespoons muesli (Swiss-style cereal) and serve.

Light Meal

BAKED BEANS AND CHEESE TOASTIE, AND APPLE
Mash 1 × 150 g/5 oz can baked beans in tomato sauce with 15 g/ ½ oz/⅛ cup grated Edam cheese. Spread the mixture on 1 × 25 g/ 1 oz slice wholemeal bread and top with another 25 g/1 oz slice wholemeal bread. Toast on both sides under a hot grill. Serve a small apple to follow.

Main Meal

Mushroom Omelette with Chips, and Fruit Salad

Metric/Imperial	American
75 g/3 oz oven/grill potato chips	¾ cup oven French fries
75 g/3 oz mushrooms, sliced	¾ cup sliced mushrooms
2 eggs, size 3	2 medium eggs
15 ml/1 tablespoon water	1 tablespoon water
salt and pepper	salt and pepper
5 ml/1 level teaspoon butter	1 level teaspoon butter
To follow	*To follow*
1 x 225 g/8 oz can fruit salad in low-calorie syrup	1 cup canned fruit salad in low-calorie syrup

Cook the potato chips (French fries) according to packet instructions. Cook the mushrooms in a little boiling, salted water for about 5 minutes until tender, then drain. Lightly beat the eggs with the water and season with salt and pepper. Melt the butter in a small non-stick omelette pan and pour in the eggs. Cook until lightly set, tilting the pan and lifting the omelette edges so that the uncooked mixture runs underneath. Place the mushrooms in the centre of the omelette, fold over and serve with the chips. Serve the fruit salad to follow.

Breakfast

TOAST AND HONEY
Toast 2 × 25 g/1 oz slices wholemeal bread and spread each with 5 ml/1 level teaspoon low-fat spread and 7.5 ml/1½ level teaspoons honey.

Light Meal

EGG SANDWICH
Hard-boil (hard-cook), shell and chop 1 size 3 (medium) egg. Mix with 15 ml/1 level tablespoon low-calorie salad dressing. Make into a sandwich with 2 × 40 g/ 1½ oz slices wholemeal bread, adding a little mustard and cress, if wished.

Main Meal

Vegetable Kebabs with Beany Baked Potato, and Yogurt

Metric/Imperial	American
1 x 175 g/6 oz potato	1 x 6 oz potato
2 courgettes, sliced	2 zucchini, sliced
2 tomatoes, skinned and quartered	2 tomatoes, peeled and quartered
2 pickled onions	2 pickled onions
8 small button mushrooms	8 small button mushrooms
4 bay leaves	4 bay leaves
15 ml/1 tablespoon lemon juice	1 tablespoon lemon juice
1 x 150 g/5 oz can baked beans in tomato sauce	1 x 5 oz can baked beans in tomato sauce
To follow	*To follow*
1 x 150 g/5 oz carton low-fat natural yogurt	⅔ cup low-fat natural yogurt

Bake the potato in its jacket in a preheated moderately hot oven (200°C/ 400°F/Gas Mark 6), for about 50 minutes, until soft when pinched. Boil the courgettes (zucchini) for 1–2 minutes, then drain. Thread the courgettes (zucchini), tomatoes, onions, mushrooms and bay leaves alternately on 2 kebab skewers. Brush with lemon juice. Cook under a hot grill (broiler), turning frequently and brushing with more lemon juice, for 10–15 minutes, until cooked. Halve the baked potato, scoop out the flesh carefully, and mash with the baked beans. Pile back into the potato skins and reheat for 10 minutes in the oven. Serve with the vegetable kebabs. Serve the yogurt to follow.

Note

Where calorie-reduced crispbreads are mentioned, choose any brand of crispbread that has 20 Calories or under per crispbread.
   Unless otherwise stated, the vegetables used in the recipes can be fresh or frozen.

The Super-speedy Health Farm Diet

Use the Super-speedy Health Farm Diet to rid yourself of those few lingering pounds, to make a fast start on a larger weight problem or to compensate for a binge. It is amazingly effective, the perfect emergency plan, and the ideal diet to follow if you are able to devote several days to your Home Health Farm treatments. It is designed to be followed for no more than four days at a time.

Decide whether you have a liquid day using any one of our lovely liquid mixes, or opt for a salad day, using one of our crunchy creations. Make up the liquid mix or salad in the morning, refrigerate it and dip into it whenever you have time for a meal break.

Each recipe is generous enough to last you from breakfast through to bedtime and adds up to just 600 Calories. Consume 275 ml/½ pint/1¼ cups skimmed milk in drinks throughout the day and you will add an additional 100 Calories to your total. But for the calorie conscious, sip ice-cold water instead – delicious.

For good nutrition vary your choice of liquid mixes or salady stuff each day *but don't be tempted to follow the diet for more than four days*.

If after four days on the Super-speedy Health Farm Diet you still have pounds to lose switch to one of our less stringent diets.

Salady Stuff

Ham and Vegetable Salad

Metric/Imperial	American
1 x 175 g/6 oz potato	1 x 6 oz potato
350 g/12 oz cauliflower	2 cups cauliflower
50 g/2 oz lean cooked ham	2 oz lean cooked ham
½ green pepper, cored, seeded and chopped	½ green pepper, seeded and chopped
2 spring onions, chopped	2 scallions, chopped
2 celery sticks, chopped	2 stalks celery, chopped
125 g/4 oz mushrooms, chopped	1 cup chopped mushrooms
125 g/4 oz red kidney beans, cooked or canned, drained	⅔ cup drained canned or cooked red kidney beans, drained
125 g/4 oz cooked or canned sweetcorn, drained	⅔ cup drained canned or cooked whole kernel corn
60 ml/4 tablespoons low-fat natural yogurt	4 tablespoons low-fat natural yogurt
15 ml/1 level tablespoon low-calorie salad dressing	1 level tablespoon low-calorie salad dressing

Boil the potato (with or without the skin) until tender. Drain, leave until cool and then slice. Break the cauliflower into florets and boil quickly until just cooked. Drain and cool. Discard all visible fat from the ham and chop the lean. Put the ham into a large bowl with all the vegetables. Blend the yogurt with the salad dressing and stir into the salad. Cover the bowl with plastic wrap and refrigerate until ready to eat.

Tropical Rice Salad

Metric/Imperial	American
50 g/2 oz brown rice	¼ cup brown rice
1 medium apple	1 medium apple
15 ml/1 tablespoon lemon juice	1 tablespoon lemon juice
125 g/4 oz pineapple canned in natural juice, drained and chopped	4 oz pineapple canned in natural juice, drained and chopped
125 g/4 oz peaches canned in natural juice, drained and chopped	4 oz peaches canned in natural juice, drained and chopped
175 g/6 oz slice melon, weighed with skin	6 oz slice melon, weighed with skin
1 medium mango	1 medium mango
50 g/2 oz peeled prawns	⅓ cup shelled shrimp
50 g/2 oz cooked or canned sweetcorn, drained	⅓ cup drained cooked or canned whole kernel corn

Cook the rice in boiling water. Drain and leave to cool. Core the apple, dice and sprinkle with lemon juice. Place the pineapple and peaches in a large bowl. Remove the flesh from the melon and mango and chop. Add to the bowl with the rice, apple, prawns (shrimp) and corn and mix thoroughly. Cover with plastic wrap. Keep in the refrigerator until ready to eat.

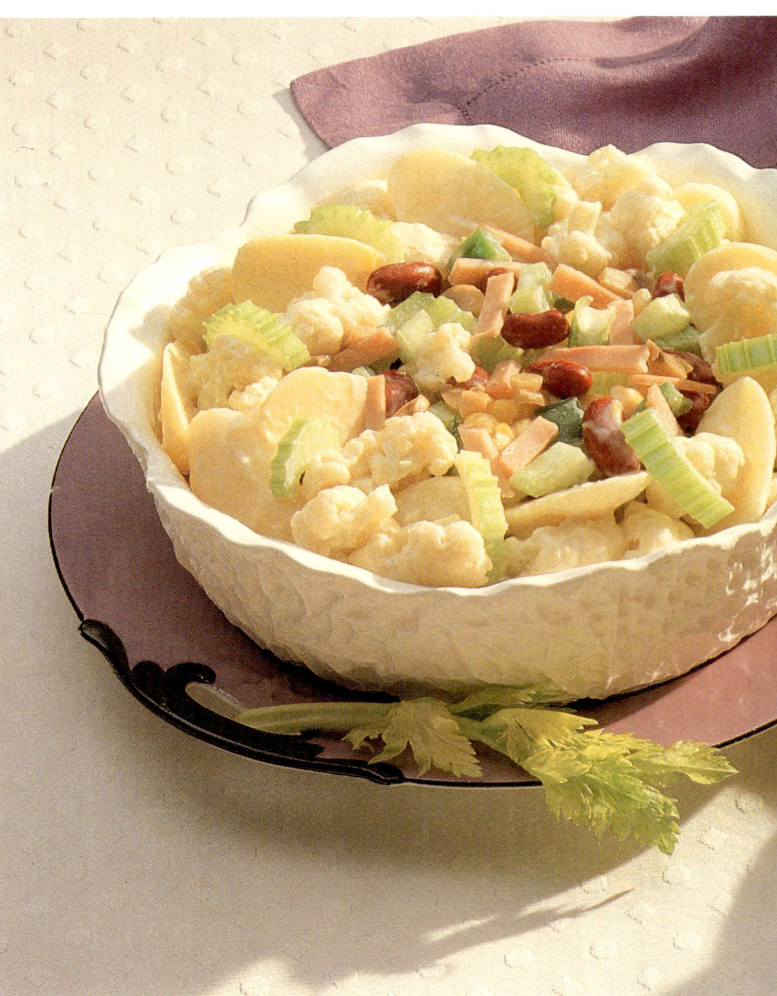

Left: A day's allowance of Ham and Vegetable Salad; Centre back: A day's allowance of Tropical Rice Salad; Centre front: A portion of Haddock Coleslaw; Right: A portion of Wheat and Pasta Salad

Haddock Coleslaw

Metric/Imperial
150 g/5 oz smoked haddock
50 g/2 oz wholewheat pasta
  shapes
1 medium apple
15 ml/1 tablespoon lemon juice
2 celery sticks, chopped
25 g/1 oz gherkins, chopped
125 g/4 oz white cabbage,
  shredded
1 x 213 g/7½ oz can mushrooms in
  brine, drained
1 x 198 g/7 oz can sweetcorn
  with peppers, drained
60 ml/4 tablespoons oil-free
  French dressing

American
5 oz smoked haddock
½ cup wholewheat pasta shapes
1 medium apple
1 tablespoon lemon juice
2 stalks celery, chopped
1 oz gherkins, chopped
1⅓ cups shredded white cabbage
1 x 7½ oz can mushrooms in
  brine, drained
1 x 7 oz can whole kernel corn
  with peppers, drained
4 tablespoons oil-free French
  dressing

Poach the haddock in simmering water for 10–15 minutes or until cooked, then flake, discarding any skin and bones. Cook the pasta in boiling water until tender, then drain. Core the apple, dice the flesh and sprinkle with lemon juice. Mix all the ingredients in a large bowl and toss with the French dressing. Cover with plastic wrap and keep in the refrigerator until ready to eat.

Wheat and Pasta Salad

Metric/Imperial
25 g/1 oz cracked wheat
25 g/1 oz wholewheat pasta
  shapes
2 medium apples
15 ml/1 tablespoon lemon juice
30 ml/2 tablespoons oil-free
  French dressing
5 ml/1 level teaspoon honey
1 x 150 g/5 oz carton low-fat
  natural yogurt
3 celery sticks, chopped
125 g/4 oz cucumber, chopped
175 g/6 oz carrots, grated
125 g/4 oz canned or cooked red
  kidney beans, drained

American
¼ cup Bulgur wheat
¼ cup wholewheat pasta shapes
2 medium apples
1 tablespoon lemon juice
2 tablespoons oil-free French
  dressing
1 level teaspoon honey
⅔ cup low-fat natural yogurt
3 stalks celery, chopped
1 cup chopped cucumber
1 cup grated carrots
⅔ cup drained canned or cooked
  red kidney beans

Soak the wheat in cold water for one hour. Drain and squeeze out as much water as possible. Cook the pasta in boiling water until tender, then drain. Core the unpeeled apples and dice the flesh. Toss in lemon juice. Blend the oil-free French dressing, honey and yogurt together in a large bowl and stir in all the other ingredients. Cover the bowl with plastic wrap and keep in the refrigerator until ready to eat.

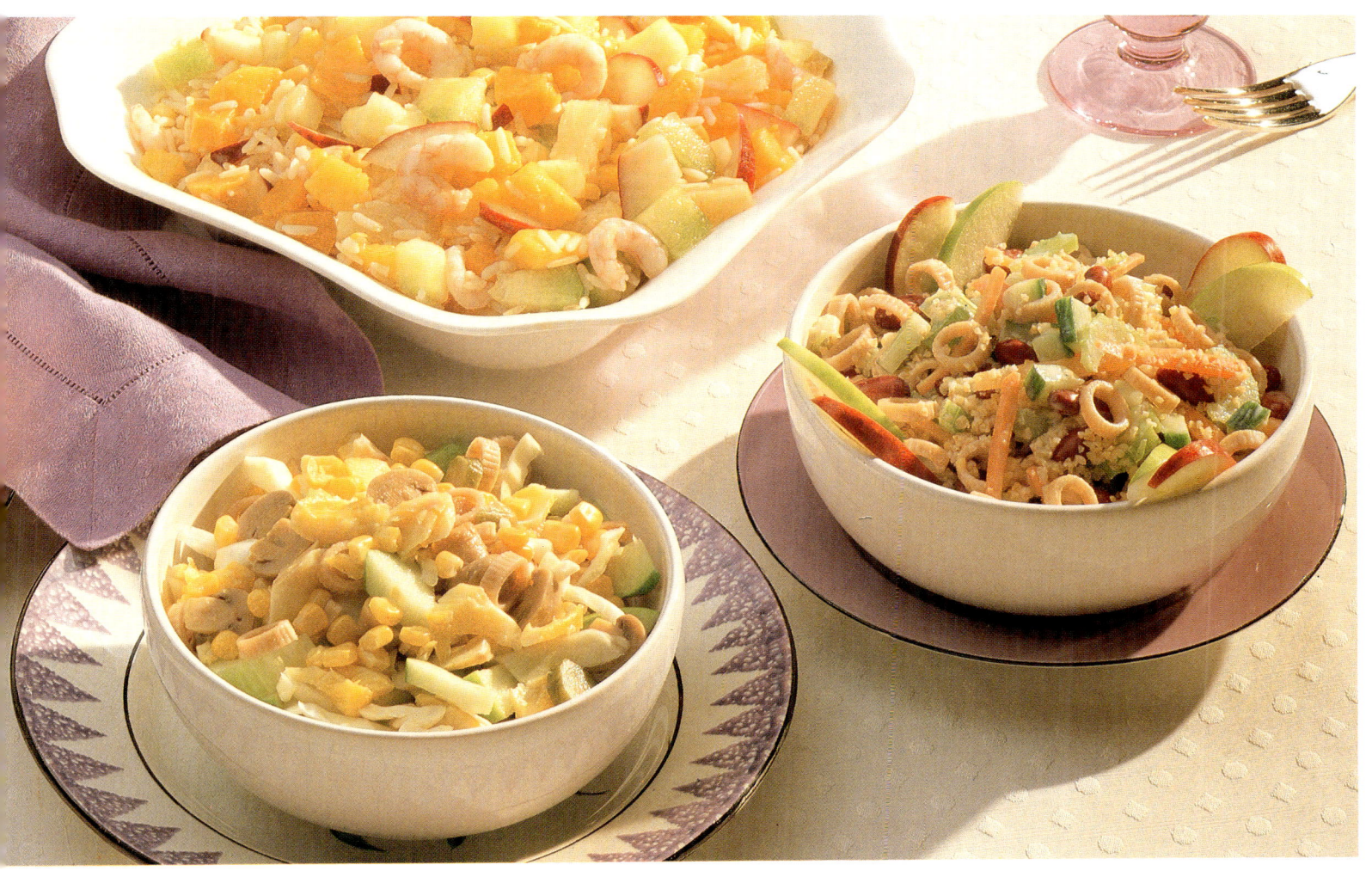

Liquid Mix

These liquid mixes consist of nutritious ingredients that are combined to create each day's delicious concoctions. Remember to select a different mix or salad for each of the four days of your Super-speedy Health Farm Diet and do not follow the diet for more than four days.

Apricot and Banana Delight

Metric/Imperial	American
25 g/1 oz semolina	2 tablespoons semolina flour
575 ml/1 pint skimmed milk	2½ cups skimmed milk
1 x 220 g/7½ oz can apricots in low-calorie syrup	1 x 7½ oz can apricots in low-calorie syrup
1 medium banana	1 medium banana
1 x 150 g/5 oz carton low-fat natural yogurt	1 x 5 oz carton low-fat natural yogurt
5 ml/1 level teaspoon honey	1 level teaspoon honey
1 Weetabix	1 wholewheat breakfast biscuit
275 ml/½ pint water	1¼ cups water

Put the semolina in a saucepan with the skimmed milk and bring to the boil. Reduce heat and simmer for 20 minutes, stirring all the time. The semolina should be clear but not thick. Leave to cool. Put into a food processor or blender with apricots and their juice, banana, yogurt, honey, Weetabix and water. Blend well. Pour into a jug or bowl and keep in the refrigerator until ready to drink.

Cheese and Vegetable Special

Metric/Imperial	American
1 x 175 g/6 oz potato, peeled weight	1 x 6 oz potato, peeled weight
2 celery sticks, chopped	2 stalks celery, chopped
50 g/2 oz watercress, chopped	1 cup watercress, chopped
125 g/4 oz carrots, peeled and chopped	⅔ cup chopped carrots
75 g/3 oz lettuce leaves	1½ cups lettuce
½ medium onion, peeled and chopped	½ medium onion, peeled and chopped
50 g/2 oz cucumber, chopped	½ cup chopped cucumber
50 g/2 oz boiled beetroot, chopped	⅓ cup chopped peeled beet
125 g/4 oz cottage cheese	½ cup cottage cheese
700 ml/24 fl oz tomato juice	3 cups tomato juice
1 x 150 g/5 oz carton low-fat natural yogurt	⅔ cup low-fat natural yogurt
5 ml/1 level teaspoon yeast extract	1 level teaspoon yeast extract
275 ml/½ pint water	1¼ cups water
10 ml/2 teaspoons Worcestershire sauce	2 teaspoons Worcestershire sauce
a dash of Tabasco	a dash of hot pepper sauce
salt and pepper	salt and pepper

Boil the potato, chop it roughly and put into a food processor or blender with all the other ingredients. Blend thoroughly and adjust seasoning if necessary. Pour into a jug or bowl and keep in the refrigerator until ready to drink. Stir before serving.

Lentil and Vegetable Cup

Metric/Imperial	American
50 g/2 oz red lentils	¼ cup red lentils
1 x 150 g/5 oz potato, peeled weight	1 x 5 oz potato, peeled weight
25 g/1 oz fine oatmeal	⅓ cup fine oatmeal
1 x 425 g/15 oz can consommé	1 x 15 oz can consommé
1 celery stick, chopped	1 stalk celery, chopped
50 g/2 oz carrots, peeled and chopped	⅓ cup chopped carrots
575 ml/1 pint tomato juice	2½ cups tomato juice
a pinch of dried tarragon	a pinch of dried tarragon
150 ml/¼ pint water	⅔ cup water
5 ml/1 teaspoon Worcestershire sauce	1 teaspoon Worcestershire sauce
salt and pepper	salt and pepper

Put the lentils in a small saucepan and just cover with water. Bring to the boil and cook rapidly for 10 minutes, then reduce heat and simmer for 15 minutes until the lentils have absorbed the water. If necessary add a little more water to prevent sticking. Boil the potato. Put the oatmeal and consommé into a saucepan and bring to the boil. Cook for 10 minutes. Put all the ingredients into a food processor or blender and blend thoroughly. Season to taste, pour into a jug or bowl and keep in the refrigerator until ready to drink.

Fruit and Wheatgerm Whizz

Metric/Imperial	American
175 g/6 oz strawberries, fresh or frozen	1½ cups strawberries, fresh or frozen
1 medium peach	1 medium peach
50 g/2 oz white grapes	½ cup white grapes
1 medium mango	1 medium mango
575 ml/1 pint skimmed milk	2½ cups skimmed milk
1 x 150 g/5 oz carton low-fat natural yogurt	⅔ cup low-fat natural yogurt
25 g/1 oz wheatgerm	⅓ cup wheatgerm
275 ml/½ pint water	1¼ cups water
a few drops of vanilla essence	a few drops of vanilla extract

Hull the strawberries if fresh; discard stone (pit) and skin from the peach; halve the grapes and remove pips (seeds); discard the skin and stone (pit) from the mango. Put the fruit in a food processor or blender with all the other ingredients and process until blended. Pour into a jug or bowl and keep in the refrigerator until ready to drink.

Front: Lentil and Vegetable Cup; Back left: Cheese and Vegetable Special; Back right: Apricot and Banana Delight; Right: Preparing Fruit and Wheatgerm Whizz

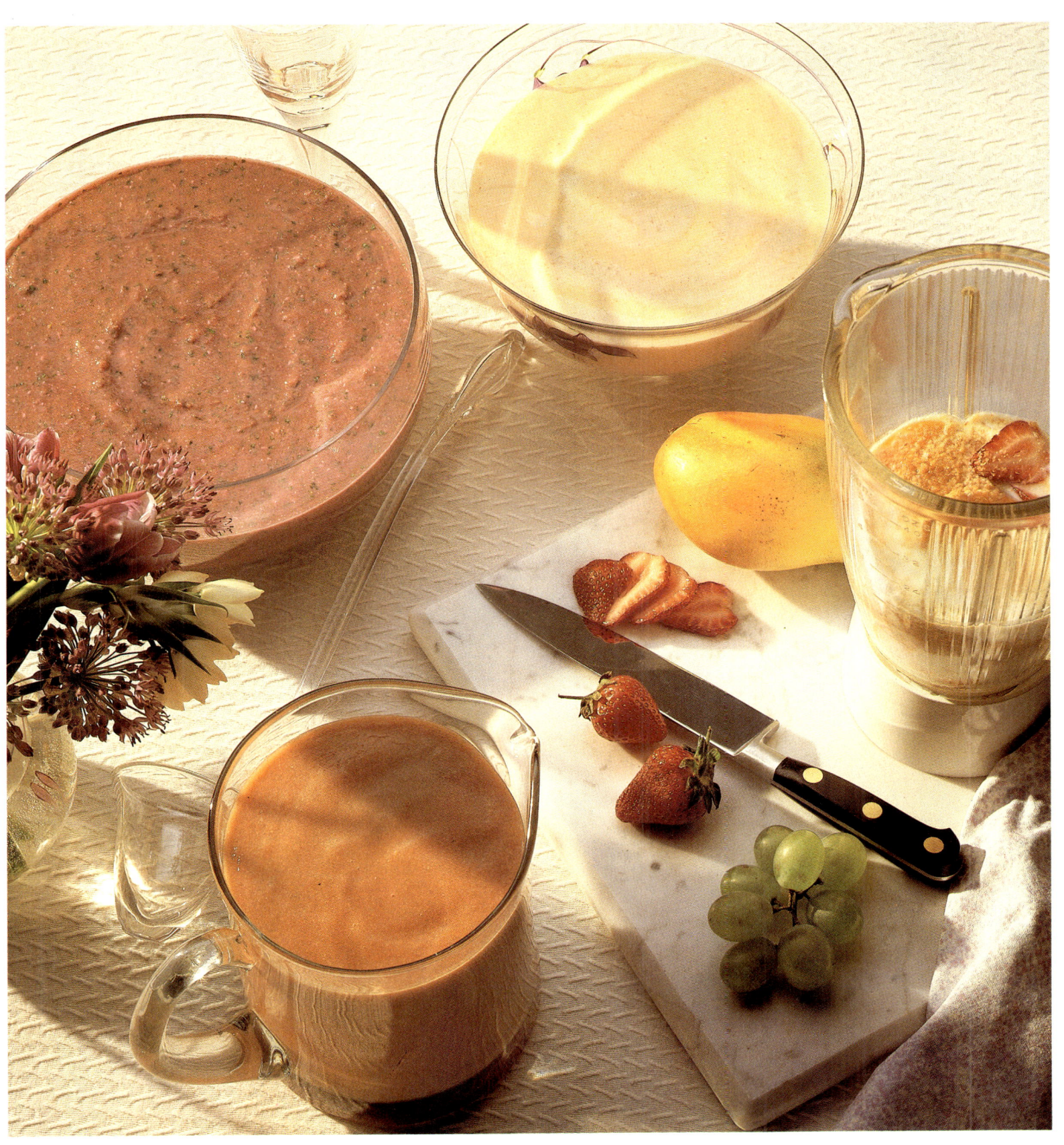

This guide to the calorie content of basic foods will prove invaluable to slimmers following one of our calorie-controlled diets. If we suggest a food in the diet that you do not enjoy you can use this chart to find a suitable substitute with the same calorie content.

ALMONDS

Shelled, per 28g/1oz	160
Ground, per 15 ml/1 level tablespoon	40

ANCHOVIES

Per anchovy fillet	5

APPLES

Medium whole eating, 150g/5oz	50
Medium whole cooking, 225g/8oz	80
Applesauce, unsweetened per 15ml/1 level tablespoon	10

APRICOTS

Per 28g/1oz	
Canned in natural juice	13
Dried	52
Fresh with stone	7
Per dried apricot	10
Per whole fresh fruit	5

ARTICHOKES

Globe, boiled, per 28g/1oz	4
1 medium globe artichoke	10
Jerusalem, boiled, per 28g/1oz	5

ASPARAGUS

Raw or boiled, soft tips, per 28g/1oz	5
Per asparagus spear	5

AUBERGINES (EGGPLANT)

Raw, per 28g/1oz	4

AVOCADOS

Flesh only, per 28g/1oz	63

BACON

1 streaky rasher, well grilled or fried, 20g/¾oz raw weight	50
1 back rasher, well grilled or fried, 35g/1¼oz raw weight	80
1 bacon steak, well grilled 100g/3½oz raw weight	105

BANANAS

Small whole fruit, 115g/4oz	55
Medium whole fruit, 175g/6oz	80
Large whole fruit, 200g/7oz	95
Dried, per 28g/1oz	140

BEAN SPROUTS

Canned, per 28g/1oz	3
Raw, per 28g/1oz	8
Boiled, per 28g/1oz	7

BEANS

Per 28g/1oz	
Aduki, raw weight	92
Aduki, boiled	40
Baked, canned in tomato sauce	20
Black eye, raw weight	93
Black eye, boiled	38
Broad, boiled	14
Butter, boiled	27
Butter, raw weight	77
Cannellini, canned	25
Flageolet, boiled	32
French, frozen	10
Haricot, boiled	26
Haricot, raw weight	77
Lima, raw, dry weight	92
Mung, raw, dry weight	92
Red kidney, canned	25
Red kidney, raw, dry weight	77
Runner, boiled	5
Runner, raw	7
Snap, raw, green	10
Soya, raw, dry weight	108
Soya, boiled	50

BEEF

Per 28g/1oz unless otherwise stated	
Fillet steak, medium grilled 175g/6oz raw	305
Ground beef, lean, raw	45
Ground beef, lean, fried and drained of fat, 28g/1oz raw weight	40
Minced beef, raw	74
Minced beef, well fried and drained of fat, 28g/1oz raw weight	60
Rump steak, medium grilled, 175g/6oz raw	290
Sirloin, roast, lean and fat	80
Sirloin, roast, lean only	55
Stewing steak, raw, lean only	35
Stewing steak, raw, lean and fat	50
Topside, roast, lean and fat	61
Topside, roast, lean only	44

BEEFBURGER

Average 50g/2oz, grilled	115
Average 115g/4oz, grilled	240

BEETROOT

Raw, per 28g/1oz	8
Boiled, per 28g/1oz	12

BISCUITS

Per 28g/1oz	
Digestive, plain	134
Rich Tea	126

BLACKBERRIES

Raw or Frozen, per 28g/1oz	8

BLACKCURRANTS

Raw or frozen, per 28g/1oz	8

BRAN

Per 28g/1oz	58

BRAZIL NUTS

Shelled, per 28g/1oz	175

BREAD

Per 28g/1oz	
Black Rye	90
Bran	65
Brown or Wheatmeal	63
Currant	70
Enriched, eg Cholla	110
Fried bread, 28g/1oz unfried weight	160
French	85
Fruit Sesame	120
Granary	70
Light Rye	70
Malt	70
Milk	80
Pumpernickel	60
Soda	75
Vogel	65
Wheatgerm, eg Hovis and VitBe	65
White	66
Wholemeal (100%)	61

BREADSTICKS (GRISSINI)

Each	15

BROCCOLI

Raw, per 28g/1oz	7
Boiled, per 28g/1oz	5

BRUSSELS SPROUTS

Raw, per 28g/1oz	7
Boiled, per 28g/1oz	5

BUCKWHEAT

Whole grain, per 28g/1oz	100

BUTTER

All brands, per 28g/1oz	210
Per 15ml/1 level tablespoon	105
Per 5ml/1 level teaspoon	35

CABBAGE

Raw, per 28g/1oz	6
Boiled, per 28g/1oz	4

CARROTS

Raw, per 28g/1oz	6
Boiled, per 28g/1oz	5
Canned, per 28g/1oz	5

CASHEW NUTS

Dry roasted, per 28g/1oz	125
Shelled, per 28g/1oz	160

CAULIFLOWER

Raw, per 28g/1oz	4
Boiled, per 28g/1oz	3

CELERIAC

Raw, per 28g/1oz	8
Boiled, per 28g/1oz	4

CELERY

Raw, per 28g/1oz	2
Boiled, per 28g/1oz	1

CHEESE

Per 28g/1oz	
Austrian Smoked	78
Brie	88
Caerphilly	120
Camembert	88
Cheddar	120
Cheese spread	80
Cheshire	110
Cotswold	105
Cottage cheese	27
Cream cheese	125
Curd cheese	54
Danish Blue	103
Derby	110
Dolcellata	100
Double Gloucester	105
Edam	90
Emmental	115
Fetta	54
Fromage blanc	35
Gorgonzola	112
Gouda	100
Gruyere	117
Lancashire	109
Leicester	105
Lymeswold	120
Mozzarella, Danish	98
Mozzarella, Italian	87
Norwegian Blue	100
Norwegian Gjeost	133
Parmesan	118
Processed	88
Riccotta	55
Roquefort	88
Sage Derby	112
St Paulin	98
Shape	77
Skimmed milk soft cheese	25
Stilton, Blue	131
Stilton, White	108
Tendale	70
Wensleydale	115

CHERRIES

Canned, per 28g/1oz	20
Fresh, with stones, per 28g/1oz	12

CHESTNUTS

Shelled, per 28g/1oz	48
With shells	40

CHICK PEAS

Boiled, per 28g/1oz	40
Raw, per 28g/1oz	91

CHICKEN

Per 28g/1oz unless otherwise stated	
On the bone, raw	25
Meat only, raw	34
Boiled, meat only	52
Roast, meat only	42
Roast, meat and skin	61

CHICORY

Raw, per 28g/1oz	3

CHILLIES

Dried, per 28g/1oz	85
Fresh, flesh only	6

CHIVES

Per 28g/1oz	10

CHINESE LEAVES

Raw, per 28g/1oz	3
Boiled, per 28g/1oz	2

CHOCOLATE

Per 28g/1oz	
Milk or Plain	150

Cooking	155
Vermicelli, per 5ml/1 level teaspoon	20
COCKLES	
Without shells, boiled, per 28g/1oz	14
COCONUT	
Per 28g/1oz	
Fresh	100
Desiccated	171
COD	
Per 28g/1oz	
Fillet, raw	22
On the bone, raw	15
COFFEE	
Per 28g/1oz	
Coffee beans, roasted and ground, infusion	0
Instant	28
Coffee and chicory essence, per 5ml/1 teaspoon	10
COLEY	
Per 28g/1oz	
Fillet, raw	21
CORNED BEEF	
Per 28g/1oz	62
CORNFLOUR	
Per 28g/1oz	100
CORN OIL	
Per 15ml/1 tablespoon	120
COURGETTES	
Raw, per 28g/1oz	4
CRAB	
Meat only, per 28g/1oz boiled	36
Average crab with shell	95
CRANBERRY SAUCE	
Per 15ml/1 level tablespoon	45
CRANBERRY JELLY	
Per 28g/1oz	40
CREAM	
Per 28g/1oz	
Clotted	165
Double	127
Half Cream	35
Imitation	85
Non-dairy	80
Single	60
Soured	60
Sterilized, canned	65
Whipping	94
Per 15ml/1 level tablespoon	
Clotted	105
Double	55
Single or soured	30
Whipping	45
CUCUMBER	
Raw, per 28g/1oz	3
CURRANTS, DRIED	
Per 28g/1oz	69
Per 15ml/1 level tablespoon	20
CURRY PASTE	
Per 28g/1oz	40
CURRY POWDER	
Per 5ml/1 level teaspoon	12

DAMSONS	
Fresh, with stones, per 28g/1oz	11
DATES	
Per 28g/1oz	
Dried, with stones	60
Dried, without stones	70
Fresh, with stones	30
DUCK	
Per 28g/1oz	
Roast, meat only	54
Roast, meat, fat and skin	96

EGGS each	raw	fried
Size 1	95	115
Size 2	90	110
Size 3	80	100
Size 4	75	95
Size 5	70	90
Size 6	60	80
Yolk of size 3 egg	65	
White of size 3 egg	15	

ENDIVE	
Raw, per 28g/1oz	3
FENNEL	
Raw, per 28g/1oz	6
Boiled, per 28g/1oz	8
FIGS	
Dried, per 28g/1oz	60
Fresh, green, per 28g/1oz	12
FISH CAKES	
Average, grilled, each	65
FISHFINGERS	
Average, grilled, each	50
FLOUR	
Per 28g/1oz	
Wheatmeal	93
White, plain	99
White, self-raising	96
White, strong	96
Wholemeal	90
Buckwheat	100
Cassava	97
Granary	99
Maizemeal or Cornmeal (96%)	103
Maizemeal or Cornmeal (60%)	100
Rice	100
Rye (100%)	95
Soya, low fat	100
Soya, full fat	127
Per 15ml/1 level tablespoon	
White	32
Wholemeal	29
FLOUNDER	
On the bone, raw, per 28g/1oz	20
FRANKFURTER	
Each	80
FRENCH DRESSING	
Per 15ml/1 tablespoon	75
Oil-free, per 15ml/1 tablespoon	3

FRUIT SUGAR	
Per 28g/1oz	105
GARLIC	
One clove	0
GHERKINS	
Per 28g/1oz	5
GINGER	
Ground, per 28g/1oz	73
Root, raw, peeled, per 28g/1oz	18
GOLDEN SYRUP	
Per 28g/1oz	84
Per 15ml/1 level tablespoon	60
GOOSEBERRIES	
Fresh ripe dessert, per 28g/1oz	10
GRAPEFRUIT	
Medium whole fruit, 350g/12oz	35
Juice, unsweetened, per 150ml/¼ pint	45
Juice, sweetened, per 150ml/¼ pint	55
GRAPES	
Black, per 28g/1oz	14
White, per 28g/1oz	17
GRAVY	
Per 30ml/2 tablespoons	
Thick, made with meat dripping	30
Thick, made without fat	10
Thin, made without fat	5
GREENGAGES	
Fresh, with stones, per 28g/1oz	13
GROUND RICE	
Per 28g/1oz	100
GUAVAS	
Fresh, with seeds, per 28g/1oz	16
Canned, per 28g/1oz	17
HADDOCK	
Per 28g/1oz unless otherwise stated	
Fillet, raw	21
On the bone, raw	15
Smoked, raw	25
HAKE	
Per 28g/1oz	
Fillet, raw	20
Fillet, steamed	30
Fillet, fried	60
HAM	
Per 28g/1oz	
Chopped ham roll or loaf	75
Ham, boiled, lean	47
Ham, boiled, fatty	90
Honey Roast ham	50
Old smokey ham	65
Maryland ham	55
Parma ham, lean and fat	85
Parma ham, lean only	60
Virginia ham	40

HAZEL NUTS	
Shelled, per 28g/1oz	108
Per nut	5
HEART	
Per 28g/1oz unless otherwise stated	
Lamb's, raw	34
Ox, raw	31
Pig's, raw	26
HERRING	
Per 28g/1oz unless otherwise stated	
Fillet, raw	66
On the bone, grilled	38
Rollmop herring	47
HONEY	
Per 5ml/1 level teaspoon	20
HORSERADISH	
Sauce, per 15ml/1 level tablespoon	13
ICE CREAM	
Vanilla, per 28g/1oz	45
JAM	
Per 5ml/1 level teaspoon	15
KIDNEY	
All types, raw, per 28g/1oz	25
KIPPERS	
Fillet, raw, per 28g/1oz	75
KIWI FRUIT	
1 medium	30
LAMB	
Per 28g/1oz unless otherwise stated	
Leg, raw, lean and fat, without bone	68
Leg, raw, lean only, without bone	46
Leg, roast, lean and fat, without bone	75
Leg, roast, lean, without bone	54
Shoulder, boned, raw, lean and fat	83
Shoulder, boned, roast, lean	56
Chump chop, well grilled, 150g/5oz raw weight	205
Loin chop, well grilled, 150g/5oz raw weight	175
LARD	
Per 28g/1oz	253
LEEKS	
Raw, per 28g/1oz	9
Average whole leek, raw	25
LEMON	
Flesh and skin, per 28g/1oz	4
Lemon juice, per 15ml/1 tablespoon	0
LENTILS	
Raw, per 28g/1oz	86
Boiled, per 28g/1oz	28
LETTUCE	
Fresh, per 28g/1oz	3

LIVER
Per 28g/1oz
Calves', raw	43
Chicken's, raw	38
Lamb's, raw	51
Ox, raw	46
Pig's, raw	44
Turkey's, raw	37

LOBSTER
With shell, boiled, per 28g/1oz	12
Meat only, boiled, per 28g/1oz	34

LOGANBERRIES
Fresh, per 28g/1oz	5

LOW-FAT SPREAD
Per 28g/1oz	105
Per 5ml/1 level teaspoon	15

LUNCHEON MEAT
Per 28g/1oz	89

LYCHEES
Fresh, flesh only, per 28g/1oz	18
Canned, per 28g/1oz	19
Per lychee	8

MACARONI
Per 28g/1oz
White, raw	105
White, boiled	33
Wholewheat macaroni, raw	95
Wholewheat macaroni, boiled	34

MACEDONIA NUTS
Shelled, per 28g/1oz	188

MACKEREL
Per 28g/1oz unless otherwise stated
Fillet, raw	63
Kippered mackerel	62
Smoked mackerel	70

MANDARINES
Whole fruit, 70g/2½oz	20

MANGO
Medium whole fruit, 285g/10oz	100
Mango chutney, per 15ml/1 level tablespoon	40

MARGARINE
All brands including those labelled 'high in polyunsaturates', per 28g/1oz	210
Per 5ml/1 level teaspoon	35

MARMALADE
Per 5ml/1 level teaspoon	15

MARROW
Raw, per 28g/1oz	5
Boiled, per 28g/1oz	2

MAYONNAISE
Per 15ml/1 level tablespoon	120

MELON
Per 28g/1oz
Cantaloupe, with skin	4
Charentais, fresh only	5
Honeydew or Yellow, with skin	4
Ogen, with skin	5
Watermelon, with skin	3
Melon seeds, coat removed	165

MILK
Per 568ml/1 pint unless otherwise stated
Buttermilk	232
Channel Island or Gold Top	445
Evaporated milk, full cream, reconstituted	360
Goat's	415
Homogenized	380
Instant spray dried low-fat skimmed milk, reconstituted	200
Instant dried skimmed milk with vegetable fat, reconstituted	280
Instant low-fat milk, dry, per 28g/1oz	100
Longlife or UHT	380
Pasteurized or Silver Top	380
Semi-skimmed milk	300
Skimmed	200
Soya milk, diluted as directed	370
Sterilized	380

MINT
Fresh, per 28g/1oz	3

MINT SAUCE
Per 15ml/1 tablespoon	5

MUESLI
Per 28g/1oz	105
Per 15ml/1 level tablespoon	30

MULLLET
Raw, per 28g/1oz	40

MUSHROOMS
Raw, per 28g/1oz	4
Dried, per 28g/1oz	40

MUSSELS
With shells, boiled, per 28g/1oz	7
Without shells, boiled, per 28g/1oz	25

MUSTARD AND CRESS
Raw, per 28g/1oz	3

MUSTARD
Dry, per 28g/1oz	128
Made, per 5ml/1 level teaspoon	10

NECTARINES
Medium whole, 115g/4oz	50

NOODLES
Cooked, per 28g/1oz	33
Raw, per 28g/1oz	102

NUTMEG
Ground, per 2.5ml/½ level teaspoon	0

OATMEAL
Raw, per 28g/1oz	114

OATS
Rolled, per 28g/1oz	115

OLIVE OIL
Per 15ml/1 tablespoon	120

OLIVES
Stoned, in brine, per 28g/1oz	29
With stones, in brine, per 28g/1oz	23

ONIONS
Per 28g/1oz unless otherwise stated
Raw	7
Boiled	4
Fried	98

ORANGES
Whole fruit, small, 150g/5oz	35
Whole fruit, medium, 225g/8oz	60
Whole fruit, large, 275g/10oz	75

ORANGE JUICE
Unsweetened, per 28ml/1floz	11

OYSTERS
With shells, raw, per 28g/1oz	2
Without shells, raw, per 28g/1oz	14

PARSLEY
Fresh, per 28g/1oz	6

PARSNIPS
Per 28g/1oz
Raw	14
Roast	30

PASSION FRUIT
Flesh only, per 28g/1oz	10
With skin, per 28g/1oz	4

PASTA
Per 28g/1oz
White, raw, all shapes	105
White, boiled, all shapes	33
Wholewheat, raw, all shapes	95

PAW PAW (PAPAYA)
Canned, per 28g/1oz	18
Whole medium-sized fruit	100

PEACHES
Canned in natural juice, per 28g/1oz	13
Dried, per 28g/1oz	60
Whole fruit, 115g/4oz	35

PEANUTS
Per 28g/1oz unless otherwise stated
Shelled, fresh	162
Dry roasted	160
Roasted and salted	162

PEANUT BUTTER
Per 5ml/1 level teaspoon	35

PEARS
Per 28g/1oz unless otherwise stated
Cooking pears, raw, peeled	10
Dried	45
Whole fruit, 150g/5oz	40

PEAS
Per 28g/1oz
Fresh, raw	19
Frozen, raw	15
Canned, garden	13
Canned, processed	23
Dried, raw	81
Dried, boiled	29
Mange tout, raw	16
Mange tout, boiled	12
Split, raw	88
Split boiled	33

PECANS
Per nut	15

PEPPER
Powdered, per pinch	0

PEPPERS (PIMENTOS)
Red or green, per 28g/1oz	4

PHEASANT
Meat only, roast, per 28g/1oz	65

PILCHARDS
Canned in tomato sauce, per 28g/1oz	36

PINEAPPLE
Canned in natural juice, per 28g/1oz	15
Slice of fresh pineapple, weight with skin and core, 150g/5oz	35
Ring of canned pineapple in natural juice, drained	20

PISTACHIO NUTS
Shelled, per 28g/1oz	180

PLAICE
Per 28g/1oz unless otherwise stated
Fillet, raw or steamed	26
Fillet, in breadcrumbs, fried	65

PLUMS
Per 28g/1oz unless otherwise stated
Cooking plums, with stones	7
Fresh dessert plums, with stones	10

POLONY
Per 28g/1oz	80

POMEGRANATE
Whole pomegranate, 200g/7oz	65

POPCORN
Per 28g/1oz	110

PORK
Per 28g/1oz unless otherwise stated
Fillet (tenderloin), raw, lean only	42
Leg, raw, lean and fat, without bone	76
Leg, raw, lean only, without bone	42
Leg, roast, lean and fat	81
Leg, roast, lean only	52
Pork chop, well grilled, 185g/6½oz raw weight	240
Pork chop, well fried, 185g/6½oz raw weight	290

POTATOES
Per 28g/1oz unless otherwise stated
Raw, peeled	25

Baked, weighed with skin	24	**SARDINES**		
Boiled, old potatoes	23	Raw, per 28g/1oz	55	
Boiled, new potatoes	22	Canned in oil, drained, per		
Canned, new potatoes,		28g/1oz	62	
drained	15	Canned in tomato sauce, per		
Chips (average thickness)	70	28g/1oz	50	
Crisps	150	**SAUERKRAUT**		
Roast, medium chunks	45	Canned, per 28g/1oz	5	
Sauté	40	**SAUSAGES**		

PRAWNS
With shells, per 28g/1oz — 12
Without shells, per 28g/1oz — 30
Per shelled prawn — 2

Instant mashed potato powder, dry — 90
Jacket-baked potato, 200g/7oz raw weight — 170

SAUSAGES
Beef chipolata, well grilled, each — 50
Beef large, well grilled, each — 120
Beef skinless, well grilled, each — 65
Pork chipolata, well grilled, each — 65
Pork large, well grilled, each — 125
Pork skinless, well grilled, each — 95
Pork and beef chipolata well grilled, each — 60
Pork and beef large, well grilled, each — 125

SOLE (DOVER)
Per 28g/1oz
Fillet, raw — 23

SOY SAUCE
Per 15ml/1 tablespoon — 13

SOYA BEAN CURD (TORFU)
Per 28g/1oz — 15

SPAGHETTI
Per 28g/1oz
White, raw — 107
Wholewheat, raw — 97
Boiled — 33
Canned in tomato sauce — 17

SPINACH
Boiled, per 28g/1oz — 9
Raw, per 28g/1oz — 7

SPRING ONIONS
Raw, per 28g/1oz — 10

SQUID
Flesh only, raw, per 28g/1oz — 25

STRAWBERRIES
Fresh or frozen, per 28g/1oz — 7

SUGAR
White, brown, Demerara, icing, caster or granulated, per 28g/1oz — 112
Per 5ml/1 level teaspoon — 17

SULTANAS
Dried, per 28g/1oz — 71
Per 15ml/1 level tablespoon — 25

SUNFLOWER SEED OIL
Per 28g/1oz — 255

SUNFLOWER SEEDS
Per 28g/1oz, coats removed — 170

SWEDES
Per 28g/1oz
Raw — 6
Boiled — 5

SWEETCORN
Canned, in brine, per 28g/1oz — 22
Fresh Kernels only, boiled, per 28g/1oz — 25
Frozen, per 28g/1oz — 25
Whole medium cob — 155

SWEET PICKLE
Per 28g/1oz — 35

SWEET POTATOES
Raw, per 28g/1oz — 26
Boiled, per 28g/1oz — 24

TANGERINES
Whole fruit, 75g/3oz — 20

TARAMASALATA
Per 28g/1oz — 135

TARTARE SAUCE
Per 28g/1oz — 80

TEA
All brands, per cup, no milk or sugar — 0

TOMATOES
Per 28g/1oz unless otherwise stated
Raw — 4
Canned — 3

PRUNES
Per 28g/1oz unless otherwise stated
Dried, raw, with stones — 38
Dried, no stones — 46
Prune juice — 25

PUMPKIN
Per 28g/1oz
Flesh only, raw — 4
Pumpkin seeds, seed coat removed — 173

RABBIT
Per 28g/1oz
Meat only, raw — 35

RADISHES
Fresh, per 28g/1oz — 4

RAISINS
Dried, per 28g/1oz — 70
Per 15ml/1 level tablespoon — 25

RASPBERRIES
Fresh or frozen, per 28g/1oz — 7

RICE
Brown, raw, per 28g/1oz — 99
Brown, boiled, per 28g/1oz — 33
White, raw, per 28g/1oz — 102
White, boiled, per 28g/1oz — 35
Per 15ml/1 level tablespoon
Boiled — 20
Fried — 35

SAGO
Raw per 28g/1oz — 101

SALAMI
Belgian — 130
Danish — 160
German — 120
Hungarian — 130

SALMON
Per 28g/1oz
Canned — 44
Raw — 52
Smoked — 40

SALMON TROUT
Raw, flesh only, per 28g/1oz — 50

SALT
Per 28g/1oz — 0

SAUSAGES, DELICATESSEN
Per 28g/1oz
Belgian Liver Sausage — 90
Bierwurst — 75
Bockwurst — 180
Cervelat — 140
Chorizo — 140
Continental Liver Sausage — 85
French Garlic Sausage — 90
Garlic Sausage — 70
Ham Sausage — 50
Kabanos — 115
Krakowska — 80
Mettwurst — 120
Mortadella, Italian — 105
Pastrami — 65
Polish Country Sausage — 60
Polony — 80
Smoked Dutch Sausage — 105
Smoked Ham Sausage — 65
Smoked Pork Sausage — 130

SCALLOPS
Raw, per 28g/1oz — 20

SCAMPI
Fried in breadcrumbs, per 28g/1oz — 90
Peeled, raw, per 28g/1oz — 30

SESAME SEEDS
Per 28g/1oz — 168
Per 15ml/1 level tablespoon — 55

SHRIMPS
Per 28g/1oz
Canned, drained — 27
Fresh, with shells — 11
Fresh, without shells — 33

SKATE
Fillet, in batter, fried, per 28g/1oz — 57

SNAILS
Flesh only, per 28g/1oz — 25

Chutney — 45
Per 15ml/1 level teaspoon
Ketchup — 15
Purée — 10

TOMATO JUICE
Per 115ml/4 fl oz — 25

TREACLE
Black, per 28g/1oz — 73
Per 15ml/1 level tablespoon — 50

TROUT
Per 28g/1oz
Fillet, smoked — 38
On the bone, poached or steamed — 25

TUNA
Per 28g/1oz
Canned in brine, drained — 30
Canned in oil, drained — 60

TURKEY
Per 28g/1oz
Raw, meat only — 30
Roast, meat only — 40
Meat and skin, roast — 48

TURNIPS
Per 28g/1oz
Raw — 3
Boiled — 4

VEAL
Per 28g/1oz
Fillet, raw — 31
Fillet, roast — 65

VENISON
Per 28g/1oz
Raw, meat only — 42
Roast, meat only — 36

VINEGAR
Per 28ml/1floz — 1

WALNUTS
Shelled, per 28g/1oz — 149
Per walnut half — 15

WATERCHESTNUTS
Canned, per 28g/1oz — 10

WATERCRESS
Per 28g/1oz — 4

WATERMELON
Flesh only, per 28g/1oz — 6
Flesh with skin, per 28g/1oz — 3

WHEATGERM
Per 28g/1oz — 100
Per 15ml/1 level tablespoon — 18

WHITEBAIT
Fried, per 28g/1oz — 149

YAMS
Per 28g/1oz
Raw — 37
Boiled — 34

YOGURT
Per 28g/1oz
Low-fat natural — 15
Whole milk — 25
Low-fat, per 15ml/1 level tablespoon — 10

Index

Recipe Index

Acknowledgements

Special Photography
Chris Harvey: 1–61 and 88/9
Duncan McNicol: 91–153

Illustrations
Lucy Su

Photographic styling
Maggi Heinz: 1–61 and 88/9
Alison Williams: 91–153

Food prepared by Clare Gordon Smith
and Gill McCormick

The publishers would like to thank
Barbara Dale of the Bodyworkshop
Exercise Studio, Lambton Place,
London W11 for her valuable
assistance with the exercise section
of this book.

The publishers would also like to
thank the following companies for
kindly lending accessories for the
food photography:
Harrods, Way In Living Department,
Knightsbridge, London SW1; David
Mellor, 4 Sloane Square, London
SW1; and Equinox, 43 Neal Street,
London, WC2.

The illustrations on pages 82–83,
84–85, 86–87 are based upon
illustrations from Principles and
Techniques for the Beauty Specialist
2nd Edition by Ann Gallant.
Used by kind permission of the
publisher Stanley Thornes
(Publishers Ltd)
Old Station Drive,
off Leckhampton Road,
Cheltenham GL53 0DN

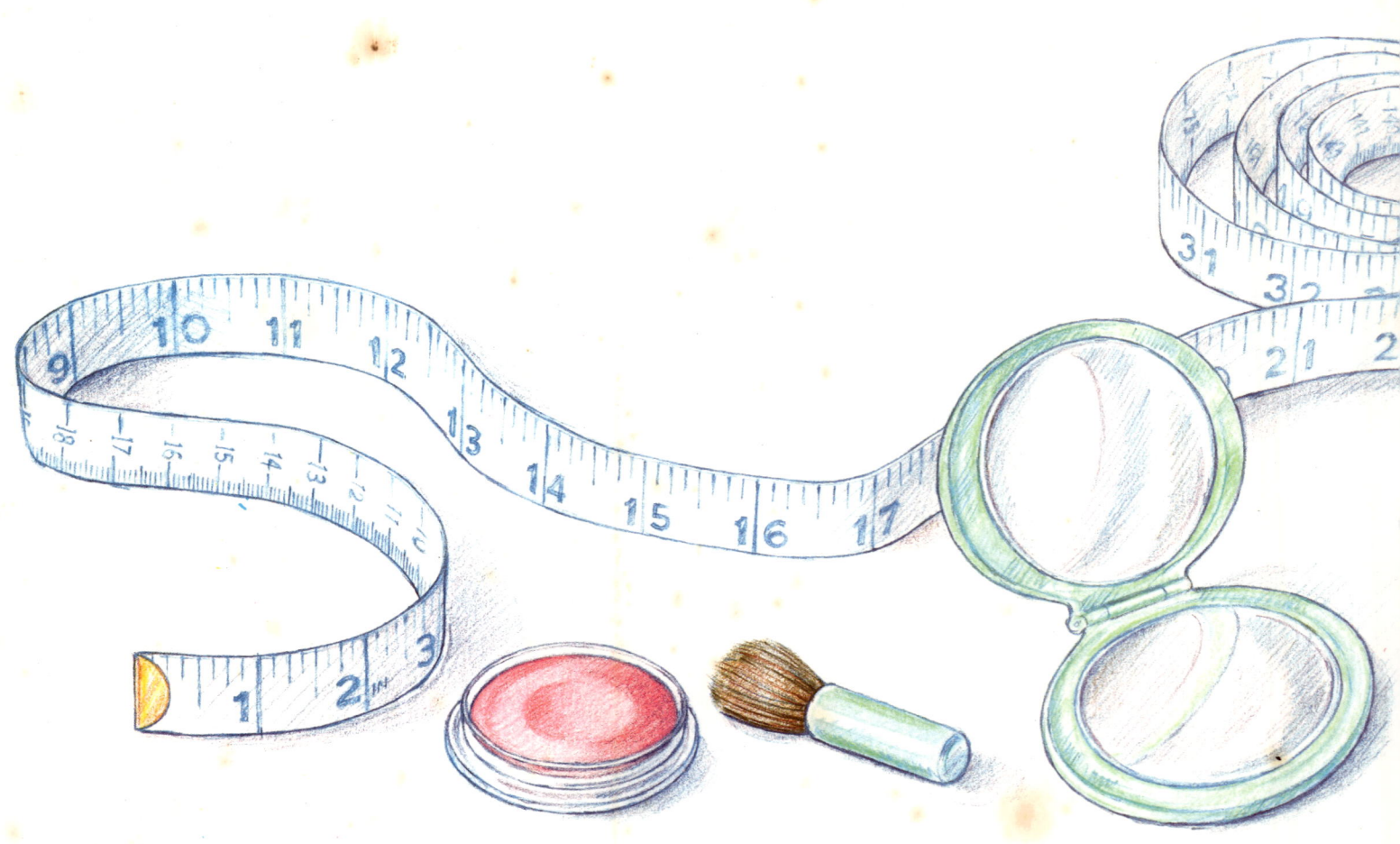